Practical Cardiac Diagnosis

Cardiac Pacing
Second Edition

General Series Editor

Stephen C. Vlay, M.D., F.A.C.P., F.A.C.C.
  Associate Professor of Medicine
Director, The Stony Brook Arrhythmia Study
  and Sudden Death Prevention Center
Director, The Coronary Care Unit
  University Hospital
Division of Cardiology, Department of Medicine
  State University of New York at Stony Brook

Other titles in the series:

Practical Cardiac Diagnosis

Cardiac Pacing
Second Edition

edited by

Kenneth A. Ellenbogen, M.D.

Director, Electrophysiology and Pacing
Medical College of Virginia and
Hunter Holmes McGuire VA Medical Center
Richmond, Virginia

**Blackwell
Science**

Blackwell Science

Editorial offices:

238 Main Street, Cambridge, Massachusetts
  02142, USA
Osney Mead, Oxford OX2 0El, England
25 John Street, London WC1N 2BL, England
23 Ainslie Place, Edinburgh EH3 6AJ, Scotland
54 University Street, Carlton, Victoria 3053,
  Australia
Arnette Blackwell SA, 224, Boulevard Saint
  Germain, 75007 Paris, France
Blackwell Wissenschafts-Verlag GmbH
  Kurfürstendamm 57, 10707 Berlin, Germany
Feldgasse 13, A-1238 Vienna, Austria

Distributors:

USA
Blackwell Science, Inc.
238 Main Street
Cambridge, Massachusetts 02142
(Telephone orders: 800-215-1000 or
  617-876-7000)

Canada
Copp Clark, Ltd.
2775 Matheson Blvd. East
Mississauga, Ontario
Canada, L4W 4P7
(Telephone orders: 800-263-4374 or
  905-238-6074)

Australia
Blackwell Science Pty, Ltd.
54 University Street
Carlton, Victoria 3053
(Telephone orders: 03-9347-0300;
fax orders 03-9349-3016)

Outside North America and Australia
Blackwell Science, Ltd.
c/o Marston Book Services, Ltd.
P.O. Box 269
Abingdon
Oxon OX14 4YN
England
(Telephone orders: 44-01235-465500;
fax orders 44-01235-465555)

Acquisitions: Chris Davis
Development: Kathleen Broderick
Production: Irene Herlihy
Manufacturing: Lisa Flanagan
Typeset by Best-set Typesetter Ltd., Hong Kong
Printed and bound by Quebecor Printing/
  Fairfield
©1996 by Blackwell Science, Inc.
Printed in the United States of America
  97 98 99 5 4 3 2

Library of Congress Cataloging-in-Publication
Data
Cardiac pacing / edited by Kenneth A.
Ellenbogen. — 2nd ed.
      p.   cm. — (Practical cardiac diagnosis)
      Includes bibliographical references and index.
      ISBN 0-86542-471-3
      1. Cardiac pacing.   I. Ellenbogen, Kenneth
A. II. Series.
      [DNLM: 1. Cardiac Pacing, Artificial.
2. Pacemaker, Artificial.   3. Defibrillators,
Implantable.   WG 168 C2623 1996]
RC684.P3C29   1996
617.4'120645—dc20
DNLM/DLC
for Library of Congress   96-19016
                                                CIP

to my wife Phyllis,
whose support and encouragement
helped make this
project successful, and to my children,
Michael, Amy, and Bethany for their
patience and love

Contents

Contributors

Jeffrey Brinker, MD
The Johns Hopkins Hospital
Baltimore, Maryland

Kenneth A. Ellenbogen, MD
Director, Electrophysiology and
  Pacing
Medical College of Virginia
Richmond, Virginia

Michael R. Gold, MD
Division of Cardiology
University of Maryland
  Hospital
Baltimore, Maryland

David L. Hayes, MD
Cardiovascular Diseases and
  Internal Medicine
Mayo Clinic
Rochester, Minnesota

G. Neal Kay, MD
University of Alabama
Birmingham, Alabama

Paul A. Levine, MD
Vice President and Medical
  Director
Pacesetter Systems, Inc.
Sylmar, California

Mark Midei, MD
Assistant Professor of Medicine
The Johns Hopkins University
  School of Medicine
Baltimore, Maryland

Robert W. Peters, MD
VA Medical Center
Baltimore, Maryland

Dwight W. Reynolds, MD
Cardiology–5SP300
University of Oklahoma
Oklahoma City, Oklahoma

Mark H. Schoenfeld, MD,
  FACC
Director, Cardiac
  Electrophysiology and Pacer
  Laboratory
Hospital of Saint Raphael

Associate Clinical Professor of
Medicine
Yale University School of
Medicine
Arrhythmia Center of C. T.,
P. C.
New Haven, Connecticut

Mark Wood, MD
Medical College of Virginia
Richmond, Virginia

Preface to the Second Edition

In the four years since we published the first edition, many new and exciting developments in cardiac pacing have occurred. We have succeeded in including much of this new information in our second edition. *Cardiac Pacing* has retained its focus of providing a readable, richly illustrated introductory text on cardiac pacemakers and implantable cardioverter defibrillators to physicians, nurses, technicians, and engineers. We have been fortunate to have many of the same contributors from the first edition rewrite and update their chapters.

Once again, the "saintly" patience of my wife and children was paramount to successfully completing this project. Without their support, the time necessary to read, write, and edit would never be possible.

Finally, we hope this book will continue to reach out to a wide variety of students of cardiac pacing. The real benefit of this book is to make us all better health care providers, and to help maximize the benefit our patients receive from their implanted device(s).

Kenneth A. Ellenbogen, M.D.

Preface to the First Edition

Approximately 115,000 permanent pacemakers are implanted each year in this country. With the development of multiprogrammable pacemakers, as well as single and dual chamber rate responsive pacing, this field continues to require more sophistication and knowledge. The majority of physicians who implant or follow pacemaker patients are involved in the busy clinical practice of general cardiology. The purpose of this book is to provide a clinically practical and useful text for these cardiologists. In addition, it is hoped that implanting surgeons, primary care physicians, general internists, cardiology fellows, clinical nurses and pacemaker technicians make use of this volume which stresses the basic aspects of permanent and temporary cardiac pacing.

This text is structured to provide the cardiologist with information in the same sequence as it becomes relevant during the evaluation of a potential pacemaker patient. The first chapter summarizes the current clinical indications for temporary and permanent cardiac pacing. Chapter 2 is a discussion of the basic concepts of cardiac pacing; leads, batteries, and sensors. Chapter 3 discusses how to select an appropriate pacing mode for an individual patient. Chapter 4 covers the methods and complications of temporary cardiac pacing. The surgical aspects of pacemaker implantation and potential complications are discussed in Chapter 5. Chapter 6 reviews the timing cycles for single chamber, dual chamber and rate responsive single and dual chamber pacemakers, while Chapter 7 covers pacemaker troubleshooting. The practical aspects and indications for antitachycardia pacing and implantable defibrillators are discussed in Chapter 8. Finally, pacemaker followup is reviewed in Chapter 9. Throughout the text, we have tried to include as many clinical examples and electrocardiographic tracings as possible, to make the material clinically relevant. In addition, there are many tables and figures summarizing the essential elements of each chapter as well as providing easy reference. Whenever possible, figures were darkened to improve clarity, and to allow for optimal reproduction.

Finally, each author is an authority in one or more aspect of pacemaker and/or implantable defibrillator implantation and followup. They have each drawn upon their own clinical practice and experience to provide information that is as up to date and clinically useful as possible.

This book was made possible by the excellent help and patience of Victoria Reeders, M.D. and Patricia Tyler from Blackwell Scientific Publications. I would also like to thank Steve Vlay, M.D., the series editor, for asking me to write this volume. Finally, the success of this volume is largely due to the excellent contributions from each of the authors. Their hard work has made this volume possible.

Kenneth A. Ellenbogen, M.D.

Notice

The indications and dosages of all drugs in this book have been recommended in the medical literature and conform to the practices of the general medical community. The medications described do not necessarily have specific approval by the U.S. Food and Drug Administration for use in the diseases and dosages for which they are recommended. The package insert for each drug should be consulted for use and dosage as approved by the FDA. Because standards for usage change, it is advisable to keep abreast of revised recommendations, particularly those concerning new drugs.

Practical Cardiac Diagnosis

Cardiac Pacing

Indications for Permanent and Temporary Cardiac Pacing

Kenneth A. Ellenbogen and Robert W. Peters

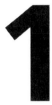

ANATOMY

To understand the principles and concepts involved in cardiac pacing more completely, a brief review of the anatomy and physiology of the specialized conduction system is warranted[1] (Table 1.1).

Sinoatrial node

The sinoatrial (SA) node is a subepicardial structure located at the junction of the right atrium and superior vena cava. It has abundant autonomic innervation and a copious blood supply, often being located within the adventitia of the large SA nodal artery, a proximal branch of the right coronary artery (55 percent of the time) or the left circumflex coronary artery. Histologically, the SA node consists of a dense framework of collagen that contains a variety of cells, among them the large, centrally located P cells, thought to initiate impulses; transitional cells, intermediate in structure between P cells and regular atrial myocardial cells; and Purkinje-like fiber tracts, extending through the perinodal area and into the atrium.

Atrioventricular node

The atrioventricular (AV) node is a small subendocardial structure within the interatrial septum located at the convergence of the specialized conduction tracts that course through the atria. Like the SA node, the AV node has extensive autonomic innervation and an abundant blood supply from the large AV nodal artery, a branch of

Table 1.1 The Specialized Conduction System

Structure	Location	Histology	Arterial Blood Supply	Autonomic Innervation	Physiology
SA node (pacemaker)	Subepicardial; junction of SVC and HRA	Abundant P cells	SA nodal artery RCA 55% LCX 45%	Abundant	Normal impulse generator
AV node	Subendocardial; interatrial septum transitional	Fewer P cells, Purkinje cells, "working" myocardial cells	AV nodal artery RCA 90% LCX 10%	Abundant	Delays impulses; subsidiary pacemaker
His bundle	Membranous septum	Narrow tubular structure consisting of Purkinje fibers in longitudinal compartments; few P cells	AV nodal artery Branches of LAD	Sparse	Conducts impulses from AV node to bundle branches
Bundle branches	Starts in muscular septum and branches out into ventricles	Purkinje fibers; very variable anatomy	Branches of LAD, RCA	Sparse	Activates ventricles

Key: SA node = sinoatrial node, AV node = atrioventricular node, RCA = right coronary artery, LCX = left circumflex coronary artery, LAD = left anterior descending coronary artery.

the right coronary artery in 90 percent of cases, and also from septal branches of the left anterior descending coronary artery. Histologic examination of the AV node reveals a variety of cells embedded in a loose collagenous network including P cells (although not nearly as many as in the SA node), atrial transitional cells, ordinary myocardial cells, and Purkinje cells.

His bundle

Purkinje fibers emerging from the area of the distal AV node converge gradually to form the His bundle, a narrow tubular structure that runs through the membranous septum to the crest of the muscular septum, where it divides into the bundle branches. The His bundle has relatively sparse autonomic innervation, although its blood supply is quite ample, emanating from both the AV nodal artery and septal branches of the left anterior descending artery. Longitudinal strands of Purkinje fibers, divided into separate parallel compartments by a collagenous skeleton, can be discerned by histologic examination of the His bundle. Relatively sparse P cells can also be identified, embedded within the collagen.

Bundle branches

The bundle branch system is an enormously complex network of interlacing Purkinje fibers that varies greatly between individuals. It generally starts as one or more large fiber bands that split and fan out across the ventricles until they finally terminate in a Purkinje network that interfaces with the myocardium. In some cases, the bundle branches clearly conform to the tri- or quadrifascicular system identified by Rosenbaum and refined by others. In other cases, however, detailed dissection of the conduction system has failed to delineate separate fascicles. The right bundle is usually a single, discrete structure that extends down the right side of the interventricular septum to the base of the anterior papillary muscle, where it divides into three or more branches. The left bundle more commonly originates as a very broad band of interlacing fibers that spread out over the left ventricle, sometimes in two or three distinct fiber tracts. There is relatively little autonomic innervation of the bundle branch system, but the blood supply is extensive, with most areas receiving branches from both the right and left coronary systems.

PHYSIOLOGY

The SA node has the highest rate of spontaneous depolarization (automaticity) in the specialized conduction system and under ordinary circumstances is the major generator of impulses. Its unique location astride the large SA nodal artery provides an ideal milieu for continuous monitoring and instantaneous adjustment of heart rate to meet the body's changing metabolic needs. The SA node is connected to the AV node by several specialized fiber tracts, the function of which has not been fully elucidated. The AV node appears to have three major functions: It delays the passing impulse for a period of 0.04 second under normal circumstances, permitting complete atrial emptying with appropriate loading of the ventricle; it serves as a subsidiary impulse generator because its concentration of P cells is second only to that of the SA node; and it acts as a type of filter, preventing ventricular rates from becoming too rapid in the event of an atrial tachyarrhythmia.

The His bundle arises from the convergence of Purkinje fibers from the AV node, although the exact point at which the AV node ends and the His bundle begins has not been delineated either anatomically or electrically. The separation of the His bundle into longitudinally distinct compartments by the collagenous framework allows for longitudinal dissociation of electrical impulses. Thus a localized lesion below the bifurcation of the His bundle (into the bundle branches) may cause a specific conduction defect (e.g., left anterior fascicular block). The bundle branches arise as a direct continuation of the His bundle fibers. Disease within any aspect of the His bundle branch system may cause conduction defects that may affect AV synchrony or prevent simultaneous ventricular activation. The accompanying hemodynamic consequences have considerable clinical relevance. These consequences have provided the impetus for some of the advances in pacemaker technology, which will be addressed in later chapters of this book. Although a detailed discussion of the histopathology of the conduction system is beyond the scope of the present chapter, it is worth noting that conduction system disease is often *diffuse* and that, for example, normal AV conduction cannot necessarily be assumed when a pacemaker is implanted for a disorder seemingly localized to the sinus node. Similarly, normal sinus node function cannot be assumed when a pacemaker is implanted in a patient with AV block.

The decision to implant a permanent pacemaker is an important one and should be based on solid clinical evidence. A joint committee of the American College of Cardiology and the American Heart Association was formed in the 1980s to provide uniform criteria for pacemaker implantation.[2,3] These guidelines were first published in 1984 and recently revised.[3] It must be realized, however, that medicine is a constantly changing science, and absolute and relative indications for permanent pacing may change as a result of advances in the diagnosis and treatment of arrhythmias. It is useful to keep these ACC/AHA guidelines in mind when evaluating a patient for pacemaker implantation. When approaching a patient with bradycardia, it is also important to take into account several extenuating circumstances. The patient's overall general medical condition must be considered as well as his or her occupation or desire to operate a motor vehicle or equipment where the safety of other individuals may be at risk.

In the ACC/AHA classification, there are three classes of indications for permanent pacemaker implantation. These classes are defined below.

Class I

These are conditions under which implantation of a permanent pacemaker is considered necessary and acceptable. There is general agreement among physicians that a permanent pacemaker should be im-planted. This implies that the condition(s) is (are) chronic or recurrent, but not due to drug toxicity, acute myocardial ischemia or infarction, or electrolyte imbalance.

Class II

These are conditions for which cardiac pacemakers are generally found acceptable or necessary, but there is some divergence of opinion.

Class III

These are conditions that are considered to be unsupported by present evidence to benefit adequately from permanent pacemakers, and there is general agreement that a pacemaker is *not* indicated.

ACQUIRED ATRIOVENTRICULAR BLOCK

Acquired atrioventricular block with syncope (e.g., Stokes-Adams attacks) was historically the first indication for cardiac pacing. The

5

site of AV block (e.g., AV node, His bundle, or distal conduction system) will to a great extent determine the adequacy and reliability of the underlying escape rhythm (Figure 1.1). It is worth noting that in the presence of symptoms documented to be due to AV block, permanent pacing is *indicated*, regardless of the site of the block (e.g., above the His bundle as well as below the His bundle). The indications for permanent pacing with AV block are as follows:

Class I

Permanent or intermittent AV block with symptoms of
a) Syncope or presyncope
b) Congestive heart failure
c) Mental confusion, especially when it improves with temporary pacing
d) Symptomatic ventricular ectopy, nonsustained or sustained ventricular tachycardia or ventricular fibrillation; related to heart block or lack of an adequate escape rhythm
e) Asymptomatic, but with a ventricular escape rate less than 40 beats per minute (ppm)
f) Asymptomatic, with documented asystole greater than 3 seconds
g) Chronotropic incompetence of the escape pacemaker, accompanied by symptoms due to the inability to increase heart rate with exercise or stress

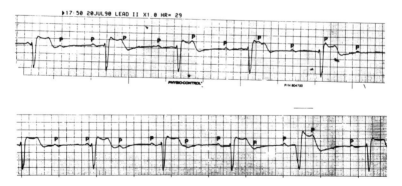

Figure 1.1 An elderly woman presented with syncope and complete heart block after being treated for ventricular tachycardia with amiodarone for three years. The patient is in complete heart block with a wide complex escape rhythm; ventricular rate 29 ppm, atrial rate 75 ppm.

Second-degree AV block with symptoms of syncope or presyncope:
a) Type I (Wenckebach, Mobitz I)
b) Type II (Mobitz II)

Atrial flutter, atrial fibrillation, or atrial tachycardia with advanced symptomatic AV block.

Class II

Asymptomatic complete AV block with a ventricular rate greater than 40 ppm.

Asymptomatic type II second-degree AV block.

Asymptomatic type I second-degree AV block within the His–Purkinje system (rare, requires invasive electrophysiology study for definitive diagnosis).

Class III

First-degree AV block.

Asymptomatic type I second-degree AV block.

The majority of these diagnoses can be made from the surface electrocardiogram. Invasive electrophysiology studies are only rarely necessary but may be helpful or of interest in elucidating the site of AV block (Figure 1.2). Regarding the first two items in Class II, it is likely that permanent pacemakers are more frequently implanted in patients with wide QRS complexes and/or documented infranodal block than in patients with narrow QRS complex escape rhythms.

The next category of patients to be evaluated include those patients with *AV block associated with myocardial infarction*. In these patients, a decision about permanent pacing must be made following the course of a myocardial infarction and prior to discharge. Unfortunately, there is some uncertainty regarding permanent pacing in patients in this category because large, prospective controlled trials have not been performed. Instead, much of our information about pacing in these patients is based on the results of small clinical trials and information in clinical databases. Finally, unlike other indications for permanent cardiac pacing, the criteria for pacing in patients with myocardial infarction do not necessarily require the presence of symptoms.

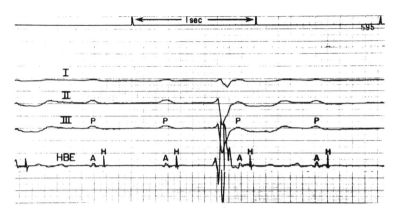

Figure 1.2 A 67-year-old man was admitted complaining of weakness and lightheadedness. A 12-lead ECG showed complete AV block with a wide QRS complex escape rhythm. Intracardiac recordings revealed the site of block below the His bundle. A permanent pacemaker was implanted, and the patient's symptoms resolved. From top to bottom, standard surface ECG leads I, II, III, and intracardiac recording of the His bundle electrogram (HBE). Abbreviations: P = P wave, A = atrial depolarization, H = His bundle depolarization. Paper speed is 100 mm/sec.

Class I

Persistent complete heart block.

Persistent type II second-degree AV block.

Class II

Newly acquired bundle branch block with transient high-grade AV or complete heart block.

Newly acquired bundle branch block with first-degree AV block.

Newly acquired bifascicular bundle branch block.

Class III

First-degree AV block.

Asymptomatic type I second-degree AV block.

Transient AV block without bundle branch block.

Table 1.2 Differential Diagnosis of 2:1 AV Block

	Block Above AV Node	Block Below AV Node
Exercise	+	+/− or −
Atropine	+	+/− or −
Carotid sinus massage	−	+ or +/−
Isoprenaline	+	+ or +/−

+ Represents improved AV conduction.
− Represents worsened AV conduction.

Preexisting right or left bundle branch block.

Acquired left anterior or posterior hemiblock without AV block.

It is important to realize that the indications for *temporary* cardiac pacing in the setting of acute myocardial infarction are different from those for *permanent* pacing following a myocardial infarction (prior to discharge).

It is also worth emphasizing that 2:1 AV block may be either type I or type II, but this cannot always be discerned from the surface ECG (Table 1.2). As a rough approximation, if the QRS complex is narrow, the block is most likely localized to the AV node and considered type I. If the QRS complex is wide, the level of block may be in the AV node or His bundle, and the site of block can best be determined from an invasive electrophysiologic study (His bundle recording). The causes of acquired high-grade AV block are listed in Table 1.3.

CHRONIC BIFASCICULAR OR TRIFASCICULAR BLOCK

Patients with chronic bifascicular block (right bundle branch block and left anterior hemiblock, right bundle branch block and left posterior hemiblock, or complete left bundle branch block) and patients with trifascicular block (any of the above and first-degree AV block) are at an increased risk of progression to complete AV block.

In the 1980s, the results of several prospective studies of the role of His bundle recordings in *asymptomatic* patients with *chronic* bifascicular block were published.[4–7] In these studies, more than 750 patients were followed for three to five years.

Table 1.3   Causes of Acquired High-Grade AV Block

Ischemic
  Acute myocardial infarction
  Chronic ischemic heart disease
Nonischemic cardiomyopathy
  Hypertensive
  Idiopathic dilated
Fibrodegenerative
  Lev's disease
  Lenègre's disease
Postcardiac surgery
  Following coronary artery bypass grafting
  Following aortic valve replacement
  Following ventricular septal defect repair
  Following septal myomectomy (for IHSS surgery)
Other iatrogenic
  After His bundle (AV junction) ablation
  After ablation of septal accessory pathways, AV nodal reentry
  After radiation therapy (e.g., lung cancer, Hodgkin's lymphoma)
Infectious
  Bacterial endocarditis
  Chagas' disease
  Lyme disease
  Other (viral, rickettsial, fungal, etc.)
Neuromuscular disease
  Myotonic dystrophy
  Muscular dystrophies (fascioscapulohumeral)
  Kearns–Sayre syndrome
  Friedreich's ataxia
Infiltrative disease
  Amyloid
  Sarcoid
  Hemochromatosis
  Carcinoid
  Malignant
Connective tissue disease
  Rheumatoid arthritis
  Systemic lupus erythematosus
  Systemic scleroderma
  Ankylosing spondylitis
  Other

The incidence of progression from bifascicular to complete heart block varied from 2 to 5 percent. Most important, the total cardiovascular mortality and the mortality from sudden cardiac death were 19 to 25 percent and 10 to 20 percent, respectively. In these patients, the presence of bifascicular block on the ECG should be taken as a sign of coexisting organic heart disease. These studies concluded that patients with *chronic asymptomatic bifascicular block* and a prolonged HV interval (HV interval represents the shortest conduction time from the His bundle to the endocardium over the specialized conduction system) have more extensive organic heart disease and an increased risk of sudden cardiac death. The risk of spontaneous progression to complete heart block is small, although probably slightly greater in patients with a prolonged HV interval, but rarely leads to cardiac death. Routine His bundle recordings are therefore of little value in evaluating patients with chronic bifascicular block and *no* associated symptoms (e.g., syncope or presyncope) (Figure 1.3).

In patients with bifascicular or trifascicular block and associated *symptoms* of syncope or presyncope, electrophysiologic testing is useful.[8] A high incidence of sudden cardiac death and inducible ventricular arrhythmias is noted in this group of patients. Electrophysiologic testing is useful for identifying the disorder responsible for syncope, and potentially avoiding implantation of a

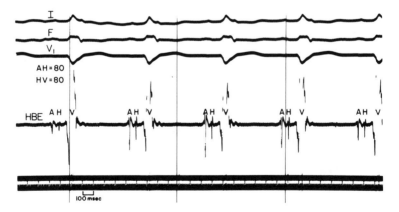

Figure 1.3   An intracardiac recording in a patient with left bundle branch block. The prolonged HV interval (80 msec) is indicative of infranodal disease, but in the absence of transient neurologic symptoms (syncope, dizzy spells, etc.), no specific therapy is indicated. Abbreviations as in Figure 1.2.

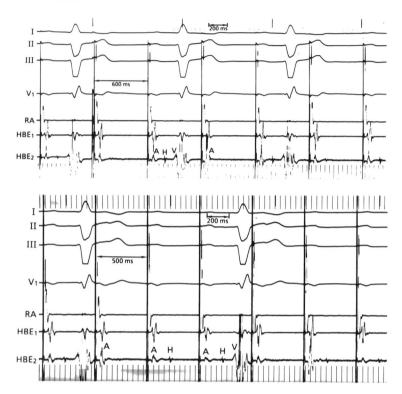

Figure 1.4 A 68-year-old man was admitted complaining of recurrent dizziness and syncope. His baseline 12-lead ECG showed a PR interval of 0.20 second and a right bundle branch block QRS morphology. During electrophysiologic study, the patient's baseline HV interval was 90 msec. (top) During atrial pacing at 600 msec (100 ppm) there is block in the AV node, and (bottom) during pacing at 500 msec (120 ppm) there is block below the AV node, in the His bundle. These findings are indicative of severe diffuse conduction system disease. A permanent dual-chamber pacemaker was implanted, and the patient's symptoms resolved. From top to bottom, standard surface ECG leads I, II, III, V₁, and intracardiac recordings from the right atrial appendage (RA) and His bundle (HBE₁ is proximal His bundle, and HBE₂ is distal His bundle). Abbreviations: A = atrial depolarization, H = His bundle depolarization, V = ventricular depolarization.

pacemaker (Figure 1.4). In patients with a markedly prolonged HV interval (>100 msec), there is a high incidence of subsequent development of complete heart block, and permanent pacing is indicated. However, these patients make up a relatively small percentage of patients undergoing electrophysiologic testing with cardiac symptoms and bifascicular block. In the majority of patients, the HV interval is normal (HV: 35–55 msec) or only *mildly* prolonged, and His bundle recording does not effectively separate out high- and low-risk subpopulations with bifascicular block who are likely to progress to complete heart block. Electrophysiologic testing will often provoke sustained ventricular arrhythmias, which are the cause of syncope in many of these patients.

In a recent review, Barold pointed out that the standard definition of trifascicular block is often too loosely applied.[9] Thus, in patients with right bundle branch block and either left anterior or left posterior fascicular block or in patients with left bundle branch block and first-degree AV block, the *site* of block could be located either in the His–Purkinje system *or* in the AV node. The term "trifascicular block" should be reserved for alternating right and left bundle branch block or for block of either bundle in the setting of a prolonged HV interval.

Class I

Bifascicular block and intermittent third-degree AV block associated with a symptomatic slow escape rhythm.

Bifascicular or trifascicular block with asymptomatic intermittent second-degree AV block.

Symptoms suggestive of intermittent bradycardia in patients with trifascicular block during 1:1 AV conduction (e.g., alternating RBBB and LBBB; RBBB with alternating left anterior or posterior fascicular block)

Class II

Symptomatic patients with bifascicular or trifascicular block and no identifiable cause of syncope.

Block distal to the His bundle at atrial paced rates <150 ppm.

HV prolonged >100 msec.

Class III

Asymptomatic fascicular or bifascicular block.

Asymptomatic fascicular or bifascicular block and first-degree AV block.

SINUS NODE DYSFUNCTION

Sinus node dysfunction, or sick sinus syndrome and its variants, is a heterogeneous clinical syndrome of diverse etiologies.[10,11] This disorder includes sinus bradycardia, sinus arrest, sinoatrial block, and various supraventricular tachycardias (atrial or junctional) alternating with periods of bradycardia or asystole. Sinus node dysfunction is quite common and its incidence increases with advancing age. In patients with sinus node dysfunction, the correlation of symptoms with the bradyarrhythmia is critically important. This is because there is a great deal of disagreement about the absolute heart rate or length of pause required before pacing is indicated. If the symptoms of sinus node disease are dramatic (e.g., syncope, recurrent dizzy spells, seizures, or severe heart failure), then the diagnosis may be relatively easy, but often the symptoms are extremely nonspecific (e.g., easy fatigability, depression, listlessness, early signs of dementia) which, in the elderly, may be easily misinterpreted.[12,13] Instead, many of these patients have symptoms as a result of an abrupt change in heart rate (e.g., termination of tachycardia with a sinus pause or sinus bradycardia) (Figure 1.5). It is important to realize that the degree of bradycardia that may produce symptoms will vary depending on the patient's physiologic status, age, and activity at the time of bradycardia (e.g., eating, sleeping, or walking). In patients with sinus node dysfunction whose symptoms have not been shown to correlate with electrocardiographic abnormalities, a simple exercise test may be helpful (to assess the degree of chronotropic incompetence, especially in

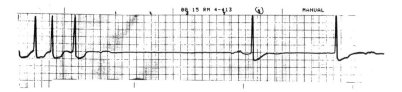

Figure 1.5 An ECG rhythm strip from an elderly woman with recurrent palpitations and syncope. In the left portion of this strip, her rhythm is atrial fibrillation with a ventricular response of about 120 ppm. This is followed by a symptomatic five-second pause with termination in a sinus beat, followed by a junctional escape beat, and then reversion to sinus bradycardia. This patient was asymptomatic during sinus bradycardia and atrial fibrillation; she became symptomatic only when tachycardia termination was followed by a long pause.

the individual with vague symptoms), or electrophysiologic study may be considered.

More permanent pacemakers are implanted for sinus node disease than for any other indication in the United States. Patients with alternating periods of bradycardia and tachycardia (i.e., tachy–brady syndrome) are especially likely to require permanent pacing because medical treatment of the tachycardia often worsens the bradycardia and vice versa. Up to 30 percent of patients with sinus node disease will also have distal conduction system disease. Thus, atrial fibrillation, which is a common complication of sinus node disease, may be accompanied by a slow ventricular response, even in the absence of medications that depress AV conduction. Other important complications of sinus node disease include systemic emboli, especially in the setting of alternating periods of bradycardia and tachycardia, and congestive heart failure, usually related to the slow heart rate.

In addition, many commonly used medications may exacerbate sinus node dysfunction (Table 1.4). For many patients, an acceptable alternative cannot be found, and pacing is necessary so the patient can continue these medications.

A group of patients has been identified with a relatively fixed heart rate during exercise; this condition is referred to as chronotropic incompetence. These patients frequently have other symptoms of sinus node dysfunction. Some of these patients may have symptoms at rest (generally nonspecific), but most will note symptoms, such as fatigue or shortness of breath with exercise. In some cases the diagnosis is straightforward; there is no or only a very slight increase in heart rate with exercise. In other cases the

---

Table 1.4 Commonly Used Medications That May Cause Sinus Node Dysfunction or AV Block

1. Digitalis (especially in the setting of hypokalemia)
2. Antihypertensive agents (clonidine, methyldopa, guanethidine)
3. Beta-adrenergic blockers (inderal, metoprolol, nadolol, atenotol)
4. Calcium channel blockers (verapamil, diltiazem)
5. Type 1A antiarrhythmic drugs (quinidine, procainamide, disopyramide)
6. Type 1C antiarrhythmic drugs (flecainide, propafenone)
7. Type III antiarrhythmic drugs (amiodarone sotalol)
8. Psychotropic medications
   a) Tricyclics
   b) Phenothiazines
   c) Lithium

---

diagnosis is difficult and will require comparison of the patient's exercise response with that of age- and sex-matched patients using specific exercise protocols.

The indications for pacemaker implantation in patients with sinus node dysfunction are as follows:

Class I

Sinus node dysfunction with symptoms due to associated bradycardia, even when exacerbated or due to long-term drug therapy for which an acceptable alternative is *not* available.

Symptomatic sinus bradycardia.

Symptomatic chronotropic incompetence (of the sinus node or AV junction).

Class II

Sinus bradycardia persistently or intermittently less than 40 to 50 ppm, or asystole >3 seconds and suggestive symptoms not documented to be due to bradycardia.

Class III

Asymptomatic sinus bradycardia.

Neurocardiogenic syncope

Neurally mediated syncope is a form of abnormal autonomic control of the circulation. It may take one of three forms:[14,15]

1. the cardioinhibitory type, characterized by ventricular asystole of at least 3 seconds due to sinus arrest or (occasionally) complete heart block;
2. the pure vasodepressor response, marked by a decrease in arterial pressure of ≥ 20 to 30 mmHg but little or no change in heart rhythm;
3. the mixed type, having features of both the cardioinhibitory and vasodepressor types.

Syncope is a common disorder that is estimated to account for approximately 6 percent of all hospital admissions in the United States annually.[16] Despite extensive evaluation, the cause of syncope may not be found in up to 50 percent of cases.[16,17] It is believed that a substantial proportion of these may be due to neurally mediated syncope. The exact mechanism of neurally mediated syncope has not been fully elucidated but appears to be initiated by an exaggerated response of the sympathetic nervous system to a variety of stimuli. Although most often an isolated event with an obvious precipitating cause such as severe fright or emotional upset, in some individuals these episodes are recurrent and without apparent trigger factors.

One variant is the hypersensitive carotid sinus syndrome. A mildly abnormal response to vigorous carotid sinus massage may occur in up to 25 percent of patients, especially if coexisting vascular disease is present. Some patients with an abnormal response to carotid sinus massage may have no symptoms suggestive of carotid sinus syncope. On the other hand, the typical history of syncope—blurred vision and lightheadedness or confusion in the standing or sitting position, especially during movement of the head or neck—should be suggestive of this entity. Classical triggers of carotid sinus syncope are head turning, tight neckwear, shaving, and neck hyperextension. Syncopal episodes usually last only several minutes and are generally reproducible in a given patient. Symptoms associated with this syndrome may wax or wane over several years. Carotid sinus hypersensitivity is most often predominantly cardioinhibitory in nature so that permanent pacing may be very helpful. In contrast, other forms of neurocardiogenic syncope often have a prominent vasodepressor component, so that permanent pacing has a more limited role.

A variety of other stimuli may give rise to cardioinhibitory or mixed cardioinhibitory responses. These conditions, when recurrent, may also be treated by permanent pacemakers. The conditions include pain, coughing, micturition, swallowing, defecation, and the relatively common vasovagal syndrome. In general, pacemakers are implanted in these patients when symptoms are recurrent, severe, and cannot be controlled by more conservative measures (e.g., avoidance of stimuli, beta blookers, and/or florinef). Pacemaker therapy tends to be most successful in patients who predominantly experience the cardioinhibitory type of response.

The advent of head-upright tilt testing has had a major impact on the area of neurocardiogenic syncope.[18] Vasodepressor and/or cardioinhibitory responses may be elicited, which appear to correlate well with the clinical symptomatology. As with the abovementioned clinical syndromes, permanent pacemakers are most effective in patients whose tilt test displays a prominent cardioinhibitory component. The indications for pacemaker implantation are:

Class I

Patients with recurrent syncope, a suggestive clinical setting, and in whom tilt testing or carotid sinus pressure produces asystole of 3 seconds or longer in duration, or heart block of 3 seconds or longer in duration.

Patients with recurrent syncope and clear-cut clinical situation suggestive of a vasoinhibitory response.

Class II

Patients with recurrent syncope, with neither a clear clinical setting nor precipitating feature(s), but with an abnormal response to carotid sinus pressure or tilt testing.

Class III

Patients with vasodepressor syncope.

Asymptomatic or vaguely symptomatic patients with dizziness or lightheadedness and a negative response to carotid sinus massage or tilt testing.

INDICATIONS FOR PERMANENT CARDIAC PACING

As stated earlier, the indications for permanent pacemaker implantation may change as new ones evolve. Permanent pacemakers have also shown promise in relief of symptoms in patients with obstructive hypertrophic cardiomyopathy.[19] The mechanism is presumably the induction of paradoxical septal motion with the ventricular septum moving away from, rather than toward, the anterior leaflet of the mitral valve and left ventricular outflow tract during systole. This is generally best achieved with dual-chamber pacing with a short PR interval (i.e., usually 50–125 msec), ensuring early right ventricular and septal activation and a maximum amount of wall motion dysynchrony. The hemodynamic effects of dual-chamber pacing may be quite dramatic with a major reduction in left ventricular cavity obliteration and a concomitant decrease in left ventricular outflow tract gradient (Figure 1.6).

More intriguing is the suggestion that the beneficial effects of dual-chamber pacing in this condition do not dissipate immediately once the pacing has been terminated.[19] However, the mechanism of the beneficial effects of pacing is incompletely understood and the population that would most reliably benefit has not been fully

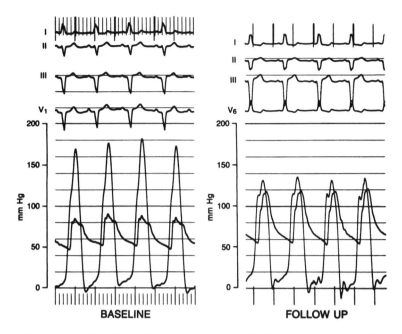

Figure 1.6 Tracings show reduction of left ventricular outflow tract obstruction after chronic dual-chamber pacing during sinus rhythm. At baseline (left panel), the left ventricular systolic pressure and left ventricular outflow tract gradient were 280 mmHg and 90 mmHg, respectively. At follow-up cardiac catheterization (right panel), the left ventricular systolic pressure and left ventricular outflow tract gradient, measured also in sinus rhythm, were reduced to 135 mmHg and 15 mmHg, respectively. From top to bottom, I, II, III, V_1, and V_6 surface electrocardiographic leads.

elucidated. Long-term results of DDD pacing in this condition suggest that further improvement in hemodynamic indices continues to occur a year after pacing and baseline pacing studies are not necessary to identify who will benefit from pacing.[20] Ongoing multicenter randomized trials of different pacing modes will provide further confirmation of the efficacy of this therapy. Since prolongation of life has not been documented with this therapy, permanent pacemakers should be reserved for patients whose symptoms are unresponsive to medical management with the understanding that surgical myotomy–myectomy is still considered the gold standard for treatment of this condition.[21]

A related area in which permanent pacing may be of benefit is dilated cardiomyopathy. Some studies have demonstrated that dual-chamber pacing, especially with a short AV delay, may have important beneficial hemodynamic benefit in patients with severe congestive heart failure.[22,23] Although the exact mechanism has not been determined, it has been postulated that the improvement in hemodynamics may be related to optimization of ventricular filling or reduction of diastolic mitral regurgitation.[24] Other groups, more recently, however, have failed to confirm these beneficial effects.[25] There has also been interest in the use of right ventricular outflow tract pacing and biventricular permanent pacing for congestive heart failure, but these areas are still in the early stages of development.

Another indication for permanent pacemaker implantation is to provide a stable rhythm following electrical or radiofrequency catheter ablation of the AV node–His bundle for refractory supraventricular tachycardias. Many of these patients will have an underlying narrow or wide QRS escape rhythm. Nevertheless, until we know more about the long-term reliability and chronotropic responsiveness of these subsidiary pacemakers, permanent pacemakers should be implanted in all these patients. In contrast, patients who undergo selective ablation of a "slow" or "fast" pathway (AV nodal modification) may have no interruption of AV conduction and should not be considered for pacemaker implantation.

Several small reports have documented a benefit of atrial or AV sequential pacing in patients with idiopathic orthostatic hypotension refractory to salt and steroid therapy.[26] The rationale for pacing for this condition is that by increasing the pacing heart rate (i.e., the programmed lower pacing rate in series varies from 80 to 100 ppm), the cardiac output increases, and potentially leads to more vasoconstriction. This therapy usually results in some clinical improvement, which varies considerably from patient to patient.

Permanent pacing may also be of help in patients with the long QT syndrome, especially for bradycardic patients who have a history of ventricular arrhythmias or syncope.[27] The pacing-induced increase in ventricular rate tends to shorten the QT interval and decreases or eliminates early afterdepolarizations, which may serve as initiating factors in the genesis of ventricular arrhythmias. Permanent pacing may also permit the use of beta blockers, known to be of benefit in this syndrome, without worsening resting bradycardia.

A prospective study of patients with congenital complete heart block followed into adult life has provided some recommendations regarding permanent pacing in this condition.[28] On the basis of this prospective study, the authors recommended prophylactic, permanent pacing for patients, even if they are symptom-free, because of the high incidence of unpredictable Stokes-Adams attacks with considerable mortality. These authors showed that sudden death may be the initial manifestation in congenital AV block, and exercise testing is of limited value in risk assessment for future sudden cardiac events, such as syncope or presyncope. Early intervention with pacing therapy in the asymptomatic patient may prevent the development of myocardial dysfunction and mitral regurgitation in later life.[28,29]

A study of 58 patients with a variety of diagnoses (sick sinus syndrome in 41 percent, chronic bifascicular block in 11 percent, and carotid hypersensitivity in 11 percent) and a history of transient neurologic symptoms (presyncope, syncope), but no previous *documented* relationship between their symptoms and bradycardia had permanent pacemakers implanted.[30] These patients had a high rate of relief of symptoms (94 percent) following pacemaker implantation. The ACC/AHA guidelines would have classified many of these pacemaker implants as class II or class III. This study emphasizes that the ACC/AHA scheme should serve as only a guide for pacemaker implantation. The importance of experienced clinical judgment to help further determine when pacemaker implantation is likely to be beneficial should not be underestimated. Many factors determine whether a patient benefits from pacing, and the individual patient and her or his clinical problem may not always fit neatly into a defined indication for pacing.

CLINICAL USE

Since the advent of implantable permanent cardiac pacing almost 30 years ago, the indications for implantation have changed considerably. This procedure was initially reserved for patients with syncope and complete heart block. In many current series, the most common indication for permanent cardiac pacing is sick sinus syndrome. The indications for permanent pacing in a consecutive series (1994–1995) from the VA National Registry are shown in Table 1.5 and Figure 1.7.

INDICATIONS FOR TEMPORARY CARDIAC PACING

The following section reviews the clinical settings in which temporary cardiac pacing is indicated. Chapter 4 reviews the techniques and complications of temporary cardiac pacing.

Table 1.5   Indications for Pacemaker Implantation: VA National Registry (June 1994–June 1995), N = 915

Sick Sinus Syndrome	**335**
SSS + AV block	20
SSS + bradycardia/tachycardia	73
SSS + sinus bradycardia	110
SSS + SA arrest or exit block	40
SSS (unspecified)	92
AV Block	
Complete heart block	326
Wide QRS	62
Narrow QRS	43
Intermittent	81
Unspecified QRS	140
Second-degree heart block	126
Mobitz II	69
Wenckebach	20
Unspecified	37
Atrial flutter/atrial fibrillation/with high-grade heart block	89
Asystole	**20**
Carotid Sinus Syndrome	**19***

*Included in above categories according to type of conduction abnormality occurring with carotid sinus syndrome.

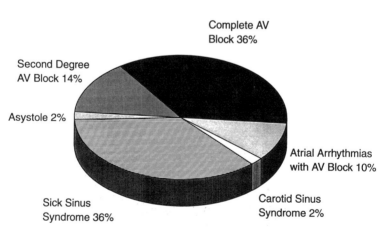

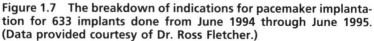

Figure 1.7   The breakdown of indications for pacemaker implantation for 633 implants done from June 1994 through June 1995. (Data provided courtesy of Dr. Ross Fletcher.)

Acute myocardial infarction

In the setting of an acute myocardial infarction, several different types of conduction disturbances may become manifest. They include abnormalities of sinus impulse formation or conduction, disorders of atrioventricular conduction, and disorders of intraventricular conduction. In general, any patient with bradyarrhythmias that are associated with symptoms or cause hemodynamic compromise must be treated. Ways of identifying patient populations at greatest risk for the development of a significant bradyarrhythmia during acute myocardial infarction and in whom temporary pacing can be performed prophylactically to avoid the increased risk of temporary pacemaker insertion in an emergency situation are discussed below.

Sinus node abnormalities: Sinus node dysfunction may include sinus bradycardia, sinus arrest, and/or sinoatrial exit block. The incidence of these electrocardiographic abnormalities is quite variable, ranging from 5 to 30 percent in different series.[31,32] In addition, it is not uncommon to see concomitant AV nodal block in these patients. These abnormalities of sinus rhythm are more common with inferoposterior infarction because either the right or left circumflex coronary artery is occluded—these arteries most commonly supply the sinus node. Another potential reason is chemically mediated activation of receptors on the posterior left ventricular wall—these receptors are supplied by vagal afferents. Treatment of sinus bradycardia, sinus pauses, or sinoatrial block is not necessary, unless symptoms such as worsening myocardial ischemia, heart failure, or hypotension are documented. If sinus abnormalities are intermittent, atropine may be administered with subsequent resolution of symptoms. Atropine, however, may cause unpredictable increases in heart rate. If bradycardia is prolonged and severe, or is not responsive to atropine, temporary cardiac pacing is indicated.

Disorders of atrioventricular conduction: Atrioventricular block occurs *without* associated intraventricular conduction system abnormalities in 12 to 25 percent of patients with acute myocardial infarction.[32,33] The incidence of this finding depends largely on the patient population and the site of infarction. First-degree AV block occurs in 2 to 12 percent of patients, second-degree AV block in 3 to 10 percent of patients, and third-degree AV block in 3 to 7 percent of patients. The majority of patients with abnormalities of atrioventricular conduction without bundle branch block have evidence of an inferoposterior infarction (approximately 70 percent).[34] In fact, about 12 to 20 percent of patients with inferior infarction demonstrate evidence of conduction system disease more advanced than first-degree block. The reasons for the increased incidence of AV conduction system abnormalities are related to the coronary blood supply to the AV node. The coronary artery supplying the inferoposterior wall of the left ventricle is typically the right or left circumflex coronary, which is occluded during an inferior infarction. In addition, as mentioned above, activation (directly or indirectly) of cardiac reflexes with augmentation of parasympathetic tone during inferior ischemia (infarction) may also be responsible. In some cases, AV block may be due to release of adenosine caused by inferior ischemia or during inferior infarction.[35]

The risk of progression from first-degree AV block to high-grade AV block (during inferior infarction) varies from 10 to 30 percent, and that of second-degree AV block to complete heart block is about 35 percent. As would be expected, the development of high-grade AV block in the setting of acute inferoposterior infarction is usually associated with narrow QRS complex escape rhythms[36,37] (Figure 1.8). The junctional escape rhythm usually remains stable at 50 to 60 ppm, and can be increased by intravenous atropine, so that even complete AV block may not require specific therapy in this situation.

Type I second-degree AV block with a narrow QRS almost always represents conduction block in the AV node, and temporary cardiac pacing is rarely required unless the patient has concomitant symptoms. Type I second-degree AV block with a wide QRS complex may represent conduction block in the AV node or His bundle or contralateral bundle branch block. In these patients,

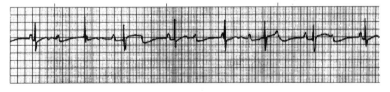

Figure 1.8 Rhythm strip of high-grade AV block with occasional capture beats (third and sixth QRS) later in the course of an acute inferior wall myocardial infarction. The narrow QRS complex escape rhythm (shown here at a rate of 47 ppm) tends to be reliable, and if the patient is asymptomatic, no specific therapy is required.

especially in the setting of anterior myocardial infarction, temporary prophylactic pacing must be considered. In patients with type II second-degree AV block and a wide QRS complex in the setting of inferior infarction, or with a wide or narrow QRS complex during an anterior myocardial infarction, a temporary pacemaker should be inserted. Patients with a narrow QRS complex and type II second-degree AV block in the setting of inferior infarction rarely progress to complete heart block.

Several special situations are worthy of consideration. Patients with high-grade AV block occurring in the setting of right ventricular infarction tend to be less responsive to intravenous atropine and demonstrate markedly improved hemodynamics during AV sequential pacing.[38-40] The mechanism for this hemodynamic improvement is probably a reflection of the restrictive physiology the infarcted right ventricle demonstrates. Another group of patients who may benefit from prophylactic temporary pacing are patients with acute inferior wall infarction with alternating Wenckebach periods.[41] This electrocardiographic finding is rare (<2 percent) but frequently leads to hemodynamic embarrassment without temporary pacing. Alternating Wenckebach periodicity occurs in the setting of 2:1 AV conduction when there is a progressive increase in the PR intervals of the conducted sinus beats until two or more consecutive atrial impulses fail to be conducted (Figure 1.9). This pattern generally repeats and probably reflects multilevel AV block. Isoproterenol and atropine rarely are associated with improvement of conduction in this condition, and temporary pacing is often required.

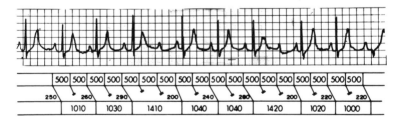

Figure 1.9 Monitor lead from a 53-year-old man with an acute inferior wall infarction and alternating Wenckebach periodicity. Ladder diagram shown below the figure illustrates 2:1 AV conduction with progressive prolongation of the PR intervals of conducted P waves and eventual failure of alternate atrial impulses. (Reproduced with permission of J. Marcus Wharton from *Electrical Therapy of Cardiac Arrhythmias*, WB Saunders, 1990.)

In contrast to inferior wall infarction, high-grade AV block complicating anterior wall infarction is usually located within the His–Purkinje system. Transition from the first nonconducted P wave to high-grade AV block is often abrupt, and the resulting escape rhythm is typically slow and unreliable. Conducted beats usually have a wide QRS complex (Figure 1.10). In general, interruption of the blood supply to the anterior wall and the interventricular septum severe enough to cause AV block usually causes severe left ventricular dysfunction and results in high mortality. Emergency temporary pacing and prophylactic pacing are indicated, although survival may not be significantly improved because of the extent of myocardial damage.

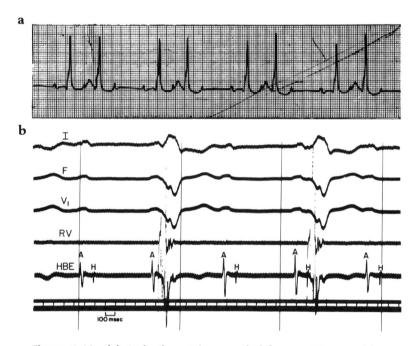

Figure 1.10 **(a) A rhythm strip recorded from a 47-year-old man with an acute anterior wall myocardial infarction, complicated by an intraventricular conduction defect and congestive heart failure, revealing type I second-degree AV block. In contrast to the patient with inferior wall infarction, second-degree AV block here warrants immediate investigation. (b) Surface and intracardiac recordings verify that the site of block is infranodal. The P waves are blocked below the AV node (block in the His bundle). Immediate temporary pacing is warranted.**

Disorders of intraventricular conduction system: A number of studies have examined the incidence of development of new bundle branch block in the setting of acute myocardial infarction and determined it to vary between 5 and 15 percent, depending on the site of infarction. New bundle branch block is three times more likely during anterior infarction than during inferior infarction, because the left anterior descending coronary artery provides the major blood supply to the His bundle and the bundle branches. In addition, not surprisingly, there is a high incidence of heart failure; the resulting high cardiac mortality leads to controversy as to whether temporary or permanent cardiac pacing improves the poor prognosis in these patients.

Multiple studies have shown that patients with acute infarction and bundle branch block have a four- to fivefold increased risk of progression to high-grade AV block (e.g., increase from 4 to 18 percent).[33,42-44] Both in-hospital and out-of-hospital mortality are higher in patients presenting with bundle branch block during acute infarction. The etiology of the increase in mortality may be due to a variety of causes.[35,36] These include an increased risk of congestive heart failure and pump failure, an increased risk of ventricular tachyarrhythmias, an increased risk of infarct extension, and an increased risk of progression to high-grade AV block in the hospital. The mortality of patients with bundle branch block and acute infarction is 30 to 40 percent, compared with 10 to 15 percent in patients without bundle branch block. Most of the increase in cardiac mortality appears to be related to the degree of heart failure, reflecting the amount of infarcted myocardium.

Several large studies have attempted to identify groups of patients that may be at increased risk of progression to high-grade heart block.[33,42-44] Unfortunately, many of these studies are limited by their retrospective nature, their small sample size, or their ascertainment bias. In one large study of patients with bundle branch block during acute infarction, the percentage of patients presenting with different bundle branch morphologies was

38 percent for left bundle branch block;

34 percent for right bundle branch block and left anterior fascicular block;

11 percent for right bundle branch block;

10 percent for right bundle branch block and left posterior fascicular block;

and 6 percent for alternating bundle branch block.

On the basis of the results of several studies, patients with the following conduction system abnormalities are generally recommended to have temporary pacemakers inserted prophylactically:

	Risk of High-Grade AV Block
First-degree AV block and new bifascicular BBB	38–43%
First-degree AV block and old bifascicular BBB	20–50%
New bifascicular BBB	15–31%
Alternating BBB	44%

Patients with new bundle branch block and first-degree AV block are at intermediate risk of progression (19–29 percent) to high-grade AV block and may or may not be recommended to undergo prophylactic pacing depending on the availability of facilities for emergency placement of a temporary pacemaker. In patients with known prior bifascicular block or old bundle branch block, His bundle recording may be useful to help determine whether temporary pacing is necessary. Finally, because the greatest risk of progression to complete heart block occurs in the first five days following infarction, these decisions should be made promptly so that temporary cardiac pacing may be instituted.

The recent Multicenter Investigation of the Limitation of Infarct Size (MILIS) study suggested a simpler method of risk stratification.[47] A "risk score" for development of complete heart block was devised. Patients with any of the following conduction disturbances were given one point: first-degree AV block, type I second-degree AV block, type II second-degree AV block, left anterior fascicular block, left posterior fascicular block, right bundle branch block, and left bundle branch block. The presence of no risk factors was associated with a 1.2 percent risk of third-degree AV block, one risk factor with a 7.8 percent risk, two risk factors with a 25 percent risk, and three risk factors with 36.4 percent risk of complete heart block. These findings were validated by testing the risk score in over 3000 patients from previously published studies. The risk score appears to be an alternative to risk stratification using combinations of conduction disorders.

The effect of thrombolytic therapy—both pharmacologic and mechanical—on the subsequent development of high-grade AV block in patients presenting with acute infarction and intraventricular conduction system disease has been poorly studied. In the Italian Group for the Study of Streptokinase in Myocardial Infarction (GISSI) study, using streptokinase, there was no statistically significant difference in the incidence of AV block in patients undergoing thrombolysis.[48] It is probably best to follow the guidelines listed above until more information is available regarding the effects of reperfusion.

PACING DURING CARDIAC CATHETERIZATION

During catheterization of the right side of the heart, manipulation of the catheter may induce a transient right bundle branch block in up to 10 percent of patients. This block generally lasts for seconds or minutes but can occasionally last for hours or days. Trauma induced by right ventricular endomyocardial biopsy also may result in temporary or, rarely, long-lasting right bundle branch block. This is a problem only in patients with preexisting left bundle branch block, in whom complete heart block may result. We therefore recommend placement of a temporary transvenous pacing wire in patients undergoing right heart catheterization or biopsy in the presence of previously known left bundle branch block. Catheterization of the left side of the heart in patients with known preexisting right bundle branch block only rarely gives rise to complete heart block because of the short length of the left bundle branch.

Significant bradycardia and asystole can occur during injection of the right coronary artery. This complication is extremely rare, and the placement of a temporary pacing catheter does not alter the morbidity or mortality of catheterization. The bradycardia usually resolves after several seconds. The same comments apply in general to placement of a temporary pacing wire during angioplasty.

PREOPERATIVE PACING

One of the questions most frequently asked of a consulting cardiologist by both surgeons and anesthesiologists is whether it is necessary to insert a temporary pacing catheter in patients with bifascicular block undergoing general anesthesia.[49] The results of several studies have shown that the incidence of intraoperative and perioperative complete heart block is quite low. There does not appear to be any benefit from preoperative prophylactic pacemaker insertion. Even in patients with first-degree AV block and bifascicular block, there is a very low incidence of perioperative high-grade heart block.

In patients who have bifascicular block and also type II second-degree AV block or a history of unexplained syncope or presyncope, however, the risk of development of high-grade AV block is higher, and a temporary pacemaker should be inserted. The appearance of new bifascicular block in the immediate post-operative period should also lead to insertion of a temporary pacemaker and should raise suspicion of an intraoperative infarct.

OTHER TEMPORARY PACING

Temporary pacing is indicated in patients with new AV or bundle branch block in the setting of acute bacterial endocarditis. The development of a new conduction system abnormality generally suggests that there is a perivalvular (ring) abscess that has extended to involve the conduction system near the AV node and/or the His bundle. The endocarditis generally involves the noncoronary cusp of the aortic valve. In one study, 22 percent of patients with aortic valve endocarditis and new first-degree AV block developed high-grade or complete heart block. Although these studies are retrospective, the patient with development of new AV block or bundle branch block, especially in the setting of aortic valve endocarditis, should probably undergo temporary pacing while cardiac evaluation continues.

Treatment of tumors of the head and/or neck or around the carotid sinus may in some circumstances give rise to high-grade AV block. Temporary pacing may be required during surgical treatment, radiation therapy, or chemotherapy. If the tumor responds poorly, permanent pacing may be necessary in some cases. The long-term risk for subsequent heart block due to tumor recurrence is difficult to predict in some cases.

Lyme disease, a tick-borne spirochete infection, causes a systemic infection with arthritis, skin lesions, myalgias, meningoencephalitis, and cardiac involvement in 5 to 10 percent of patients.[50,51] Lyme disease is epidemic in the summer months in the northeastern United States. Carditis typically occurs relatively late in the course of the illness, usually 4 to 8 weeks after the onset of symptoms. AV block is the most common manifestation of carditis and tends to be transient. Block is most commonly at the level of the AV node and fluctuation between first-degree and higher degrees of AV block is frequent. Temporary cardiac pacing may be required, but the conduction disturbances usually resolve spontaneously, especially with antibiotic treatment, so that permanent cardiac pacing rarely is necessary. Similar conduction disturbances can occasionally be seen in patients with viral myocarditis, as well as with other tick-borne infections.

Finally, a number of medications may produce transient bradycardia that may require temporary pacing until the drug has been stopped (see Table 1.4). These drugs may cause sinus node dysfunction and/or AV block; if used in combination, their effects may potentiate each other and exacerbate mild or latent conduction system disease. If long-term therapy with these agents is necessary for an underlying disorder and a substitute cannot be found, permanent pacing may be required.

TREATMENT OF TACHYCARDIAS

The use of temporary cardiac pacing for the treatment and/or prophylaxis of arrhythmias is discussed extensively in Chapter 8. Type I atrial flutter, paroxysmal supraventricular tachycardia, and ventricular tachycardia can often be terminated by cardiac pacing.

In patients with torsades de pointes, a polymorphic ventricular tachycardia, seen in association with a number of clinical conditions (Table 1.6), overdrive atrial, and/or ventricular pacing may be central to treatment. Torsades de pointes is a polymorphic tachycardia with a sinusoidal electrocardiographic appearance because the QRS complex undulates about the baseline. This condition results from prolonged myocardial repolarization, which is often reflected on the surface ECG by a prolonged QT or QT-U interval. Tachycardia is often preceded by short–long–short series of changes in cycle length. Importantly, episodes tend to be recurrent, paroxysmal, and nonsustained initially, but may become sustained later unless the underlying condition is identified and corrected. Therefore it is critical that the clinical syndrome be recognized, any offending drugs or toxins be stopped, and any electrolyte deficiencies be corrected. In some patients these treatments will be adequate, but in others temporary atrial pacing (if AV node conduction is adequate) or ventricular pacing should be initiated. Such pacing will be effective because it provides more uniform repolarization and an increased heart rate, which will shorten the QT interval. Pacing and intravenous magnesium is the mainstay of therapy for this problem. Finally, isoproterenol infusion will also increase heart rate and thus shorten repolarization, but it

Table 1.6 Causes of Torsades de Pointes

Electrolyte abnormalities
  Hypokalemia
  Hypomagnesemia
Antiarrhythmic agents
  Quinidine
  Procainamide
  Disopyramide
  Amiodarone
Hereditary long QT syndrome(s)
Bradyarrhythmias
Liquid protein diets
Myocardial ischemia/infarction
Neurologic events
  Subarachnoid hemorrhage
  Head trauma
Other drugs – antihistamines (astemizole, terfenadine), bepridil
Neuroleptics
  Tricyclic and tetracyclic antidepressants
  Phenothiazines
Antibiotics
  Erythromycin
  Trimethoprim sulfamethoxazole
  Chloroquine
  Amantidine
Toxins
  Organophosphates
  Arsenic

tends to be associated with significant side effects, especially in patients with organic heart disease.

As indicated by the above discussion, there is a wide variety of clinical circumstances during which temporary or permanent cardiac pacing is indicated.

REFERENCES

1. Schlant RC, Silverman ME. Anatomy of the heart. In JW Hurst (ed.), *The Heart* (6th ed). New York: McGraw-Hill, 1986; pp 16–37.
2. Dreifus LS, Fisch C, Griffin JC, et al. Guidelines for implantation of cardiac pacemakers and antiarrhythmia devices: A report of the American College of Cardiology/American Heart

Association Task Force on Assessment of Diagnostic and Therapeutic Cardiovascular Procedures (Subcommittee on Pacemaker Implantation). *J Am Coll Cardiol* 1991;18:1–13.

3. Phibbs B, Friedman HS, Graboys TB, et al. Indications for pacing in the treatment of bradyarrhythmias: Report of an independent study group. *JAMA* 1984;252:1307–1311.

4. Dhingra RC, Denes P, Wu D, et al. Prospective observations in patients with chronic branch block and H-V prolongation. *Circulation* 1976;53:600–604.

5. McAnulty JH, Rahimtoola SH, Murphy E, et al. Natural history of "high-risk" bundle branch block: Final report of a prospective study. *N Engl J Med* 1982;307:137–143.

6. McAnulty JH, Rahimtoola SH. Bundle branch block. *Prog Cardiovasc Dis* 1984;26:333–354.

7. Scheinman MM, Peters RW, Sauve MJ, et al. Value of the H-Q interval in patients with bundle branch block and the role of prophylactic permanent pacing. *Am J Cardiol* 1982;50:1316–1322.

8. Morady F, Higgins J, Peters RW, et al. Electrophysiological testing in bundle branch block and unexplained syncope. *Am J Cardiol* 1984;54:587–591.

9. Barold SS. ACC/AHA guidelines for implantation of cardiac pacemakers: How accurate are the definitions of atrioventricular and intraventricular conduction blocks? *PACE* 1993;16:1221–1226.

10. Sutton R, Kenny R. The natural history of sick sinus syndrome. *PACE* 1986;9:1110–1114.

11. Simon AB, Zloto AE. Symptomatic sinus node disease: Natural history after permanent ventricular pacing. *PACE* 1979;2:305–314.

12. Hilgard J, Ezri MD, Denes PB. Significance of the ventricular pauses of three seconds or more detected on 24-hour Holter recordings. *Am J Cardiol* 1985;55;1005–1008.

13. Ector H, Rolies L, De Geest H. Dynamic electrocardiography and ventricular pauses of 3 seconds and more: Etiology and therapeutic implications. *PACE* 1983;6:548–551.

14. Morley CA, Sutton R. Carotid sinus syncope. *Int J Cardiol* 1984;6:287–293.

15. Thomas JE. Hyperactive carotid sinus reflex and carotid sinus syncope. *Mayo Clin Proc* 1969;44:127–139.

16. Kapoor WN. Evaluation and management of the patient with syncope. *JAMA* 1992;268:2553–2560.

17. Manolis AS, Linzer M, Estes NAM. Syncope: Current diagnostic evaluation and management. *Ann Intern Med* 1990;112: 850–863.
18. Abboud FM. Neurocardiogenic syncope. *N Engl J Med* 1993;328:1117–1119.
19. Fananapazir L, Canno RO, Tripodi D, Panza JA. Impact of dual-chamber permanent pacing in patients with obstructive hypertrophic cardiomyopathy with symptoms refractory to verapamil and beta-adrenergic blocker therapy. *Circulation* 1992;85:2149–2161.
20. Fananapazir L, Epstein ND, Curiel RV, et al. Long-term results of dual-chamber (DDD) pacing in hypertrophic cardiomyopathy: Evidence for progressive symptomatic and hemodynamic improvement and reduction of left ventricular hypertrophy. *Circulation* 1994;90:2731–2742.
21. Maron BJ. Therapeutic strategies in hypertrophic cardiomyopathy: Considerations and critique of new treatment modalities. *Heart Failure* 1995; February/March: 27–32.
22. Hochleitner M, Hortnagel H, Ng C-K, et al. Usefulness of physiologic dual-chamber pacing in drug-resistant idiopathic dilated cardiomyopathy. *Am J Cardiol* 1990;66:198–202.
23. Hochleitner M, Hortnagel H, Fridich L, Gschnitzer F. Long-term efficacy of physiologic dual-chamber pacing in the treatment of end-stage idiopathic dilated cardiomyopathy. *Am J Cardiol* 1992;70:1320–1325.
24. Nishimura RA, Hayes DL, Holmes DR Jr, Tajik AJ. Mechanism of hemodynamic improvement by dual-chamber pacing for severe left ventricular dysfunction: An acute Doppler and catheterization study. *J Am Coll Cardiol* 1995;25:281–288.
25. Gold MR, Feliciano Z, Gottlieb SS, Fisher ML. Dual-chamber pacing with a short atrioventricular delay in congestive heart failure: A randomized study. *J Am Coll Cardiol* 1995;26:967–973.
26. Weissmann P, Chin MT, Moss AJ. Cardiac tachypacing for severe refractory idiopathic orthostatic hypotension. *Ann Intern Med* 1992;116:650.
27. Moss AJ, Liu JE, Gottlieb S, et al. Efficacy of permanent pacing in the management of high risk patients with long QT syndrome. *Circulation* 1991;84:1530.
28. Michaelsson M, Jonzon A, Riesenfeld T. Isolated congenital complete atrioventricular block in adult life. A prospective study. *Circulation* 1995;92:442–449.

29. Friedman RA. Congenital AV block. Pace me now or pace me later? *Circulation* 1995;92:283–285.
30. Lamas GA, Dawley D, Splaine K, et al. Documented symptomatic bradycardia and symptoms relief in patients receiving permanent pacemakers: An evaluation of joint ACC/AHA pacing guidelines. *PACE* 1988;11:1098–1104.
31. Parameswaran R, Ohe T, Goldberg H. Sinus node dysfunction in acute myocardial infarction. *Br Heart J* 1976;38:93–96.
32. Rotman M, Wagner GS, Wallace AG. Bradyarrhythmias in acute myocardial infarction. *Circulation* 1972;45:703–722.
33. DeGuzman M, Rahimtoola SH. What is the role of pacemakers in patients with coronary artery disease and conduction abnormalities? *Cardiovasc Clin* 1983;13(1):191–201. (Also in SH Rahimtoola (ed.), *Current Controversies in Coronary Heart Disease.* Philadelphia: FA Davis, 1983, pp 191–207.)
34. Sclarovsky S, Strasberg B, Hirshberg A, et al. Advanced early and later atrioventricular block in acute inferior myocardial infarction. *Am Heart J* 1984;108:19–24.
35. Wesley RC, Lerman BB, DiMarco JP, et al. Mechanism of atropine-resistant atrioventricular block during inferior myocardial infarction; possible role of adenosine. *J Am Coll Cardiol* 1986;8:1232–1234.
36. Tans AC, Lie KI, Durrer D. Clinical settings and prognostic significance of high degree atrioventricular block in acute inferior myocardial infarction: A study of 144 patients. *Am Heart J* 1980;99:48.
37. Feigl D, Ashkenazy J, Kishon Y. Early and late atrioventricular block in acute inferior myocardial infarction. *J Am Coll Cardiol* 1984;4:35–38.
38. Topol EJ, Goldschlager N, Ports TA, et al. Hemodynamic benefit of atrial pacing in right ventricular myocardial infarction. *Ann Intern Med* 1982;96:594–597.
39. Braat SH, de Zwaan C, Brugada P, et al. Right ventricular involvement with acute interior wall myocardial infarction identifies high risk of developing atrioventricular node conduction disturbances. *Am Heart J* 1984;107:1183–1187.
40. Bilbao FJ, Zabalza IE, Vilanova JR, Froufe J. Atrioventricular block in posterior acute myocardial infarction: A clinicopathologic correlation. *Circulation* 1987;75:733–736.
41. Lewin RF, Kusniec J, Sclarovsky S, et al. Alternating Wenckebach periods in acute inferior myocardial infarction:

Clinical, electrocardiographic, and therapeutic characterization. *PACE* 1986;9:468–475.

42. Hindman MC, Wagner GS, JaRo M, et al. The clinical significance of bundle branch block complicating acute myocardial infarction. 1. Clinical characteristics, hospital mortality, and one year follow up. *Circulation* 1978;58:679–688.

43. Hindman MC, Wagner GS, JaRo M, et al. The clinical significance of bundle branch block complicating acute myocardial infarction. 2. Indications for temporary and permanent pacemaker insertion. *Circulation* 1978;58:689–699.

44. Nimetz AA, Shubrooks SJ, Hutter AM Jr, DeSanctis RW. The significance of bundle branch block during acute myocardial infarction. *Am Heart J* 1975;90:439–444.

45. Hauer RNW, Lie KI, Liem RL, Durrer D. Long-term prognosis in patients with bundle branch block complicating acute anteroseptal infarction. *Am J Cardiol* 1982;49:1581–1585.

46. Gann D, Balachandran PK, El-Sherif N, Samet P. Prognostic significance of chronic versus acute bundle block in acute myocardial infarction. *Chest* 1975;67:298–303.

47. Lamas GA, Muller JE, Turi ZG, et al. A simplified method to predict occurrence of complete heart block during acute myocardial infarction. *Am J Cardiol* 1986;57:1213–1219.

48. Italian Group for the Study of Streptokinase in Myocardial Infarction (GISSI). Effectiveness of intravenous thrombolytic treatment in acute myocardial infarction. *Lancet* 1986;1:397–401.

49. Bellocci F, Santarelli P, DiGennaro M, et al. The risk of cardiac complications in surgical patients with bifascicular block: A clinical and electrophysiological study in 98 patients. *Chest* 1980;77:343–348.

50. Rahn DW, Malawista SE. Lyme disease: Recommendations for diagnosis and treatment. *Ann Intern Med* 1991;114:472–481.

51. Cox J, Krajden M. Cardiovascular manifestations of Lyme disease. *Am Heart J* 1991;122:1449–1455.

Basic Concepts of Pacing

G. Neal Kay

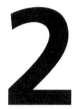

MYOCARDIAL STIMULATION

An artificial electrical pacing stimulus excites cardiac tissue by the creation of an electrical field at the interface of the stimulating electrode with the underlying myocardium. Although a pacing stimulus can be applied to any portion of the body, a tissue response occurs only in cells that are excitable. For an artificial polarizing pulse to induce a response in excitable tissue, the stimulus must be of sufficient amplitude and duration to initiate a self-regenerating wavefront of action potentials that propagate away from the site of stimulation. Myocardial stimulation is dependent on an intact source of the electrical pulse (the pulse generator), a conductor between the source of the electrical pulse and the stimulating electrode (the lead conductor), an electrode for delivery of the pulse, and an area of myocardium that is excitable. In this section, the basic properties of myocardial stimulation will be reviewed in detail.

BASIC ELECTROPHYSIOLOGY

The property of biologic tissues such as nerve and muscle to respond to a stimulus with a response that is out of proportion to the strength of the stimulus is known as excitability.[1] Excitable tissues are characterized by a separation of charge across the cell membrane that results in a resting transmembrane potential. For cardiac myocytes, the concentration of Na^+ ions outside the cell exceeds the concentration inside the cell. In contrast, the inside of the cell has a 35-fold greater concentration of K^+ ions than the outside of the cell. The resting transmembrane potential is maintained by the high resistance to ion flow that is an intrinsic property of the lipid bilayer of the cell membrane. Because there is a passive leak of ions through membrane-bound ion channels, the resting potential is further maintained by two active transport mechanisms that exchange Na^+ ions for K^+ and Ca^{2+} ions. The Na^+–K^+ ATPase exchange "pump" extrudes 3 Na^+ ions for 2 K^+ ions that are moved into the cell.[2–4] The Na^+–Ca^{2+} transport mechanism exchanges 3 Na^+ ions toward the outside of the cell for each Ca^{2+} ion that is moved into the cell.[5,6] Because both these transport mechanisms result in the net movement of three positive charges out of the cell in exchange for two positive charges that are moved in, a net polarization of the cell membrane is produced such that the inside of the cell is maintained electrically negative with respect to the outside. These transport mechanisms are dependent on the expenditure of energy in the form of high-energy phosphates and are susceptible to disruptions in aerobic cellular metabolism during myocardial ischemia.

Excitable tissues are further characterized by their ability to generate and propagate a transmembrane action potential.[1] The action potential is triggered by depolarization of the membrane from a resting potential of approximately -90 mV to a threshold potential of approximately -70 to -60 mV. Upon reaching the threshold transmembrane potential, specialized membrane-bound protein channels change conformation from an inactive state to an active state, allowing the free movement of Na^+ ions through the channel.[7–9] The upstroke of the action potential (phase 0) is a consequence of this sudden influx of Na^+ into the myocyte and is associated with a change in transmembrane potential from -90 mV to approximately $+20$ mV[10–12] (Figure 2.1). It is estimated that the opening of a single Na^+ channel allows approximately 10^4 Na^+ ions to enter the cardiac myocyte.[13] The number of Na^+ channels is estimated to be on the order of 5 to 10 channels per square micron of cell membrane.[13–15] In addition to Na^+ channels, specialized proteins are also suspended in the membrane that have differential selectivity for K^+, Ca^{2+}, and Cl^- ions.[16–19] The channels may remain in the open configuration for less than 1 msec (characteristic of the Na^+ channel) to hundreds of milliseconds (typical of K^+ channels). The rapid upstroke of the action potential is followed by a short period of hyperpolarization when the transmembrane potential is transiently positively charged. The overshoot potential is quickly abolished (phase 1); and the cell enters the plateau phase

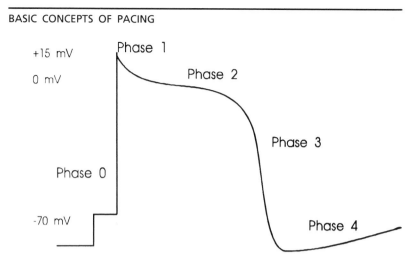

Figure 2.1 The action potential of a Purkinje fiber is illustrated. The resting transmembrane potential is approximately −90 mV. Upon depolarization of the membrane to a threshold potential of −70 to −60 mV, the upstroke of the action potential is triggered (phase 0), carried predominantly by an influx of Na+ ions into the cell. The transmembrane potential reaches approximately +15 mV (overshoot potential) and is repolarized to approximately 0 mV during phase 1. The plateau phase of the action potential (phase 2) is produced by a complex interaction of inward Ca²⁺ and Na+ currents and outward K+ currents. Repolarization of the cell occurs during phase 3, during which the cell regains the capability of responding to a polarizing electrical stimulus with another action potential. Phase 4 of the action potential is characterized by a slow upward drift in the transmembrane potential.

(phase 2), during which Ca^{2+} is triggered[20] to enter the cell and the outward K^+ current is activated.[21-23] The cardiac cell is refractory to further electrical stimulation by a stimulus of any strength during the plateau phase. After the plateau phase, which lasts several hundred milliseconds, the cardiac cell begins the process of repolarization with regeneration of the resting membrane potential and the capability for responding to an electrical stimulus with another action potential (phase 3). During the repolarization phase, an action potential may be induced if the myocyte is challenged by an electrical stimulus of sufficient strength. Following complete repolarization of the membrane, the cell enters a diastolic period of gradual upward drift in transmembrane potential, during which it is fully excitable (phase 4).[24,25]

The response of excitable membranes to electrical stimuli is an active process that results in a response exceeding that of simple passive conductance along the membrane. Gap junctions that provide low-resistance intercellular connections conduct the action potential between myocytes.[26–28] The action potential at the site of stimulation results in the depolarization of neighboring areas of the myocyte membrane to threshold voltage, triggering the Na^+ channels to open and regeneration of the action potential. The action potential is not only passively conducted but also actively regenerated at each segment of membrane.[29] However, propagation of the action potential away from the site of electrical stimulation is also dependent on certain passive cable properties of the myocardium, including the axis of myofiber orientation and the geometry of the connections between fibers.[30,31] For example, a wavefront of depolarization is conducted with a conduction velocity that is three to five times greater along the longitudinal axis of a myofiber than along the transverse axis.[32,33] These anisotropic conduction properties may be further exaggerated in the presence of myocardial fibrosis in which the intercellular collagen matrix is increased with decreased cell-to-cell communication. Such fibrosis is often present in patients with disorders of the cardiac conduction system. In addition, the safety factor for successful propagation is greater at sites where sheets of myocardium of similar size are joined than where a narrow isthmus of tissue joins a larger mass.[34]

STIMULATION THRESHOLD

Cardiac pacing involves the delivery of a polarizing electrical impulse from an electrode in contact with the myocardium with the generation of an electrical field of sufficient intensity to induce a propagating wave of cardiac action potentials.[35] The stimulating pulse may be either anodal or cathodal in polarity, though with differing stimulation characteristics. In addition, the stimulation characteristics are related to the source of the stimulating pulse, with constant-voltage and constant-current generators exhibiting somewhat different stimulation properties. The minimum energy necessary to initiate a propagated depolarizing wavefront reliably from an electrode is defined as the stimulation threshold. In this section, the factors that determine stimulation threshold will be discussed.[36]

Strength–duration relation

The intensity of an electrical stimulus that is required to capture atrial or ventricular myocardium is dependent on the duration of the stimulating pulse (pulse width).[37–40] The stimulus amplitude for endocardial stimulation has an exponential relation to the duration of the pulse, with a rapidly rising strength–duration curve at pulse widths less than 0.25 msec and a relatively flat curve at pulse widths greater than 1.0 msec (Figure 2.2). As can be appreciated by examining the hyperbolic strength–duration curve, a small change in pulse duration is associated with a significant change in the threshold amplitude at short pulse durations but a small change at longer pulse durations. Because of the exponential relationship between stimulus amplitude and pulse width, the entire strength–duration curve can be described relatively accurately by two points on the

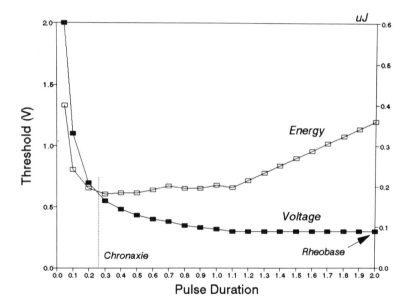

Figure 2.2   Strength–duration curve for constant-voltage stimulation obtained at the time of permanent pacing lead implantation in a patient with complete AV block. The strength–duration relation is characterized by a steeply rising portion at short pulse widths and a relatively flat portion at pulse durations greater than 1 msec. The stimulus energy at each point on the strength–duration curve is also demonstrated. The rheobase voltage of a constant-voltage strength–duration curve is defined as the lowest stimulation voltage at any pulse duration. Because the curve is essentially flat at a pulse duration of 2 msec, rheobase can be accurately approximated as the threshold voltage at this point. Chronaxie, the threshold pulse duration at twice rheobase voltage, closely approximates the point of minimum threshold stimulation energy.

curve, rheobase and chronaxie.[37] Rheobase of a constant-voltage strength–duration curve is defined as the least stimulus voltage that will electrically stimulate the myocardium at any pulse duration. For practical purposes, rheobase voltage is usually determined as the threshold stimulus voltage at a pulse width of 2.0 msec. The chronaxie pulse duration is defined as the threshold pulse duration at a stimulus amplitude that is twice rheobase voltage. Using the rheobase and chronaxie points, Lapicque[37] constructed the following mathematical equation, which can be used to derive the strength–duration curve for constant-current stimulation:

$$I = I_r(1 + t_c/t),$$

where I is the threshold current at pulse duration t, I_r is the rheobase current, and t_c is the chronaxie pulse duration.

The relation of stimulus voltage, current, and pulse duration to stimulus energy is provided by the formula

$$E = V^2/R \times t,$$

where E is the stimulus energy, V is the stimulus voltage, R is the total pacing impedance, and t is the pulse duration. The chronaxie pulse duration is important in the clinical application of pacing, as it approximates the point of minimum threshold energy on the strength–duration curve.[41,42] With pulse durations greater than chronaxie, there is little reduction in threshold voltage. Rather, the wider pulse duration results in the wasting of stimulation energy without providing an increase in safety margin. At pulse durations less than chronaxie there is a steep increase in threshold voltage and stimulation energy. As can be appreciated from Figure 2.2, the chronaxie pulse duration is usually close to the point of minimal stimulation energy.

An appreciation of the threshold strength–duration relation is important for the proper programming of stimulus amplitude and pulse width.[43] Modern pulse generators offer two major methods for evaluating the stimulation threshold: either automatic decrementation of the stimulus voltage at a constant pulse duration or automatic decrementation of the pulse duration at a constant stimulus voltage. In order to provide an adequate margin of safety, when the stimulation threshold is determined by decrementing the stimulus amplitude, the stimulus voltage is usually programmed to approximately twice the threshold value. Similarly, for pulse generators that determine threshold by automatically decrementing pulse duration, the pulse duration is usually programmed to at least three times the threshold value. It should be recognized that the hyperbolic shape of the strength–duration curve has important implications for interpreting the results of threshold testing[43] (Figure 2.3). Although these methods provide comparable margins of safety when the threshold pulse duration is 0.15 msec or less, tripling a threshold pulse duration that is greater than 0.3 msec may not provide an adequate stimulation safety margin.

The threshold strength–duration curve is influenced by several factors, including the method of measurement, the nature of the electrode, and the duration of lead implantation. Stimulation thresholds that are measured by decrementing stimulus voltage

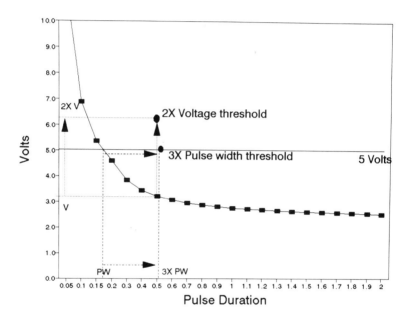

Figure 2.3 The clinical use of the strength–duration relation to determine an adequate margin of safety for stimulation is demonstrated for a patient with a chronically implanted pacing lead. Note that when the stimulation threshold is determined by decrementing pulse duration at a constant voltage (5 V), the strength–duration curve is encountered at the start of the rapidly rising portion of the curve. Tripling of the pulse duration provides an adequate safety margin. When the stimulation threshold is determined by decrementing stimulus voltage at a constant pulse duration (0.5 msec), the strength–duration curve is encountered at a relatively flat portion of the curve. Doubling the stimulation voltage results in a somewhat greater margin of safety than with the alternative method.

until loss of capture are usually 0.1 to 0.2 V lower than when the stimulus intensity is gradually increased from subthreshold until capture is achieved.[44,45] This empiric observation, known as the Wedensky effect, must be considered when accurate measurements of stimulation threshold are required. The Wedensky effect may be greater at narrow pulse durations, potentially reaching clinical significance.

Strength–duration curves for constant-voltage and constant-current stimulation

There are several differences in the shape of the strength–duration curves for constant-current and constant-voltage stimulation[41,46,47] (Figure 2.4). For example, constant-voltage stimulation usually results in a flat curve at pulse durations greater than 1.5 msec, whereas the constant-current stimulation curve may be slowly downsloping beyond this pulse duration. The strength-duration curve with constant-current stimulation increases more steeply at short pulse durations than it does with constant voltage stimulation. Small changes in pulse duration less than 0.5 msec may result in a significantly greater reduction in stimulation safety margin for constant-current than for constant-voltage pulse generators. Because of this difference in the shape of the strength–duration curves, the chronaxie pulse duration of a constant-current strength–duration relation is significantly greater than that observed with constant-voltage stimulation. Because the most efficient pulse duration for electrical stimulation is at chronaxie (in terms of threshold energy), a constant-voltage pulse generator can be set to deliver a narrower pulse width than a constant-current generator and yet provide the same safety margin.[48]

Time-dependent changes in stimulation threshold

Myocardial stimulation thresholds may change dramatically following positioning of a permanent pacing lead.[49–60] The typical course of events following implantation of an endocardial pacing lead starts with an acute rise in threshold that begins within the first 24 hours (Figure 2.5). The threshold usually continues to rise over the next several days, usually peaking at approximately one week. The typical stimulation threshold then gradually declines over the next several weeks. By six weeks, the myocardial stimulation threshold has usually stabilized at a value that is significantly greater than that measured at implantation of the lead but less than the acute peak. The magnitude of the change in threshold varies widely between

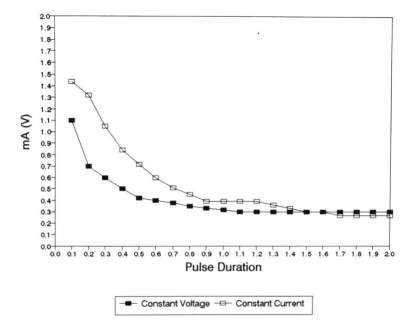

Figure 2.4 Strength–duration curves determined with constant-current and constant-voltage stimulation in a single individual are demonstrated. Note that the constant-current stimulation curve continues to decline gradually at greater pulse durations than that obtained with constant-voltage stimulation.

individuals and relates to the electrode's size, shape, chemical composition, and surface structure. The stability of the electrode–myocardial interface and the flexibility of the lead also influence the acute-to-chronic change in threshold. In addition to the typical evolution of stimulation threshold following lead implantation, certain leads may exhibit a hyperacute phase of threshold evolution. For example, active fixation electrodes utilizing a screw helix as the active electrode may produce, immediately following implantation, an increased stimulation threshold that gradually decreases over the next 20 to 30 minutes.[61] This transient increase in threshold is likely related to acute injury at the myocardial–electrode interface and is generally not observed with atraumatic passive fixation leads. Clinically, the hyperacute phase may be manifested by a current of injury in the electrogram. Both the current of injury and the stimulation threshold usually decline rapidly over the first several minutes before pursuing the typical acute-to-chronic threshold

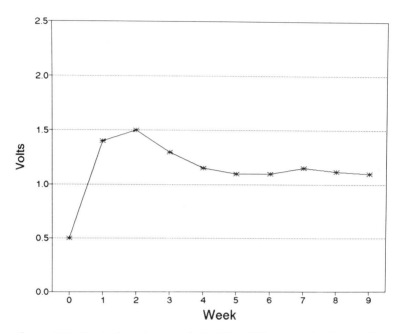

Figure 2.5 Typical evolution of the stimulation threshold over the first three months following implantation of a platinum–iridium pacing lead. The stimulation threshold increases from implantation, peaking at one to two weeks. The chronic stimulation threshold has stabilized by six weeks in this individual. Although this curve is typical of those obtained with standard (nonsteroid) permanent pacing leads, there is considerable variability among individuals in the absolute values and slope.

evolution, shown in Figure 2.5. Thus comparisons of changes in stimulation threshold between varying lead designs require an appreciation of the effects of fixation mechanism.

Proper programming of the stimulus amplitude of a permanent pacemaker requires an understanding of several factors. First, the strength–duration relation must be appreciated. Second, the safety margin that is chosen for a particular patient must be based on the degree of pacemaker dependency, that is, the likelihood of the patient's developing symptoms should loss of effective pacing occur. For patients judged to be highly pacemaker-dependent, a higher stimulation safety margin may be prudent. As an example, a patient with complete AV block with an unreliable ventricular escape rhythm may be more likely to develop symptoms with loss of ventricular capture than is a patient with intermittent sinus node dysfunction. On the other hand, the patient with AV block is likely to be less dependent on atrial than ventricular capture. Thus, a higher safety margin may be needed for the ventricular stimulus than for the atrial stimulus in such an individual. Third, an appreciation of the effect of stimulus amplitude and duration on battery longevity is required. As discussed later in this chapter in the section regarding output circuits, programming the stimulus intensity greater than 2.8 V results in a marked increase in current drain from the battery. Fourth, the overall metabolic and pharmacologic history of the patient must be considered. For example, patients requiring the addition of an antiarrhythmic drug to their medication regimen may experience an increase in pacing threshold. Similarly, patients subject to major shifts in potassium concentration or acid-base balance, such as those with renal failure, may have transient increases in pacing threshold. The safety margin that is chosen for these individuals may need to be greater than that for other patients.

Several authors have reported that pacing threshold varies inversely with the surface area of the stimulating electrode.[47,62–65] For spherical electrodes, the larger the surface area of the electrode, the lower the pacing threshold. The explanation for this observation relates to the intensity of the electric field that is generated at the surface of the electrode.[66] For a constant-voltage pulse, the smaller the electrode, the greater the intensity of the electric field and the current density at the surface. The threshold maturation process has been shown to be caused by the growth of an inexcitable capsule of fibrous tissue surrounding the electrode[67–69] (Figure 2.6). This fibrous capsule effectively increases the surface area of the electrode, thereby decreasing the intensity of the electric field at the junction of the fibrous capsule and the more normal, excitable myocardium.

The cellular events that result in the development of a fibrous capsule have been intensively studied.[46,70,71] The initial tissue reaction to the implantation of a permanent pacing lead involves acute injury to cell membranes. This is rapidly followed by the development of myocardial edema and coating of the electrode by platelets and fibrin. These events are followed by the release of chemotactic factors and the development of a typical cellular inflammatory reaction with the infiltration of polymorphonuclear leukocytes and mononuclear cells. Following the acute polymorphonuclear response, the myocardium at the interface with the stimulating electrode is invaded by macrophages. The extracellular release of

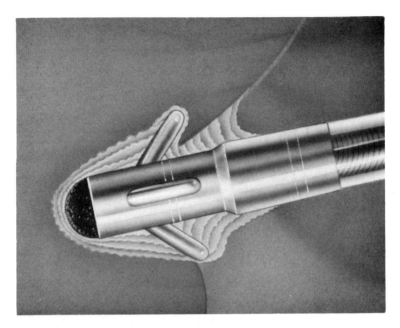

Figure 2.6 Diagrammatic illustration of a fibrous capsule surrounding a chronically implanted pacing electrode. The inexcitable capsule increases the effective radius of the stimulating electrode, reducing the current density at the interface of the capsule and excitable myocardium and increasing the stimulation threshold.

proteolytic enzymes and toxic free oxygen radicals results in an acceleration of tissue injury underlying the electrode. The acute inflammatory response is followed by the accumulation of more macrophages and the influx of fibroblasts into the myocardium. The fibroblasts in the myocardium begin producing collagen, leading to the development of the fibrotic capsule surrounding the electrode.[69]

The influences of several pharmacologic agents on the electrode–myocardial maturation process have been studied. Nonsteroidal inflammatory drugs have been shown to have minimal influence on the evolution of pacing thresholds.[46] In contrast, corticosteroids, either systemically or locally administered, may have dramatic effects on the evolution of pacing thresholds.[72–75] By the use of an infusion pump to deliver dexamethasone sodium phosphate from the center of a ring-shaped electrode, Stokes demonstrated a dramatic decrease in the expected acute-to-chronic rise in pacing threshold with both atrial and ventricular pacing leads in canines.[76] Clinical studies have confirmed these findings and have led to the development of leads that gradually elute dexamethasone from a reservoir beneath the stimulating electrode.[77–82] These corticosteroid-eluting leads have been associated with stable pacing thresholds from implantation to a follow-up period of several years. Other designs incorporate dexamethasone into a drug-eluting collar that surrounds the stimulating electrode.[83] The application of corticosteroid-eluting electrodes to active fixation leads has demonstrated that the nature of the electrode remains important to the evolution of pacing thresholds, even in the presence of anti-inflammatory drugs.[84]

Strength–interval relation

The stimulation threshold is influenced significantly by the coupling interval of electrical stimuli and the frequency of stimulation.[85–88] Figure 2.7 demonstrates a typical ventricular strength–interval curve for both cathodal and anodal stimulation. Note that the stimulus intensity required to capture the ventricle remains quite constant at long extrastimulus coupling intervals but rises exponentially at shorter intervals. The rise in stimulation threshold at short coupling intervals is related to impingement of the stimulus on the relative refractory period of the ventricular myocardium. As discussed earlier, electrical stimuli applied during the repolarization phase of the cardiac action potential may result in a propagated action potential if of sufficient intensity.[85] However, during the plateau phase of the action potential, electrical stimuli of any intensity will not be able to generate an action potential as the absolute refractory period is encountered. Figure 2.7 also illustrates the important differences in anodal and cathodal stimulation. Late diastolic stimulation thresholds are lower with cathodal than with anodal stimulation.[85] However, at relatively short extrastimulus coupling intervals, the anodal stimulation threshold may be less than the cathodal threshold.[85] During the relative refractory period, the anodal threshold may actually decline ("dip") prior to abruptly rising at shorter coupling intervals. With bipolar cardiac pacing, the stimulation threshold is generally determined by the cathode. However, with short extrastimulus coupling intervals, the bipolar stimulation threshold may actually be determined by the anode. If the stimulus intensity exceeds both the cathodal and anodal thresholds, bipolar pacing may result in stimulation at both electrode–myocardial interfaces.

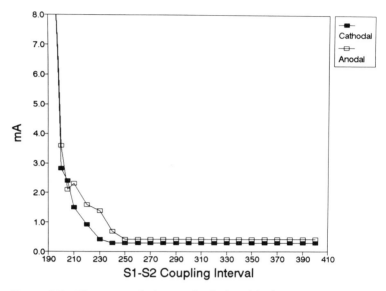

Figure 2.7 The strength–interval relationship for constant current with unipolar anodal and cathodal stimulation is demonstrated in a normal individual. Note that the shape of the curve is relatively flat at long extrastimulus coupling intervals and rises exponentially at short coupling intervals. Also note that cathodal stimulation results in a lower stimulation threshold at long coupling intervals than does anodal stimulation. At short coupling intervals, the anodal stimulation curve may transiently "dip" before rapidly rising.

Effects of pacing rate on myocardial stimulation

The stimulation frequency may have an important influence on pacing threshold.[87,89–93] At shorter stimulation cycle lengths, the action potential of atrial and ventricular myocardium shortens, resulting in a proportional decrease in the relative refractory period. At rapid pacing rates, these factors are manifested by a shift in the strength–interval curve to the left. However, at pacing rates exceeding 250 beats per minute (ppm), pacing stimuli may be delivered during the relative refractory period, resulting in an increase in threshold. The strength–duration curve is shifted upward and to the right at very rapid pacing rates (Figure 2.8), an observation that may have important implications for antitachycardia pacing.[89] Thus a stimulation amplitude that provides an adequate safety margin for pacing at slow rates may not be sufficient at rapid pacing rates. Newer antitachycardia devices provide for this possible increase in stimulation threshold by an automatic increase in the amplitude of pacing stimuli that are delivered at rapid pacing rates.

PHARMACOLOGIC AND METABOLIC EFFECTS ON STIMULATION THRESHOLD

The stimulation threshold may demonstrate considerable variability over the normal 24-hour period, generally increasing during sleep and falling during the waking hours.[94,95] The changes in threshold parallel fluctuations in autonomic tone and circulating catecholamines with decreased threshold during exercise. The stimulation threshold is inversely related to the level of circulating corticosteroids. The stimulation threshold may increase following eating, during hyperglycemia, hypoxemia, hypercarbia, and metabolic acidosis or alkalosis.[96–102] The stimulation threshold may increase dramatically during acute viral illnesses, especially in children. The concentration of serum electrolytes may also influence stimulation threshold, rising during hyperkalemia.[98–101]

Drugs may also influence stimulation threshold. As mentioned

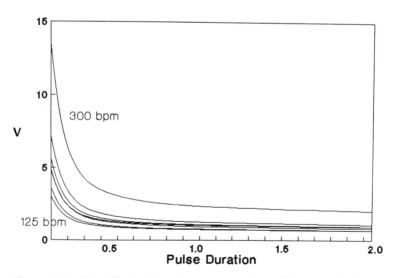

Figure 2.8 The effect of pacing rate on the atrial strength–duration relation for a normal individual is demonstrated. Threshold curves were obtained at pacing rates of 125 to 300 ppm in increments of 25 ppm. Note that the strength–duration curves largely overlap at pacing rates of 125 to 250 ppm. At pacing rates of 275 to 300 ppm, the curve is shifted upward and to the left.

above, catecholamines reduce threshold, and the infusion of isoproterenol may restore capture in some patients with exit block.[95,103] In contrast, beta-blocking drugs increase the stimulation threshold.[104] Corticosteroids, either orally or parenterally administered, may produce a dramatic decrease in stimulation threshold and are occasionally useful for the management of the acute rise in threshold that may be observed following lead implantation.[72–75] The list of drugs that raise the stimulation threshold includes the type I antiarrhythmic drugs quinidine,[105] procainamide,[106] flecainide,[107] and encainide.[108] It is not clear whether the type III drug amiodarone has similar effects.[109] Virtually all antiarrhythmic drugs may influence the pacing threshold, although they are usually clinically important only at high serum concentrations.

Occasional patients exhibit a progressive rise in stimulation threshold over time, a clinical syndrome known as exit block. Exit block seems to occur despite optimal lead positioning, as it recurs with the subsequent implantation of new pacing leads. In patients with exit block, the threshold changes in the atrium tend to parallel those in the ventricle. Exit block is best managed by the use of steroid-eluting ventricular leads, which have been associated with low thresholds in patients with this syndrome[77–82] (Figure 2.9).

IMPEDANCE

Impedance is the sum of all factors that oppose the flow of current in an electric circuit. Impedance is not necessarily the same as resistance. The relationship between voltage, current, and resistance in an electrical circuit is estimated by Ohm's law, $V = IR$. For circuits that follow Ohm's law, impedance and resistance are equal. If voltage is held constant, the current flow is inversely related to the resistance of the circuit ($I = V/R$). The leading-edge voltage of a constant-voltage pulse generator is fixed, and the lower the resistance, the greater the current flow. In contrast, the greater the resistance, the lower the current flow. Because implantable pulse generators are powered by lithium iodide batteries with a fixed amount of charge, pacing impedance is an important determinant of battery longevity.

The total pacing impedance is determined by factors that are related to the lead conductor (resistance), the resistance to current flow from the electrode to the myocardium (electrode resistance), and the accumulation of charges of opposite polarity in the myo-

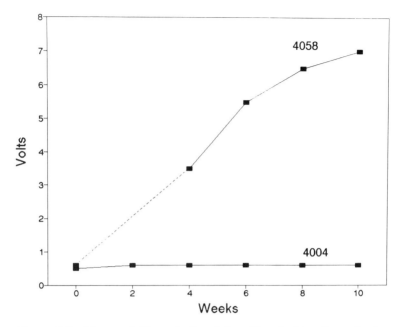

Figure 2.9 The evolution of stimulation threshold voltage (pulse duration 0.5 msec) in the right ventricular apex is demonstrated for an individual with a history of exit block. Note that the stimulation threshold increases progressively from implantation with an active fixation ventricular lead (model 4058). Following implantation of a corticosteroid-eluting electrode (model 4004) in the same patient, the stimulation threshold remains low. Exit block occurs infrequently but usually recurs with standard (nonsteroid) pacing leads.

cardium at the electrode–tissue interface (polarization).[46] Thus, the total pacing impedance $(Z_{total}) = Z_c + Z_e + Z_p$, where Z_c is the conductor resistance, Z_e is the electrode resistance, and Z_p is the polarization impedance. The resistance to current flow provided by the lead conductor results in a voltage drop across the lead with a portion of the pacing pulse converted into heat. Thus, this component of the total pacing impedance is an inefficient use of electrical energy and does not contribute to myocardial stimulation. The ideal pacing lead would have a very low conductor resistance (Z_c). *In contrast, the ideal pacing lead would also have a relatively high electrode resistance (Z_e) to minimize current flow and maximize battery* life.[110,111] The electrode resistance is largely a function of the electrode radius, with higher resistance provided by a smaller electrode.

An electrode with a small radius minimizes current flow in an efficient manner. In addition to providing a greater electrode resistance, pacing electrodes with a small radius provide increased current density and lower stimulation thresholds.[111] Because of these properties, newer pacing leads (for example, the Medtronic Capture Z series) take advantage of smaller electrodes to increase electrode resistance, allowing the total pacing impedance to exceed 1000 ohms. Compared with a standard pacing lead with a total impedance of 500 ohms, a lead with 1000 ohms of impedance would decrease current drain of the pacing pulse by 50 percent, thereby prolonging the usable battery life of the implantable pulse generator.

The third component of pacing impedance, polarization impedance, is an effect of electrical stimulation and is related to the movement of charged ions in the myocardium toward the cathode.[112] When an electrical current is applied to the myocardium, the cathode attracts positively charged ions and repels negatively charged ions in the extracellular space. The cathode rapidly becomes surrounded by a layer of hydrated Na^+ and H_3O^+ ions. Farther away from the cathode, a second layer forms of negatively charged ions (Cl^-, HPO_4^{2-}, and OH^-). Thus, the negatively charged cathode induces the accumulation of two layers of oppositely charged ions in the myocardium. Initially, the movement of charged ions results in the flow of current in the myocardium. As the cathode becomes surrounded by an inside layer of positive charges and an outside layer of negative charges, a functional capacitor develops that impedes the further movement of charge. The capacitive effect of polarization increases throughout the application of the pulse, peaking at the trailing edge and decaying exponentially following the pulse as charged layers dissolve into electrical neutrality[113] (Figure 2.10). Because polarization impedes the movement of charge in the myocardium, it is inefficient and results in an increased requirement for voltage. Thus, polarization impedance reduces the effectiveness of a pacing stimulus to stimulate the myocardium and wastes current. Polarization impedance is directly related to the duration of the pulse and can be minimized by the use of relatively short pulse widths. Polarization is inversely related to the surface area of the electrode. In order to minimize the effect of polarization (Z_p) but maximize electrode resistance (Z_e), the surface area of the electrode can be made large but the radius small by the use of a porous coating on the electrode.[114–117] Electrodes constructed with activated carbon,[118–120] or coated with plati-

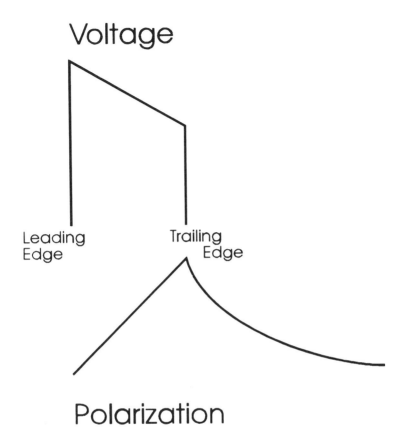

Voltage

Leading
Edge

Trailing
Edge

Polarization

Figure 2.10 The relationship between the voltage waveform of a constant-voltage pulse and the development of polarization effect at the electrode–myocardial interface is illustrated. Note that the polarization effect rises during application of the stimulating pulse and decays exponentially. The trailing edge of the output pulse is less than the leading edge as the output capacitor loses charge during discharge of the pulse.

num black[121–124] or iridium oxide, are effective in minimizing the wasteful effects of polarization and in diminishing afterpotentials, which can interfere with sensing.

The evolution of pacing impedance is usually characterized by a fall over the first one to two weeks following implantation[46,59,125] The chronic pacing impedance then rises to a stable value that is, on average, approximately 15 percent higher than at implant. Serial measurements of pacing impedance are extremely valuable for the assessment of lead integrity; low impedance measurements usually reflect a failure of conductor insulation, and high values often suggest conductor fracture or a loose set-screw at the proximal connector. It should be emphasized that the method of measurement greatly influences the impedance value. For example, if the pacing impedance is measured at the leading edge of the pulse, the value reflects Z_c and Z_e but not Z_p. In contrast, measurements near the midpoint of the pulse are a more accurate reflection of total pacing impedance. For clinical purposes, serial assessments of impedance should utilize a consistent method of measurement.

BIPOLAR VERSUS UNIPOLAR STIMULATION

The term *unipolar pacing* is technically a misnomer, as both bipolar and unipolar configurations require an anode and a cathode to complete the electrical circuit. Because both unipolar and bipolar pacing utilize an electrode in contact with the myocardium (usually as the cathode), the difference in these configurations lies in the location of the other electrode (usually the anode). For a unipolar pacing stimulus, the anode is the case of the pulse generator. The anode for bipolar stimulation is located on the pacing lead within the heart, either in contact with the endocardium or lying free within the cardiac chamber. The pacing impedance is slightly higher with bipolar than with unipolar pacing, as two conducting wires are required. However, although the stimulation threshold is slightly lower with unipolar than with bipolar pacing, this is of such a low magnitude that it is rarely of any clinical significance. The clinically important differences between bipolar and unipolar leads relate to sensing, where the advantages of bipolar leads are substantial, and to the increased diameter and reduced flexibility of bipolar leads.[126] Bipolar pacing is also devoid of the potential for pectoral muscle stimulation, which is sometimes encountered with unipolar stimulation if a high stimulus intensity is required. Bipolar pacing may be especially useful in children when a submuscular pocket is used or in patients with implantable cardioverter-defibrillators (ICDs) in whom a unipolar stimulus is more likely to be inappropriately sensed by the ICD. However, the increased size of the pacing stimulus on the surface electrocardiogram with unipolar pacing may be useful for the assessment of proper pacemaker function, especially with transtelephonic ECG tracings. With the introduction of artificial sensors for rate-adaptive cardiac pacing that measure transthoracic impedance to estimate minute ventilation, bipolar leads offer a somewhat greater range of sensors with which they can be used. Despite these advantages of bipolar leads, the track record of reliablity has been better for many unipolar than for similarly designed bipolar leads.

SENSING

Sensing of the cardiac electrogram is essential to the proper function of permanent pacemakers. In addition to responding to appropriate intrinsic atrial or ventricular electrograms, permanent pacing systems must be able to discriminate these signals from unwanted electrical interference: far-field cardiac events, diastolic potentials, skeletal muscle signals, and pacing stimuli. In this section, the basic determinants of electrogram sensing will be discussed.

Intracardiac electrograms

Intracardiac electrical signals are produced by the movement of electrical current through myocardium. An electrode that overlies a region of resting myocardium records from the outside of cardiac myocytes, which are positively charged with respect to the inside of the cell. Despite this, an electrode in one region of resting myocardium will record a charge (and no potential voltage difference) similar to that recorded by an electrode in another region of resting myocardium. During depolarization, the outside of the cell becomes electrically neutral with respect to the inside. Therefore, as a wavefront of depolarization travels toward an endocardial electrode that records from resting myocardium, the electrode becomes positively charged relative to the depolarized region. This is manifested in the intracardiac electrogram as a positive deflection. As the wavefront of depolarization passes under the recording electrode, the outside of the cell suddenly becomes negatively charged relative to resting myocardium, and a brisk negative deflection is inscribed in the intracardiac electrogram. The peak negative deflection in the intracardiac electrogram, known as the intrinsic deflection (Figure 2.11), is considered the moment of myocardial activation underlying the recording electrode.[127] The positive and negative deflections that precede and follow the intrinsic deflection represent activation in neighboring regions of myocardium relative to the recording electrode. In clinical practice, the intrinsic deflection in the intracardiac electrogram is usually biphasic, with predominantly negative or positive deflections less frequently observed.[128] Because of the greater mass of myocardium,

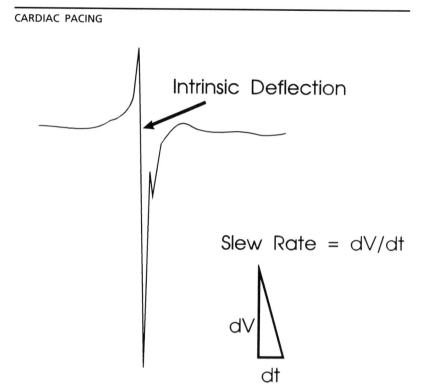

Figure 2.11 A typical bipolar ventricular electrogram in a normal individual. The sharp downward deflection in the electrogram represents the intrinsic deflection and indicates the moment of activation under the recording electrode. The slope of the intrinsic deflection (dV/dt) is expressed in volts per second and is referred to as the slew rate. In order for an electrogram to be sensed by a sensing amplifier, the amplitude and slew rate must exceed the sensing threshold.

the normal ventricular electrogram is usually of far greater amplitude than the normal atrial electrogram.

Characteristics of intracardiac electrograms: The frequency content of ventricular electrograms has been demonstrated to be similar to that of atrial electrograms.[129] By using Fourier transformation, one can express the frequency spectrum of an electrical signal as a series of sine waves of varying frequency and amplitude. Fourier transformation of ventricular electrograms demonstrates that the maximum density of frequencies for R waves is usually found between 10 and 30 Hz.[129] The effects of filtering the ventricular electrogram are shown in Figure 2.12. As can be appreciated from the figure, removing frequencies below 10 Hz markedly attenuates the T-wave amplitude without significantly influencing the R wave. The T wave is usually a slower, broader signal that is composed of lower frequencies, generally less than 5 Hz.[129] Similarly, the far-field R wave in the atrial electrogram is composed predominantly of low-frequency signals.[130] Therefore, by high-pass filtering of the intracardiac electrogram, many of the unwanted low-frequency components can be removed. In contrast, the frequency spectrum of skeletal myopotentials ranges from approximately 10 to 200 Hz, with considerable overlap with the intrinsic R wave and P wave.[129] Although the high-frequency compon-

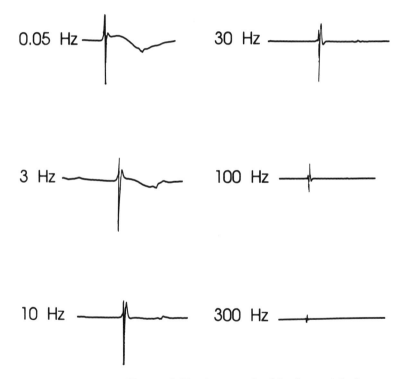

Figure 2.12 The effects of filtering on the bipolar atrial electrogram are demonstrated in an individual. Note that low-pass filtering of the electrogram below 10 Hz has the effect of attenuating the far-field R wave and T wave. Filtering of frequencies greater than 30 Hz results in marked attenuation of the electrogram amplitude. The center frequency of most sensing amplifiers is approximately 30 Hz, consistent with the typical frequency spectra of intracardiac electrograms.

ents can be removed with filtering, inappropriate sensing of myopotentials remains a potential problem with the unipolar configuration.[131,132]

In order for the intracardiac electrogram to be sensed by the sense amplifier of an implantable pulse generator, the signal must be of sufficient amplitude, measured in peak-to-peak voltage. In addition, the intrinsic deflection of the electrogram must have sufficient slope. The peak slope (dV/dt) of the electrogram (also known as the slew rate) is of critical importance to proper sensing (see Figure 2.11). The sense amplifier of most pulse generators has a center frequency (the frequency for which the amplifier is most sensitive) in the range of 30 to 40 Hz, so that frequencies greater than this are attenuated and less likely to be sensed. Components of the electrogram less than the center frequency are also attenuated, with the output of the filter proportional to the slew rate of the waveform. In general, the higher the slew rate of an electrogram, the higher the frequency content. Thus slow and broad signals with a low slew rate may not be sensed, even if the peak-to-peak amplitude of the electrogram is large. In clinical practice, the slew rate and amplitude of intracardiac electrograms are only modestly proportional.[133] Because of this, both the slew rate and the amplitude of the intracardiac electrogram should be routinely measured.

Unipolar and bipolar sensing

Although both unipolar and bipolar sensing configurations detect the difference in electrical potential between two electrodes, the interelectrode distance has a considerable influence on the nature of the electrogram.[134] If a transvenous bipolar lead is employed for sensing, both electrodes are located in the heart with an interelectrode distance that is usually less than 3 cm. A unipolar lead utilizes one electrode in contact with the heart and the other in contact with the pulse generator, often with an interelectrode distance of 30 to 50 cm. Because both electrodes may contribute to the electrical signal that is sensed, the bipolar electrode configuration is minimally influenced by electrical signals that originate outside the heart. In contrast, the unipolar electrode configuration may detect electrical signals that originate near the pulse generator pocket as well as those from inside the heart. These features of unipolar sensing make this electrode configuration much more susceptible to interference by electrical signals originating in skeletal muscle (myopotentials). The myopotentials associated with pectoral muscle contraction may be sensed by unipolar pacemakers, resulting in inappropriate inhibition or triggering of pacing output.[131,132] Bipolar sensing is relatively immune to myopotentials—a significant clinical advantage. Bipolar sensing is also less likely to be influenced by electromagnetic radiation from the environment than is unipolar sensing.[135] Electrical interference from microwaves, electrocautery, metal detectors, diathermy, or radar is more commonly observed with unipolar than with bipolar sensing.[136–138]

A bipolar electrogram is actually the instantaneous difference in electrical voltage between the two electrodes. Thus a bipolar electrogram can be constructed by subtracting the absolute unipolar voltage recorded at the cathode (versus ground) from the unipolar voltage recorded at the anode (versus ground). Because the bipolar configuration represents the signal at the cathode minus the signal at the anode, the net electrogram may be considerably different from that of either unipolar electrogram alone. For example, if an advancing wavefront of depolarization is perpendicular to the interelectrode axis of a bipolar lead, each electrode will be activated at exactly the same time. Because the unipolar electrogram at each electrode will be similar and inscribed at the same time, the instantaneous difference in voltage will be minimal. In this situation, the bipolar electrogram will be markedly attenuated. A wavefront of depolarization traveling parallel to the interelectrode axis of a bipolar lead will activate one electrode before the other. The resulting bipolar electrogram may have significantly greater amplitude than either unipolar electrogram alone. From these examples it should be recognized that bipolar sensing is more sensitive to the direction in which the depolarizing wavefront travels than is unipolar sensing. Bipolar electrograms are more likely to be influenced by phasic changes in orientation of the lead with respiration than are unipolar electrograms. Because of these considerations, the electrogram measured at the time of lead implantation should be recorded in the configuration that will be used for sensing by the pulse generator.

Another significant difference between unipolar and bipolar sensing relates to the amplitude of far-field signals.[139] Because of the significantly greater mass of the ventricles, the atrial electrogram often records a far-field R wave (Figure 2.13). For unipolar atrial leads, the far-field R wave may be equal to or of greater amplitude than the atrial deflection. In contrast, the bipolar atrial electrogram usually records an atrial deflection that is considerably larger than

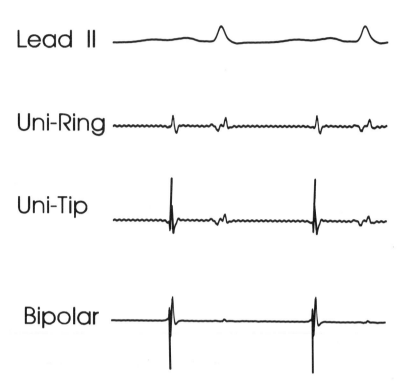

Figure 2.13 Simultaneously recorded unipolar and bipolar atrial electrograms from the ring and tip electrodes of a permanent pacing lead. Note that both of the unipolar electrograms record a far-field R wave. The bipolar electrogram records a sharp atrial deflection and markedly attenuates the far-field R wave. Bipolar sensing is characterized by a relative immunity to far-field electrical events.

the far-field R wave. The programmable postventricular atrial refractory period of dual-chamber pacemakers has effectively reduced inappropriate sensing of far-field R waves in the unipolar atrial electrogram. Despite this, far-field R wave sensing remains an important concern with AAI pacemakers and requires the use of long refractory periods in many patients. Atrial antitachycardia pacemakers (AAI-T) that are designed to interrupt atrial tachycardias require the use of short atrial refractory periods in order to detect very rapid atrial rates. Because of concerns regarding the inappropriate sensing of far-field R waves and myopotentials with unipolar sensing, antitachycardia pacing systems require the use of bipolar leads.

The problem of far-field R-wave detection in the atrial electrogram has been addressed by Goldreyer and colleagues by the development of leads incorporating a pair of closely spaced electrodes placed circumferentially around the catheter.[140–142] This concept, known as an orthogonal electrode array, uses electrodes that are separated by 180 degrees and float free within the atrial blood pool. The advantage of orthogonal sensing is that both electrodes record ventricular activation nearly simultaneously, with a marked attenuation of the far-field R wave and a greater signal-to-noise ratio. The improved signal-to-noise characteristics of orthogonal electrodes have allowed the use of more sensitive atrial amplifiers and increased reliability of atrial sensing. Orthogonal electrodes have also provided a method for dual-chamber (VDD) pacing that utilizes a single lead.[143] The single-lead concept utilizes an electrode at the tip of the catheter, which is placed at the right ventricular apex for ventricular pacing and sensing, and a pair of orthogonally arranged electrodes located more proximally along the catheter in the atrium for atrial sensing.

Polarization

Following application of a polarizing pulse, an afterpotential of opposite charge is induced in the myocardium at the interface of the stimulating electrode (Figure 2.14). Immediately after cathodal stimulation, an excess of positive charges surrounds the electrode, which then exponentially decays to electrical neutrality. This positively charged afterpotential can be inappropriately sensed by the sensing circuit of the pulse generator with resulting inhibition of the next pacing pulse.[144] The amplitude of afterdepolarizations is directly related to the amplitude and duration of the pacing stimulus. Thus afterdepolarizations are most likely to be sensed during conditions of maximum stimulus voltage and pulse duration, combined with the maximum sensitivity setting of the pulse generator.[145] The inappropriate sensing of near-field afterpotentials has been eliminated by the use of sensing refractory periods that prevent the sensing circuit from responding to electrical signals for a programmable period following the pacing stimulus. However, for dual-chamber pacing systems, afterdepolarizations of sufficient amplitude in one chamber may be sensed by the sensing amplifier in the other chamber. This is most likely to occur with the sensing of atrial afterpotentials in the AV interval by the ventricular sensing circuit, resulting in inappropriate inhibition of ventricular stimulus output (crosstalk).[146] Because of the potential for inhibition of

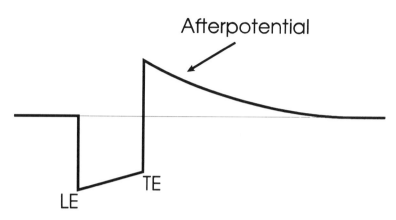

Figure 2.14 Diagrammatic illustration of a constant-voltage output pulse (downward deflection) and a resultant afterpotential of opposite polarity. (LE = leading edge, TE = trailing edge.)

ventricular pacing by the far-field sensing of atrial after-depolarizations, the ventricular sensing circuit is inactivated for a period (blanking period) following the delivery of an atrial pacing stimulus. Crosstalk is a rare clinical problem with unipolar pacing and sensing, however.

Time-related changes in intracardiac electrograms

Immediately following implantation of a transvenous lead, the ST segment usually demonstrates a typical injury current. The ST-segment elevation observed is caused by the pressure that is exerted by the distal electrode on myocardial cell membranes. The current of injury is observed with both atrial and ventricular leads and is so typical of the acute electrogram that its absence may reflect malposition of the lead with poor contact of the distal electrode and the endocardium.[147] Lack of an injury current may also reflect placement of the lead in an area of fibrotic myocardium. The injury current is observed with both active and passive fixation electrodes. The ST segment usually returns to the isoelectric line over a period ranging from several minutes to several hours.

The amplitude of the intracardiac electrogram typically declines abruptly within several days following implantation, with a gradual increase toward the acute value by six to eight weeks. The chronic R-wave amplitude of passive fixation electrodes has been shown to be approximately 85 percent of the acute value.[59,148] The attenuation of the slew rate is considerably greater, with chronic values averaging approximately 50 to 60 percent of the acute measurement. Corticosteroid-eluting leads have demonstrated minimal deterioration of the electrogram from implantation to chronic follow-up.[77-83]

Active fixation leads may be associated with a somewhat different time course than passive fixation leads in the evolution of the intracardiac electrogram, with a markedly attenuated amplitude and slew rate immediately following lead positioning.[61] Over the next 20 to 30 minutes, the electrogram amplitude typically increases. It is likely that the trauma caused by extension of a screw helix into the myocardium is responsible for this hyperacute evolution of the intracardiac electrogram.[149] Recognition of this phenomenon may prevent the unnecessary repositioning of an active fixation lead. In general, active and passive fixation leads are associated with similar chronic electrogram amplitudes.[59,149-151]

Sensing impedance

The intracardiac electrogram must be carried by the pacing lead from its source in the myocardium to the sensing amplifier of the pulse generator. The voltage drop that occurs from the origin of the electrical signal in the heart to the proximal portion of the lead is dependent on the source impedance. The components of source impedance include the resistance between the electrode and the myocardium, the resistance offered by the lead conductor, and the effect of polarization. The electrode resistance is inversely related to the surface area of the electrode.[117,152] Polarization impedance is also inversely related to electrode surface area. Thus electrodes with large surface area minimize source impedance and contribute to improved sensing.

The electrogram that is sensed by the pulse generator can also be attenuated by a mismatch in impedance between the lead (the source impedance) and the sensing amplifier (input impedance).[153,154] The greater the ratio of input impedance to source impedance, the less the electrogram is attenuated and the more accurately it reflects the true amplitude and morphology of the signal in the myocardium. Thus the drop in electrogram amplitude from the actual voltage in the myocardium to the signal that is sensed by the pulse generator is minimized by a low-source impedance and a high-input impedance. The source impedance of current pacing leads ranges from approximately 400 to 1500 ohms. The sensing amplifiers of currently available pulse generators typically have an input impedance greater than 25,000 ohms. The clinical significance of impedance mismatch (too low a ratio of input impedance to source impedance) is the failure of sensing with insulation failure or conductor fracture. An insulation failure between the conductors of a bipolar lead results in shunting across the amplifier and an effective fall in input impedance. In this situation the electrogram amplitude may be attenuated, with loss of appropriate sensing. A conductor fracture leads to a marked increase in source impedance and a similar impedance mismatch and sensing failure.

LEAD DESIGN

Permanent pacing leads have five major components: 1) the electrode(s); 2) the conductor(s); 3) insulation; 4) the connector pin; and 5) the fixation mechanism. Each of these components has critical design considerations, as well as failure modes. In this section, the factors that are important for design of leads will be reviewed.

Electrodes

As discussed previously in this chapter, the stimulation threshold is a function of the current density generated at the electrode.[42,43,46,47,62,63,65,66] In general, the smaller the radius of the electrode, the greater the current density. The resistance at the electrode–myocardial interface is higher with smaller electrodes, providing for the efficient use of a constant-voltage pulse and improving battery longevity. Both of these factors favor electrodes with small radius for myocardial stimulation. In contrast, sensing impedance and electrode polarization are decreased with electrodes of larger surface area.[42,43,117,144,145,152] Thus sensing considerations favor the use of a large electrode. The ideal pacing lead would have an electrode with a small radius (to increase current density) and a large surface area (to improve sensing).[117] The solution to these conflicting considerations for optimal stimulation and sensing characteristics has been addressed by the development of electrodes with a small radius but having a complex surface structure that provides a large surface area.[43,60,114–119,122–124,144]

Electrode shape: The effect of electrode shape on current density has been studied extensively by Irnich and colleagues.[43,66] Electrodes with a smooth, hemispherical shape produce a uniform current density. In contrast, electrodes with more complex shapes typically produce an irregular pattern of current density, with "hot spots" at the edges and points of the electrode.[122-124] Electrodes with an irregular shape enable a high current density to be maintained with a larger overall surface area. The clinical use of a ring-tipped electrode has resulted in better thresholds and sensing characteristics than use of older ball-tipped or hemispherical electrode designs. Other electrode shapes that have been introduced to produce areas of high current density include the grooved hemispherical design ("Target Tip" electrode)[122,124] (Figure 2.15) and a dish-shaped design with holes bored into the electrode ("laser-dish" electrode)[155] (Figure 2.16). Leads with helical, screw-shaped electrodes, hooks, and barbs have all been demonstrated to provide areas of increased current density and acceptable stimulation thresholds.[46,156]

Surface structure: Early pacing leads used electrodes with a polished metal surface. The use of electrodes with a textured surface has

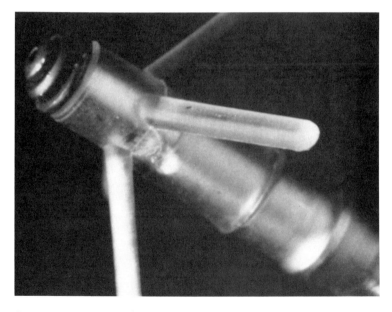

Figure 2.15 A unipolar, Target Tip electrode constructed with a grooved hemispheric shape and coated with platinum black. The combination of a complex macrostructure and a platinum-black surface coating increases current density and decreases electrode polarization.

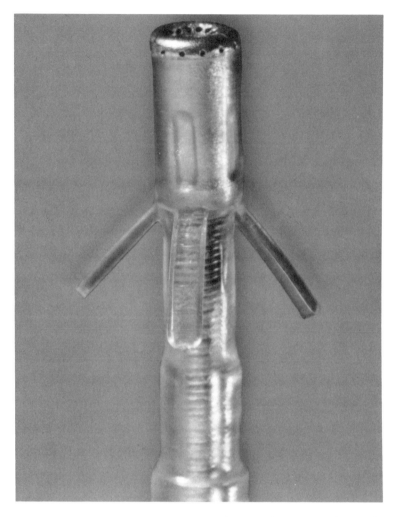

Figure 2.16 Laser-dish electrode with small holes bored into the electrode to promote ingrowth of tissue and to generate areas of increased current density. (Courtesy of Telectronics Pacing Systems, Inc.)

resulted in a dramatic increase in the surface area of the electrode without an increase in radius.[114–120,122–124,157] The textured surface of modern leads minimizes polarization and improves sensing and stimulation efficiency (Figure 2.17). The surface of an electrode may be porous, with a structure containing thousands of microscopic pores ranging from 20 to 100 microns; or the electrode's surface may consist of larger pores (130 microns) bored with a laser beam (see Figure 2.16). The surface of other leads is coated with sintered microspheres of Elgiloy or platinum. In addition, the electrode may be constructed of a woven mesh of microscopic metallic fibers enclosed within a screened basket of wire.[158,159] The performance of carbon electrodes has been improved by roughening of the surface, a process that is known as *activation* (Figure 2.17). Each of these porous or roughened surface structures has been shown to minimize polarization greatly; such a structure can lead to the ingrowth of tissue into the electrode.[123,160] The ability to differentiate an evoked intracardiac electrogram from afterpotentials is greatly influenced by the polarization characteristics of the electrode. The importance of electrodes with low polarization is likely to increase in the future as pacing systems with automatic threshold tracking and capture detection are introduced. Although sensing is improved by the porous electrode design, the improvement in chronic stimulation thresholds has been less dramatic.

Chemical composition: In order to minimize inflammation and subsequent fibrosis at the tissue interface, electrodes for permanent

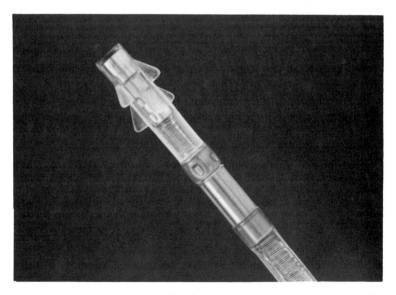

Figure 2.17 Bipolar finned lead with activated carbon electrode. The surface of the electrode has been roughened, a process known as activation. (Courtesy of Pacesetter Systems, Inc.)

pacing leads should be biologically inert and resistant to chemical degradation. Certain metals, such as zinc, copper, mercury, nickel, lead, and silver, are associated with toxic reactions in the myocardium and are unsuitable for use in the electrodes of chronically implanted leads.[161] In addition to these materials with direct tissue toxicity, metals that are susceptible to corrosion have been demonstrated to result in increased chronic stimulation thresholds. Stainless steel alloys are variably associated with the potential for corrosion. Titanium and tantalum have been shown to acquire a surface coating of oxides, which may impede charge transfer at the electrode interface.[162] However, titanium that is coated with microscopic particles of platinum or vitreous carbon has been found to have excellent long-term performance as a pacing electrode.[118–120,122–124] The polarity of the electrode may also have an important influence on its chemical stability. For example, Elgiloy is a quite acceptable electrode material when used as the cathode. However, when used as the anode, Elgiloy is susceptible to a significant degree of corrosion.[163]

The materials presently in use for the electrodes of permanent pacing leads include platinum–iridium, Elgiloy, platinum coated with platinized titanium, vitreous or pyrolytic carbon coating a titanium or graphite core, platinum, or iridium oxide. The platinized-platinum and iridium-oxide electrodes have been associated with a reduced degree of polarization. Although a small degree of corrosion may occur with any of these materials, the carbon electrodes appear to be less susceptible. The carbon electrodes have been improved by roughening the surface, a process known as activation that reduces polarization and potentially allows for ingrowth of tissue. The chronic thresholds of the activated carbon electrodes compare favorably to those observed with platinum–iridium and Elgiloy.[118,123,160,164]

Steroid-eluting electrodes: A major advance in permanent pacing lead technology has been the development of electrodes that elute small amounts of the corticosteroid dexamethasone sodium phosphate.[77–82] The steroid-eluting electrodes incorporate a silicone core that is impregnated with a small quantity of dexamethasone (Figure 2.18). The core is surrounded by a porous titanium electrode that is coated with platinum. The steroid-eluting leads are characterized by a minimal change in stimulation threshold from implantation to a follow-up period of several years. The acute peak in stimulation threshold is virtually eliminated with these leads. The variation in

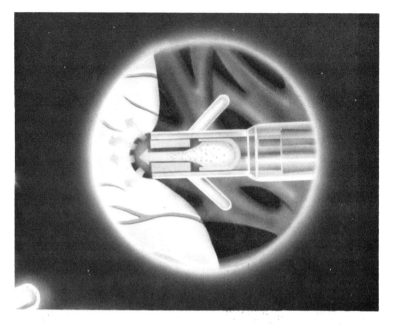

Figure 2.18 Diagrammatic representation of a steroid-eluting electrode with a reservoir of dexamethasone sodium phosphate that slowly elutes through the electrode into the underlying myocardium. (Courtesy of Medtronic, Inc.)

chronic threshold among individuals is significantly reduced, allowing the confident use of lower pacing amplitudes. It should be emphasized that the corticosteroid eluted from the lead does not affect acute stimulation thresholds. Rather, dexamethasone controls the chronic evolution of the pacing threshold. The design characteristics associated with reduced polarization and chemical stability remain important considerations, even with steroid-eluting leads.

The studies of Stokes and colleagues have indicated that the mechanism by which dexamethasone sodium phosphate prevents a rise in chronic stimulation threshold remains to be fully explained.[46] Although the thickness of the fibrous capsule that surrounds the electrode is reduced, the magnitude is less than would be expected by the evolution in stimulation threshold. This suggests that other mechanisms may be involved. In addition to studies of the steroid-eluting electrodes, clinical studies of pacing leads incorporating a drug-eluting collar surrounding the electrode are ongoing.[83] The duration that drug elution is required for sustained low thresholds remains to be fully defined. In addition, whether the impressively low chronic thresholds observed with steroid-eluting electrodes will be maintained over the entire service life of the lead remains to be proven. However, the use of steroid-eluting leads with high electrode resistance allows the use of smaller pulse generators with reduced battery capacity but acceptable longevity.

Fixation mechanism: The chronic performance of permanent pacing leads is critically dependent on stable positioning of the electrode(s). Although early pacing leads were associated with an unacceptably high risk of dislodgment, the development of active and passive fixation mechanisms has dramatically reduced the need for lead repositioning.[165] The present generation of permanent transvenous pacing leads includes several appendages at the distal end that are designed to lodge within the trabeculae of the right atrium or ventricle. These "passive" fixation mechanisms include tines, fins, helices, or conical structures that are extensions of the silicone or polyurethane insulation (Figure 2.19). However, tines are the predominant passive fixation mechanism currently used for permanent pacing leads.[166] Passive fixation leads are typically entrapped within the trabeculae of the right heart chambers immediately upon correct positioning of the lead. Effective fixation of the lead can be confirmed at the time of implantation by gentle traction or rotation of the lead. These fixation mechanisms generally add minimal technical difficulty to the implantation procedure, although tines may occasionally become entrapped in the tricuspid valve apparatus. The passive fixation devices are rapidly covered by fibrous tissue, making later removal of the lead by simple traction difficult or impossible in as short a time as three to six months. Besides the effectiveness of passive fixation devices to prevent dislodgment, the increased stability that is provided for the distal electrode serves to minimize trauma at the myocardial interface caused by motion. This added stability is likely to result in a smaller fibrous capsule surrounding the electrode and improvement of the chronic stimulation threshold. The passive fixation devices have the relative disadvantage of increasing the maximum external diameter of the lead, requiring the use of a larger venous introducer when the subclavian vein puncture technique is employed. Removability of pacing leads is an important consideration. In general, passive fixation leads are more difficult to extract than are active fixation leads.

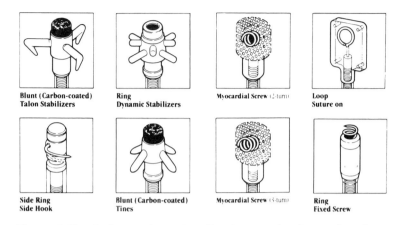

Figure 2.19 Active and passive fixation mechanisms of various types for endocardial and epicardial pacing leads.

Active fixation leads: Although several different fixation methods such as screws, barbs, or hooks have been developed, the present generation of active fixation pacing leads largely relies on a screw helix that is extended into the endocardium.[167–170] The screw helix may be permanently exposed from the tip of the lead (a fixed-screw), requiring the lead to be rotated in a counterclockwise direction during passage through the vasculature. Other leads allow the screw helix to be extended from the tip once the lead has been atraumatically passed through the venous system to the heart (an extendable–retractable screw, Figure 2.20). The design of Bisping and colleagues incorporates an extendable–retractable helical screw that is well suited for positioning at several sites in the atrium or ventricle at the time of implantation.[167] Active fixation leads may utilize the screw helix as both the fixation mechanism and the electrically active electrode (Figure 2.21). Other designs use a separate electrode at the distal end of the lead for stimulation and sensing with an electrically inactive helix. Although both devices provide similar long-term thresholds, the inactive helix leads are associated with lower acute thresholds.[53] A novel approach to active fixation leads uses a cap of mannitol or PEG over the screw helix to facilitate introduction of the lead into the vasculature.[171] After approximately five minutes in the blood pool, the mannitol or PEG dissolves, allowing the screw to engage the endocardium.

Active fixation leads offer the implanting physician the capability for stable positioning of the lead at many sites in either the

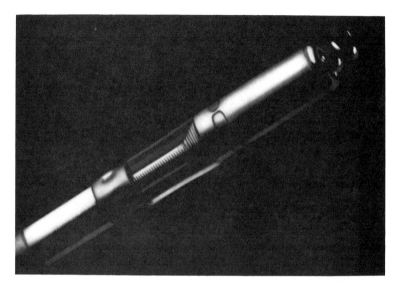

Figure 2.20 **Bipolar active fixation pacing lead with an extendable screw helix and a polished platinum-tipped electrode. (Courtesy of Pacesetter Systems, Inc.)**

atrium or the ventricle. Although active fixation leads have significantly reduced the risk of atrial lead dislodgment, the chronic pacing thresholds are somewhat higher than those of passive fixation leads. Active fixation leads may also be used in the ventricle and may have particular usefulness in rheumatic heart disease associated with important endocardial scarring. In patients with either congenital or surgically corrected transposition of the great vessels who require transvenous pacing, active fixation leads may be placed in the anatomic left ventricle, which has minimal trabeculae. However, because the stimulation thresholds of active fixation leads tend to be somewhat higher than those observed with passive fixation leads, with little difference in the rate of lead dislodgment, there appears to be little reason for the routine use of active fixation leads in the right ventricle.

Conductors

The conducting wire that connects the stimulating and sensing electrode(s) to the proximal connector pin of the lead is a critical determinant of the useable service life of permanent pacing leads. At a minimum pacing rate of 70 ppm the heart contracts and relaxes at least 36 million times a year, producing substantial mechanical stress on a permanent pacing lead. If one considers that the lead must flex with each heartbeat in a complex manner having longitudinal, transverse, and rotational components, one can appreciate the potential for metal fatigue and fracture of the conductor. The most common site for lead fracture is at the fulcrum of a freely moving conductor with a stationary point. Thus the junction of the subclavian vein and the first rib is a common site of conductor failure. In addition, leads may fail at the site of mechanical injury, such as with excessively tight fixation sutures, especially when an anchoring sleeve is not used. Although early pacing leads were made of a single conductor wire and were associated with a high rate of fracture, modern leads use multiple wires that are coiled (Figure 2.22). The use of multiple conducting coils has dramatically

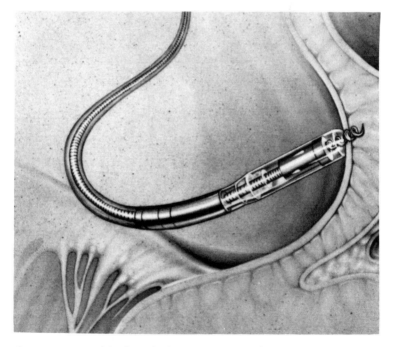

Figure 2.21 A bipolar Bisping-type active fixation that uses the screw helix as the active, distal electrode. The screw helix is extended into the endocardium by rotating the proximal connector of the lead. The screw helix is both extendable and retractable, allowing atraumatic passage through the vasculature. (Courtesy of Medtronic, Inc.)

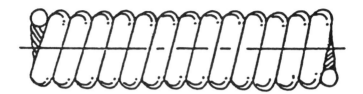

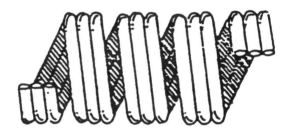

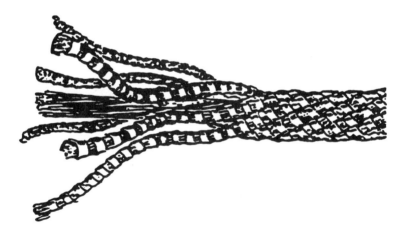

Figure 2.22   The top panel shows a unifilar conducting coil that consists of a single wire wound around a central axis. (Courtesy of Medtronic, Inc.) The middle panel shows a trifilar conducting coil constructed with three wires wound in parallel around a central axis. The bottom panel shows a braided (tinsel-type) lead conductor constructed of multiple wires woven around a central conductor wire.

improved the conductor's resistance to metal fatigue and tensile strength.[162] Stainless steel was used for the conducting coils of early multifilar leads. Stainless steel was abandoned because of the potential for corrosion, however, and was replaced by Elgiloy or MP35N, an alloy of nickel. More recently, conductors manufactured with the drawn-brazed-strand (DBS) technique have been introduced. The DBS conductor is made of six nickel alloy wires that are drawn together with heated silver. The silver forms the matrix of the conductor, occupying the central core and the spaces between the nickel alloy wires. Silver also forms a thin outer layer that conducts the conductor. DBS conductors are characterized by excellent resistance to flexion-related fracture. This conductor also has a very low ohmic resistance, allowing more efficient delivery of the stimulating pulse to the electrode and reduced sensing impedance. The Medtronic 6972 polyurethane-insulated lead was found to be associated with insulation failures that were related to internal oxidation of the polyurethane by silver chloride from the DBS conductor. Because of the potential for oxidation of polyurethane by silver complexes, DBS conductors are no longer used with polyurethane-insulated leads.[172]

Bipolar leads are usually constructed of the coaxial design, with the conductor coil to the distal electrode within the outer conductor coil, which ends at the proximal electrode (Figure 2.23a). Older bipolar leads incorporate two conductor coils wound side by side within the insulating sleeve (Figure 2.23a). The coaxial design also requires that insulation be placed around both conductors, making the overall external diameter rather large (Figure 2.23b). Coaxial bipolar leads are also less flexible than unipolar leads (Figure 2.23b). These characteristics have inhibited some physicians from using bipolar pacing leads routinely. Newer generations of bipolar pacing leads will use conductors that are coiled in parallel, allowing the external diameter of bipolar and unipolar leads to be much more comparable (Figure 2.23a, bottom).

Insulation

The materials used for the insulation of permanent pacing leads are of two varieties, silicone rubber and polyurethane (Table 2.1). Silicone rubber has proven to be a reliable insulating material in over three decades of clinical experience. Silicone is a relatively fragile material, however, with a low tear strength. Because the insulation of permanent pacing leads may be subjected to trauma

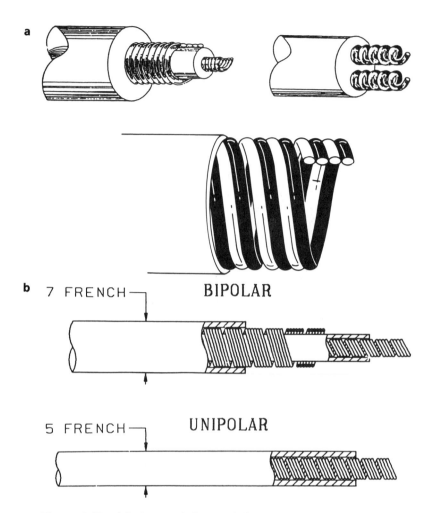

Figure 2.23 (a) The top left panel shows a bipolar lead with two conductor coils that are wound coaxially. The inner coil connects to the tip electrode, and the outer coil connects to the ring electrode. A sleeve of insulation separates the coils. The top right panel shows a bipolar lead conductor using two unifilar coils placed in parallel (side by side) with surrounding insulation. (Courtesy of Medtronic, Inc.) The bottom panel shows a schematic representation of a multiconductor lead with two Teflon-insulated conducting wires wound in parallel and encased within a polyurethane insulating sleeve. This construction provides a smaller diameter to the lead body than does the standard coaxial design. (Courtesy of Telectronics Pacing Systems, Inc.) (b) A schematic representation of a standard bipolar coaxial lead with inner and outer conductor coils and inner and outer insulation sleeves is shown on top, and a schematic representation of a unipolar lead with a quadrafilar conducting coil surrounded by a sleeve of insulation is shown on the bottom. (Courtesy of Telectronics Pacing Systems, Inc.)

Table 2.1   Pacemaker Lead Insulation

Silicone Rubber	Polyurethane
Advantages	Advantages
• 30+ years proven history	• 10+ years proven history (55D)
• Repairable	• High tear strength
• Low process sensitivity	• High cut resistance
• Easy fabrication/molding	• Low friction in blood
• Very flexible	• High abrasion resistance
Disadvantages	• Thinner walls possible (small diameter)
• Tears easily (nicks, ligatures)	• Relatively nonthrombogenic
• Cuts easily	Disadvantages
• Low abrasion resistance	• Relatively stiff (especially 55D)
• High friction in blood	• Not repairable
• Requires thicker walls (large diameter)	• Manufacturing process sensitive
• More thrombogenic and fibrotic	• Environmental stress cracking (ESC)
• Subject to cold flow failure	• Metal ion oxidation (MIO)
• Absorbs lipids (calcification)	• History of clinical failures (80A)

during or after implantation, the silicone layer must be thicker than it would be if it were stronger. Although the size of silicone-insulated unipolar leads has been clinically acceptable, coaxial bipolar leads constructed of this material have been of relatively large external diameter (often 10-Fr or greater). In addition, silicone rubber exposed to blood has a high coefficient of friction, making the manipulation of two leads in a single vein difficult. These disadvantages have been addressed by the introduction of platinum-cured silicone rubber, which is characterized by improved mechanical strength. The coefficient of friction has been greatly reduced by the development of a lubricious, "fast-pass" coating. These improved silicone leads are of smaller external diameter and are far easier to manipulate when in contact with another lead.

Polyurethane was introduced as an insulation material because of its superior tear strength and low coefficient of friction.[172] These properties allow polyurethane leads to be constructed with smaller external diameter than those made with conventional silicone rubber. The smaller polyurethane leads have contributed to the increased acceptance of bipolar pacing and have allowed two leads to be placed in a single vein, also contributing to the ease of dual-chamber pacemaker implantation.

Two major forms of polyurethane, known as P80A and

P55D, have been used to insulate permanent pacing leads. The P80A polymer, which is less stiff than the P55D variety, was used in the first polyurethane-insulated cardiac pacing leads. The P55D polymer, which has greater tensile and tear strength, has been used as the insulating material for the pacing leads of several manufacturers.[172] The P55D polymer is now the predominant form of polyurethane used for pacing leads.

Within four years of the first human implant, polyurethane insulation failures became clinically apparent.[173,174] The model 6991U unipolar atrial lead with a preformed J shape demonstrated a pattern of insulation failure in the J-region in a minority of cases.[175] The model 6972 bipolar ventricular lead was found to have surface cracks in the P80A polyurethane insulation and clinical evidence of insulation failure[173,174] (Figure 2.24). The initial polyurethane insulated leads have shown a high incidence of microscopic cracks in the outer surface of the insulation material. The extensive investigations of Stokes have shown that the surface cracks are likely related to environmental stresses rather than to biologic degradation.[172,176] The surface cracks in the polyurethane develop in the manufacturing process as the heated polyurethane cools more rapidly than the inner core, leading to opposing stresses within the insulation. Although microscopic cracks in the outer surface of the polyurethane are usually clinically unimportant, these cracks may predispose the insulation to further degradation by trauma during or after lead implantation. At sites of additional mechanical stress, such as at the anchoring suture or during stylet insertion, the surface cracks may propagate deeper into the polyurethane, leading to insulation failure. Polyurethane may also be oxidized by silver chloride. Thus, degradation of polyurethane from the inside of the lead from silver contained in DBS conductors may occur.[177]

The mechanisms of polyurethane failure have been addressed by changes in the manufacturing process (slower cooling of the heated polyurethane and the elimination of solvents) and by the recognition that conductors made with silver should not be used with leads insulated with this material. Nevertheless, the P80A polymer has had an unacceptable risk of insulation failure when used for permanent pacing leads, at least as manufactured by some manufacturers. The poor performance of the Medtronic models 6972, 4012, and 4004 bipolar, polyurethane leads has led to a shift to the P55D polymer. At this point both polyurethane P55D and silicone rubber can be considered acceptable insulating materials.

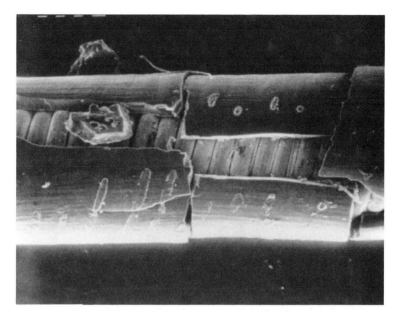

Figure 2.24   Cracking of polyurethane insulation (80 A) covering a bipolar permanent pacing lead two years after implantation. (Courtesy of Pacesetter Systems, Inc.)

The relative unsusceptibilty of unipolar leads to clinically detectable insulation failure is an important clinical advantage.

Myocardial leads

Permanent pacing leads that are sutured to the epicardium or screwed into the myocardium of either the atrium or ventricle are presently used in clinical situations involving abnormalities of the tricuspid valve, congenital heart disease, or when permanent pacing leads are implanted during intrathoracic surgical procedures (Figure 2.25). Epimyocardial electrodes utilize a fishhook shape that is stabbed into the atrial myocardium, a screw helix that is rotated into the ventricle, or loops that are placed within epicardial stab wounds in the ventricle. The chronic stimulation thresholds with myocardial leads tend to be higher than with modern endocardial electrodes, although there is considerable overlap. The use of three turns on an epicardial screw has been demonstrated to decrease the risk of exit block when compared to a two-turn screw.[178] The incorporation of corticosteroid-eluting electrodes into the design of myocardial leads is presently under investigation.[84]

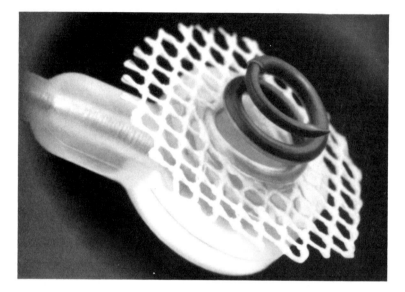

Figure 2.25 **Unipolar epicardial screw-in electrode with a screw helix that is rotated into the myocardium. (Courtesy of Pacesetter Systems, Inc.)**

Connectors

A major problem for manufacturers of pulse generators and pacing leads, as well as for implanting physicians, has been the incompatibility of lead connectors and pulse generator headers that resulted from the lack of a consistent standard. Permanent pacing leads have evolved from a standard 5- to 6-mm connector pin for unipolar and bifurcated bipolar models to an "in-line" bipolar connector with a 3.2-mm diameter (Figure 2.26). The considerable variability in the design of the in-line bipolar connector has led to considerable confusion among physicians as to whether a particular lead of one manufacturer will match the pulse generator of another. Much of this confusion is related to the location of sealing rings; some manufacturers prefer to place the sealing rings in the header of the pulse generator, and others prefer the sealing rings to be on the connector of the lead. Because of this chaotic situation (Figure 2.27), an international meeting of manufacturers agreed on a voluntary standard for leads and connectors incorporating the sealing rings on a 3.2-mm lead connector (VS-1).[179] After continued problems with universal acceptance of the VS-1 connector, the incompatibility problem has been largely resolved with an industrywide

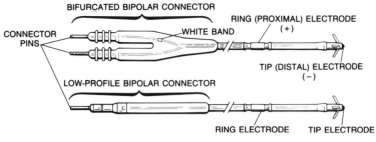

Two Designs of Bipolar Leads

Figure 2.26 A standard bifurcated bipolar lead connector with two connector pins is shown. A white band marks the conductor leading to the distal electrode. A low-profile "Medtronic" type bipolar connector that has a single pin is shown. The distal electrode connects to the pin.

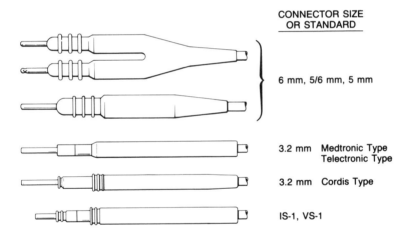

Available Connectors

Figure 2.27 Five common varieties of lead connectors. The upper connector is a bifurcated bipolar design with two connector pins, each 5 to 6 mm in diameter with sealing rings on the lead. The second connector is a standard unipolar design of 5- or 6-mm diameter incorporating sealing rings. The middle tracing represents a "Medtronic" type, low-profile connector with 3.2-mm diameter and no sealing rings. The 3.2-mm "Telectronics" type connector is similar and incorporates sealing rings on the proximal portion of the lead. The IS-1 and VS-1 connectors are incompatible with the other designs and include sealing rings on the proximal portion of the lead.

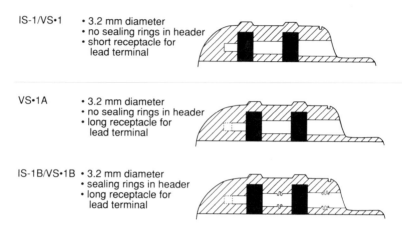

IS-1/VS•1
- 3.2 mm diameter
- no sealing rings in header
- short receptacle for lead terminal

VS•1A
- 3.2 mm diameter
- no sealing rings in header
- long receptacle for lead terminal

IS-1B/VS•1B
- 3.2 mm diameter
- sealing rings in header
- long receptacle for lead terminal

Figure 2.28 Three varieties of in-line bipolar pulse generator headers.

standard configuration known as IS-1 (Figure 2.28). Despite this vast improvement in standardization, implanting physicians encountering previously implanted leads must be aware that not all pulse generators will accept the connector pin of all 3.2-mm leads. For example, the IS-1 pulse generator will not accept an older Medtronic or Telectronics 3.2-mm or a Cordis 3.2-mm connector pin. The IS-1B connector will accept any of the VS-1, IS-1, Medtronic 3.2-mm or Cordis 3.2-mm lead connectors.

PULSE GENERATORS

All pulse generators presently used in permanent pacing systems have several basic functional elements that are critical to the operation of the device. These include a power source, an output circuit, a sensing circuit, and a timing circuit. Most pulse generators also contain a telemetry coil for sending and receiving programming instructions and diagnostic information. In addition to these basic elements, newer pulse generators often contain circuits for sensing the output of an artificial, rate-adaptive sensor. The integrated circuit of some pulse generators also contains the capability of storing information in memory—either read only memory (ROM) or random access memory (RAM)—which can be used to process diagnostic data or alter the feature set of the device following its implantation. In this section, the important aspects of each of these basic elements of pulse generators will be reviewed.

Power source

The power source of virtually all pulse generators presently in use is a chemical battery. Although mercury–zinc, rechargeable silver–modified-mercuric-oxide–zinc, rechargeable nickel–cadmium batteries[180] and radioactive plutonium[181] or promethium[147,182] have all been used as the power source of permanent pacing systems, modern pulse generators almost exclusively use lithium as the anodal element (Figure 2.29). The energy provided by a chemical battery is generated by the transfer of electrons from the anodal element to the cathodal element of the battery. In the case of lithium batteries, lithium is the anodal element and provides the supply of electrons. The cathodal element of the battery receives the electrons. In a lithium–iodine cell (most commonly used for permanent pacemakers), iodine serves as the cathodal element and

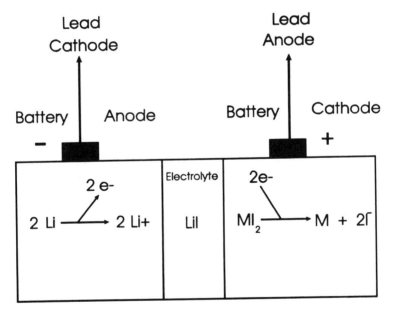

Figure 2.29 Schematic representation of a lithium–iodine battery. The anodal terminal of the battery is negatively charged as lithium releases electrons to the lead. The battery anode leads to the cathode of the pacing lead (which is also negatively charged). The anodal portion of the battery itself becomes positively charged with the reaction $2Li \rightarrow 2Li^+ + 2e^-$. The cathodal terminal of the battery is positively charged and connects to the anode of the lead. The cathodal reaction is $MI_2 + 2e^- \rightarrow M + 2I^-$, where M represents poly-2-vinyl pyridine.

accepts electrons from lithium. Poly-2-vinyl pyridine is combined with the cathodal element to assist in the transfer of electrons to iodine. At the battery terminals, the anode gives up electrons and is negatively charged, and the cathode accepts electrons and is positively charged. Internally, the anodal reaction proceeds as $2Li \rightarrow 2Li^+ + 2e^-$, with the cathodal reaction being $2I + 2e^- \rightarrow 2I^-$. Thus, within the battery, the anode is positively charged and the cathode is negatively charged; the overall chemical reaction is $2Li + 2I \rightarrow 2LiI$. The electrons are carried from the anodal terminal of the battery to the cathodal terminal when the circuit is completed by the external load. For a stimulating pulse, the output circuit of the pulse generator, the pacing lead, and the myocardium provide the external load.

The battery also contains a material separating the anodal and cathodal elements (the electrolyte); this material serves as a conductor of ionic movement but is a barrier to the transfer of electrons. The electrolyte for a lithium–iodine battery is composed of a semisolid layer of lithium iodide that gradually increases in thickness over the life of the cell. As the LiI layer grows, the internal impedance of the battery increases. A major advantage of the lithium–iodine battery is the solid nature of the material, allowing the cell to be hermetically sealed and relatively resistant to corrosion. In contrast to the solid electrolyte of lithium–iodine batteries, the lithium–cupric-sulfide battery previously manufactured by Cordis used a liquid electrolyte. Although this electrochemical cell was associated with a low impedance over 90 percent of its useable life, it has been associated with corrosion of the terminal feedthrough and early failure. The zinc–mercury battery used in early pulse generators contained sodium hydroxide as the electrolyte, a material that was corrosive and associated with the potential for sudden failure. Zinc–mercury batteries were also characterized by the production of hydrogen gas as a by-product of the battery reaction. The requirement for venting of hydrogen gas from the battery prevented hermetic sealing of the pulse generator and permitted the influx of tissue fluid, further increasing the risk of sudden failure.

The battery voltage is dependent on the chemistry of the cell. For example, the lithium–iodine cell generates approximately 2.8 V at the beginning of its life. The lithium–silver-chromate cell generates 3.2 V and the lithium–thionyl-chloride cell produces 3.6 V at beginning of life, whereas the lithium–lead-iodide cell has a voltage of only 1.9 V. Because the voltage of each of these cells is less than what may be required for chronic myocardial stimulation, a voltage multiplier in the output circuit must be used to allow output pulses of greater amplitude than the cell voltage. The voltage of the battery itself may be increased by using more than one cell in series. Using cells in series increases the output voltage of the battery but does not increase battery capacity. Electrochemical cells may also be connected in parallel to increase capacity. However, cells in parallel do not generate an increased voltage. Mallory has produced a lithium–lead-iodine battery constructed of 21 cells, arranged with seven parallel banks of three cells in series. Similarly, the Medtronic Xyrel pulse generators used two lithium–iodine cells in series to generate 5.6 V, and the Cordis lithium–cupric-sulfide battery used three cells in series to produce 6.3 V.

The capacity of an electrochemical cell is determined by several factors, including the chemical elements of the battery, the size of the battery, the external load, the amount of internal discharge, and the voltage decay characteristics of the cell. To maximize battery life, the ideal electrochemical cell would have no internal discharge. However, batteries used for permanent pacemakers have been associated with internal discharge of variable degree. For example, the initial zinc–mercury cells were associated with an internal rate of self-discharge of over 15 percent per year. The lithium–iodine cell is associated with a low rate of self-discharge following the initial reaction of lithium and iodine in the cell, generally less than 1 percent per year in chronic use.

In order for a battery to be suitable for use in permanent pacemakers, the decay characteristics of the cell should be predictable (Figure 2.30). The ideal battery should have a predictable fall in voltage near the end of life, yet provide sufficient service life after the initial voltage decay to allow time for the elective replacement indicator to be detected and for replacement to be performed. The early zinc–mercury batteries were associated with a nearly constant cell voltage until end of life, when the voltage declined abruptly. These characteristics were generally unacceptable because of the difficulty of anticipating battery depletion. Lithium cells are associated with a more predictable behavior at end of life. The lithium–silver-chromate cell is characterized by two distinct plateau phases of voltage, the first phase (3.2 V) representing approximately 70 percent of the service life and a second phase of approximately 2.5 V. This two-phase decay characteristic is an attractive feature of this cell and allows a wide period of time in which to detect the elective replacement indicator.

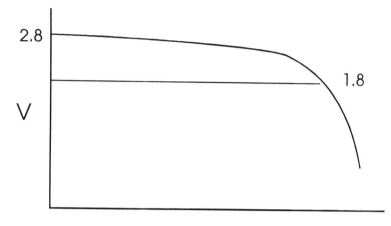

Years

Figure 2.30 Typical voltage decay characteristics of a lithium-iodine battery. At beginning of life, the lithium–iodine cell generates 2.8 V. At end of useable life (90 percent depletion), the battery voltage decreases to approximately 1.8 V.

Another battery that has been used for permanent pacemakers is the lithium–thionyl-chloride cell. This battery was associated with instances of an abrupt fall in battery voltage related to a sudden rise in cell impedance and unexpected end-of-life behavior. The voltage produced by a lithium–iodine cell is inversely related to the internal battery impedance. The internal impedance of the battery increases with the thickness of the lithium–iodide electrolyte layer, from less than 1 kohm at the beginning of life to over 15 kohms at the extreme end of life. The voltage generated by the cell declines almost linearly from the initial value of 2.8 V to 2.4 V at approximately 90 percent of the useable battery life. Following this, the voltage declines exponentially to 1.8 V at the end of life. The magnet-related pacing rate of the pulse generator is related to the cell voltage, usually declining once the voltage falls below 2.4 V. The end-of-life indicator of pulse generators is usually signalled by a decrease in the magnet-related pacing rate to a fixed percentage of the beginning-of-life rate. Unfortunately, the end-of-life magnet rate is variable between manufacturers and between models. Some manufacturers signal the end of life by a two-step process, with an initial decrease in the magnet rate to an intermediate value followed by a stepwise decrease in rate to a second, lower value in association with a change in pacing mode, such as from DDD to VVI. In addition to a decrease in the magnet rate, the cell impedance of many pulse generators can be directly telemetered from the device, allowing a more accurate estimation of the useable service life. Some manufacturers also include an automatic increase in the pulse duration of the output circuit so that the total energy of the pulse delivered remains constant. Although the output energy may remain constant by stretching of the pulse duration, loss of capture will occur if the stimulus voltage falls below rheobase.

The useable service life of a pulse generator is not only dependent on the characteristics of the battery, but is greatly influenced by the current drain of the integrated circuit, the amplitude and duration of the output pulse, the frequency of stimulation, the total impedance of the pacing lead, and the additional energy required to monitor and generate the output of a rate-adaptive sensor. Advances in the design of integrated circuits have greatly minimized the static current drain required to operate the circuit, to less than 2 to 3 microamperes. The major source of current drain for the present generation of pulse generators is the output pulses. Thus, the amplitude, duration, and frequency of stimulating pulses are major contributors to the life of the power source. The pacing impedance is another critical influence on the current drain of the output pulse. Advances in pacing leads that are likely to improve pulse generator longevity yet provide an adequate safety margin include the use of electrodes with steroid elution, high electrode–tissue impedance, and low polarization. With the introduction of these high-performance leads, the nominal output energy will be significantly reduced. The addition of automatic threshold tracking and capture verification also holds the potential to increase pulse generator longevity by optimizing the energy of the stimulating pulse for each patient.

Output circuits

The output pulse of the pulse generator is generated from the discharge of a capacitor to the anode and cathode of the pacing leads. The output capacitor is charged from the battery at a relatively slow rate to the programmed output voltage. Since the battery voltage of lithium–iodine cells is approximately 2.8 V, delivery of a stimulus of amplitude greater than this requires the use of a voltage multiplier. The voltage multiplier involves charging more than one capacitor from the battery. For example, if a

89

stimulus voltage of 5.6 V is programmed, two capacitors must be charged from the battery in parallel and discharged in series. The output voltage may be doubled by charging two pump capacitors in parallel (each to 2.8 V), with the discharge delivered to the output capacitor in series. In this way, the output capacitor is charged to 5.6 V. The cost of doubling the output voltage is a fourfold increase in current drain from the battery. If the stimulus amplitude is programmed to 8.4 V (3 times the voltage of a lithium–iodide cell), three capacitors must be charged. In this case, a threefold increase in stimulus voltage results in a ninefold increase in current drain from the battery, markedly shortening battery life.

Output pulse waveforms: Most pulse generators used for permanent cardiac pacing deliver a capacitively coupled, constant-voltage pulse of programmable duration. When the fully charged capacitor is discharged, the resulting voltage at the leading edge of the pulse is independent of the pacing impedance. However, the trailing edge of the pulse is less than that of the leading edge, with the magnitude of the voltage drop being a function of the pacing impedance (Figure 2.31). Because the capacitor stores a charge of fixed quantity, the greater the current flow, the smaller the charge (and voltage) remaining on the capacitor at the end of the pulse. Therefore, the lower the impedance, the greater the current delivered and the greater the drop in voltage from leading edge to trailing edge during the pulse. Thus, even though the term *constant voltage* is used to describe the stimulus waveform of permanent pacemakers, in reality the output voltage of the pulse is not constant from beginning to end.

Constant-current generators are no longer being implanted for permanent pacing, though some pulse generators manufactured by Cordis are still in service. However, constant-current pulse generators are typical of many external pacing systems. The constant-current pulse is typically flat, with little or no change in current from leading edge to trailing edge. However, as the polarization impedance rises during the pulse, the resulting voltage must also rise proportionally to maintain the current at a constant level. Although either constant-current or constant-voltage pulse generators are capable of providing reliable pacing in the vast majority of clinical circumstances, at extremely high lead impedances, the voltage required to maintain a constant-current pulse may exceed the capabilities of the battery.

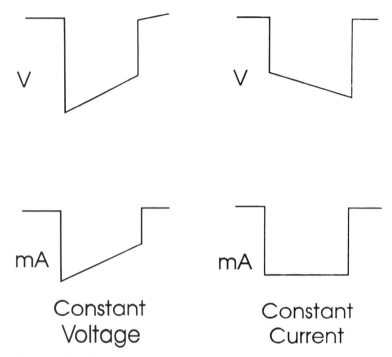

Constant Voltage

Constant Current

Figure 2.31 Output voltage and current waveforms for constant-voltage (left) and constant-current (right) stimulation. With a constant-voltage pulse, the leading-edge voltage is independent of load. The trailing-edge voltage depends on the total pacing impedance. The delivered current also declines from leading edge to trailing edge. With constant-current stimulation, the current remains constant throughout the pulse (provided that the cell can generate the required voltage). The delivered voltage increases with rising impedance during the pulse.

The output waveform of the pulse generator is followed by a low-amplitude, long-duration wave of opposite polarity known as the afterpotential. The afterpotential is caused by polarization at the electrode–tissue interface and is dependent on the stimulus amplitude and duration. The afterpotential is also influenced by the polarization characteristics of the electrode. Afterpotentials may be inappropriately sensed by the sensing circuit if the stimulus amplitude and pulse duration are great and the sensing threshold is low. In order to reduce the afterpotential, the output circuit of some manufacturers incorporates a fast recharge pulse, during which the electrode polarity is reversed for a short period following the output pulse. This diminishes the polarization at the electrode–tissue interface, although it does not eliminate the need for low-polarization electrodes.

Sensing circuits

The intracardiac electrogram is conducted from the electrodes to the sensing circuit of the pulse generator, where it is amplified and filtered. As discussed previously in this chapter, in order to minimize attenuation of the signal, the sensing amplifier must have an input impedance greatly in excess of the sensing impedance. The greater the input impedance, the less the electrogram is attenuated by the amplifier. The input impedances of the sense amplifiers used in permanent pacing systems are in excess of 25,000 ohms. The intracardiac electrogram is filtered to remove unwanted frequencies, a process that markedly affects the amplitude of the processed signal. A bandpass filter attenuates components of the electrogram on either side of the center frequency (the frequency with least attenuation) (Figure 2.32). The bandpass filters of different manufacturers vary significantly with regard to center frequency (from approximately 20 to 40 Hz), so that intracardiac electrograms measured with a pacing system analyzer of one manufacturer may produce considerably different electrogram amplitudes than will the pulse generator sensing amplifier of another manufacturer.[183,184] It is also somewhat difficult to compare the sense amplifiers of different manufacturers because the shape of the test waveform has an important influence on the amplitude of the filtered electrogram, such that square-wave and sinusoidal test pulses may produce frequency attenuation spectra that differ from those of intracardiac electrograms.[185] Following filtering of the intracardiac signal, the processed signal is compared with a reference voltage to determine if the signal exceeds a threshold detection level. Signals with amplitude greater than the sensitivity threshold level are sensed as intracardiac events, whereas signals of lower amplitude are discarded as noise. Signals that exceed the threshold level are marked by an output voltage pulse that is sent to the timing circuit.

Permanent pacemakers also contain noise reversion circuits that change the pulse generator to an asynchronous pacing mode when the sensing threshold level is exceeded at a rate faster than the noise reversion rate. The noise reversion mode prevents inhibition of pacing in the presence of electromagnetic interference. The electronic circuitry of the pulse generator must also be pro-

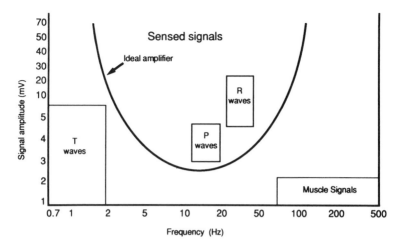

Figure 2.32 Signal processing with bandpass filtering of a sine-squared test waveform by a ventricular sensing amplifier. The curve denotes the signal amplitude required to be detected by the sensing amplifier with a threshold sensitivity value of 2.5 mV. Note that the amplitude of the signal that is needed for appropriate sensing is markedly increased at frequencies below and above the center frequency.

tected from damage caused by overwhelming electrical energy generated in the clinical environment. The input voltage to the sensing amplifier is limited by a Zener diode that is designed to protect the integrated circuit from high external voltages such as may occur during defibrillation shocks or electrocautery. When the input voltage carried by the pacing leads exceeds the Zener voltage, the excess energy is shunted back to the myocardium through the leads. In addition to these features, which are designed to manage external electromagnetic interference, the sensing amplifier must prevent the detection of unwanted intracardiac signals such as far-field R waves in the atrial electrogram, afterpotentials, T waves, and retrogradely conducted P waves.

The potential for inappropriate inhibition of the ventricular output of a dual chamber pacemaker by far-field ventricular sensing of the atrial pacing stimulus or its afterpotential can be effectively reduced by the use of a ventricular blanking period. During the ventricular blanking period, the ventricular sensing amplifier is turned off immediately following the atrial pacing pulse. Although the blanking period has been quite effective in decreasing the frequency of ventricular crosstalk (inappropriate inhibition of ven-

CARDIAC PACING

tricular pacing by far-field atrial pacing stimuli), several manufacturers also provide a nonphysiologic AV delay with delivery of a
ventricular pacing pulse on sensing a ventricular event early in the
AV interval. The inappropriate detection of intracardiac signals is
also managed by the use of sensing refractory periods, during which
the sense amplifier is not responsive to events such as T waves or
retrogradely conducted P waves. The initial portion of the refractory period is a blanking period during which the sense amplifier is
totally insensitive to electrical signals.

The remainder of the refractory period is typically a noise-
sampling period. Events in this portion of the refractory period do
not reset the timing circuit but initiate a new blanking period.
Although sensing refractory periods are extremely effective for the
management of unwanted signals, there are relative disadvantages
to this approach, such as the inability of a DDD pacing system to
track rapid atrial rates when a prolonged atrial refractory period is
required to manage retrograde ventriculoatrial conduction. Newer
pacing systems that incorporate variable refractory periods that
change in proportion to the output of a metabolic sensor are likely
to reduce the importance of these disadvantages.

Timing circuits

The pacing cycle length, sensing refractory and alert periods, pulse
duration, and AV interval are precisely regulated by the timing
circuit of the pulse generator. The timing circuit of a pulse generator is a crystal oscillator that generates a very accurate signal with a
frequency in the KHz range. The output of the crystal oscillator is
sent to a digital timing and logic control circuit that operates
internally generated clocks at divisions of the oscillator frequency.
The output of the logic control circuit is a logic pulse that triggers
the output pacing pulse, the blanking and refractory intervals, and
the AV delay. The timing circuit also receives input from the sense
amplifier to reset the escape intervals of an inhibited pacing system
or trigger initiation of an AV delay for triggered pacing modes.
The pulse generator also contains a rate-limiting circuit that prevents the pacing rate from exceeding an upper limit in the case of
a random component failure. This runaway protection rate is
typically in the range of 180 to 200 ppm.

Telemetry circuits

Programmable pulse generators have the capability of responding to
radiofrequency signals emitted from the programmer as well as

sending information in the reverse direction, from the pulse generator to the programmer. The pulse generator is capable of both transmitting information from a radiofrequency antenna and receiving information with a radiofrequency decoder. Telemetry information may be sent as radiofrequency signals or as a pulsed magnetic field. Information that is sent from an external programmer to the pulse generator is sent in coded programming sequences with a preset frequency spectrum. Most pulse generators require the radiofrequency signal to be pulsed with a specific frequency in a sequence that is typically 16 pulses in duration. Thus the radiofrequency signal is quite precise, decreasing the likelihood of inappropriate alteration of the program by environmental sources of radiofrequency energy or magnetic fields. This characteristic also prevents the programmers of one manufacturer from programming the pulse generator of another. The detected telemetry bursts from the programmer are sent as digital information from the radiofrequency demodulator to the telemetry control logic circuit of the pulse generator. This logic circuit also provides for properly timed pulses to be sent from the antenna of the pulse generator to the programmer. *Real-time telemetry* is the term used to describe the capability of a pulse generator to transmit information to the programmer regarding measurements of pulse amplitude and duration, lead impedance, battery impedance, and delivered current, charge, and energy. These measurements may provide useful information for troubleshooting pacing systems. The pulse generator may also allow telemetry of intracardiac electrograms and timing circuit markers that can be extremely valuable for the evaluation of sensing (see Chapters 7 and 9).

Microprocessors

The integrated circuit of pulse generators may contain both ROM and RAM. ROM (typically 1–2 Kbytes of 8–32 bits) is used to guide the sensing and output circuits. Devices with 8- or 16-bit processors usually require several clock cycles to decode an instruction from memory. The processors operating with larger instruction words (such as 32 bits) may load and execute an instruction in a single clock cycle, improving the efficiency of the repetitive tasks that are required for pacing and sensing. In addition, RAM is used to store diagnostic information regarding pacing rate, intrinsic heart rates, and sensor output. The amount of RAM that is included in the pulse generator varies between models and manufacturers. The amount of RAM in modern pulse generators is rapidly increasing, with some models offering up to 64 Kbytes of memory. The increased RAM of newer pulse generators allows increased collection of diagnostic data. Such data include histograms of paced and intrinsic heart rate, sensor function, trends of heart rate and sensor function over time, storage of electrograms from episodes of high atrial or ventricular rates, and mode-switching events. The rapidly expanding diagnostic capabilities of pacemakers will allow improved assessment of the physiologic condition of patients.

Almost all manufacturers offer fully RAM-based pulse generators. There are several important advantages to microprocessor-based pacemakers, including decreased production costs for an entire product line, increased flexibility to upgrade features in subsequent pacemaker models, and the capability for downloading new features into previously implanted pacemakers by telemetry. It is important to emphasize that the microprocessors used in permanent pacemakers must be custom designed in order to minimize current drain and operate with a lithium–iodine battery. Thus a microprocessor that is used in a microcomputer and has access to a virtually unlimited power supply (AC current operating at 110 V) would not be feasible for inclusion in a permanent pacemaker.

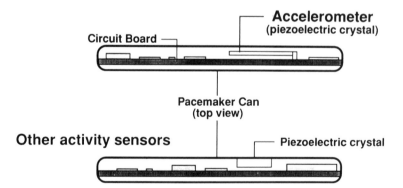

Figure 2.33 Schematic representation of two motion-sensing, rate-adaptive pacing systems. In the upper panel, an accelerometer (piezoelectric crystal) is mounted on the circuit board of the pulse generator. The bottom panel represents the alternative sensor location, with the piezoelectric crystal mounted on the inside of the pulse generator can. (Courtesy of Intermedics, Inc.)

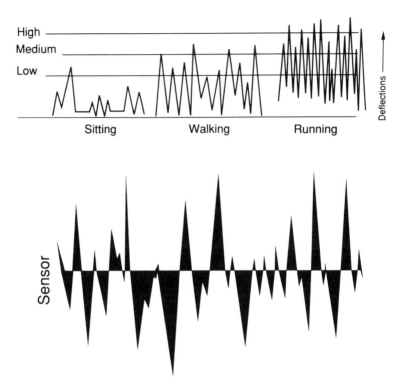

Figure 2.34 The top panel shows processing of the activity sensor signal by simple counting of the frequency of deflections above a threshold amplitude (high, medium, or low). The bottom panel shows processing of the activity signal by integration of the amplitude and frequency of sensor deflections above a threshold value.

RATE-ADAPTIVE SENSORS

Widespread appreciation of the importance of rate modulation in the augmentation of cardiac output with exercise has led to the development of a wide variety of physiologic sensors. Although the normal sinus node may be an ideal rate-adaptive sensor for many patients who require pacemakers, the frequent occurrence of sinus node dysfunction and atrial fibrillation in clinical practice limits the applicability of atrial sensing in reliably modulating pacing rate in many individuals. Thus, artificial sensors that correlate with the level of metabolic demand either directly or indirectly have assumed increased importance in the design and application of permanent pacing systems. In this section, the design considerations of these sensors will be discussed.

The ideal rate-adaptive pacing system should provide pacing rates that are proportional to the level of metabolic needs. The speed of change in the pacing rate should be similar to that of the sinus node. The ideal sensor demonstrates sensitivity and specificity. It should demonstrate sensitivity to both exercise- and nonexercise-related changes, such as mental stress. Specificity is demonstrated by the failure of the sensor to be affected by stimuli that should not cause an increase in pacing rate.

Multiple technical considerations are important in the implementation of the sensor. These include the stability of the sensor, the size of the sensor, its biocompatibility and the ease of its programming. Excessive energy consumption by a sensor will limit the life span of the pulse generator. Sensors that are large or require the placement of additional electrodes or a new type of electrode may present a technical problem. The response of the sensor is determined by its intrinsic properties in response to stimuli, the algorithm used to relate changes in the sensed parameter to changes in paced heart rate and the ease and way it is programmed.

Motion (activity) sensors

Rate-adaptive pacing systems that detect mechanical vibration are based on the clinical association of increasing body motion with increasing levels of exercise.[186] These devices are designed to detect low-frequency vibrations in the range of the resonant frequency of the human body (approximately 4 Hz). A piezoelectric ceramic crystal functioning as a strain gauge is bonded to the inside of the pulse generator case or to the circuit board (Figure 2.33, top).[186] As the ceramic crystal flexes and deforms in response to mechanical vibration or pressure, an electric current is generated. The magnitude of the electric current from the crystal is related to the frequency and amplitude of vibrations. The output of the sensor is processed electronically and used to modulate changes in pacing rate.

Early motion-sensitive pacing systems simply counted the occurrence of sensor output exceeding a programmable threshold level[186–190] (Figure 2.33, bottom). Because vibrations that greatly exceeded the threshold registered the same as those that exceeded this level only slightly, the function of these devices was frequently an all-or-none increase in pacing rate. Newer devices integrate the output of the sensor, responding to both the frequency and the amplitude of the electrical signal[191–194] (Figure 2.34). This change in signal processing has improved the proportionality of the sensor-related pacing rate to the level of exercise. The threshold level for the detection of vibrations is programmable from low to high, allowing the device to be individualized to the resonant characteristics of the individual. The slope of the relationship between sensor output and pacing rate is also programmable. Newer devices also allow separate programming of rate onset and rate offset.

Motion-sensitive, rate-adaptive pacing systems are characterized by a rapid response to the onset of exercise. Combined with simplicity of function and compatibility with any standard pacing lead, these devices have become the most widely prescribed rate-adaptive pacing systems presently in use. There are important limitations to these sensors, however, as they are related only indirectly to metabolic demand. For example, exercise that generates significant mechanical vibration (such as walking or arm motion) leads to a greater rate increase than exercise that produces less motion (such as bicycling).[194] Similarly, the pacing rate produced by descending stairs is typically greater than that produced by climbing stairs.[194,195] In addition, these sensors are susceptible to environmental noise from vibrations produced by transportation or direct pressure over the pulse generator.[196] Finally, these sensors respond poorly to some types of exercise (e.g., swimming, isometric exercise).

Accelerometers

Acceleration sensors use either piezoelectric (Intermedics, Inc., Biotronik, Inc.) or piezoresistive (CPI, Inc.) materials.[197] The piezoelectric accelerometer is mounted on the hybrid circuitry in the pulse generator rather than bonded to the pulse generator case. This allows the accelerometer to be mechanically insulated from the case, preventing increases in pacing rate as a result of simple pressure on the pulse generator. As the patient moves in the anterior–posterior axis, the mass of the accelerometer deflects in proportion to the change in velocity (acceleration = dV/dt). Accelerometers that are piezoelectric generate an electrical potential as a result of deformation of the piezoceramic material. In contrast, piezoresistive accelerometers measure changes in electrical resistance that occur with mechanical deformation of the sensor and require a somewhat greater current drain in order to power the sensor.

Although motion of the body during walking or bicycling

occurs in both the anterior–posterior and vertical axes, exercise workload is more proportional in the anterior–posterior axis than in the vertical axis. Since accelerometers tend to detect acceleration in the anterior–posterior axis to a greater extent than the vertical axis, these sensors offer the potential for greater proportionality of response than do activity sensors. Accelerometers have been shown to be somewhat less susceptible to excessive rate increases during descending stairs than activity sensors. Accelerometers have also been demonstrated to produce rate response that is closer to the expected behavior of the sinus node during bicycle exercise than is observed with activity sensors.[198] In general, accelerometers offer rate modulation that is somewhat more proportional to exercise workload than activity sensors. Whether these advantages translate into clinically significant improvements in exercise performance has not been shown.

Respiration sensors

Respiratory rate (RR), tidal volume (TV), and the product of these two parameters (minute ventilation) increase in proportion to changes in carbon dioxide production (VCO_2).[199–201] At exercise workloads less than anaerobic threshold, the minute ventilation is closely associated with oxygen consumption (VO_2). Rossi described an implantable rate-adaptive pacing system that measured respiratory rate from cyclic changes in impedance between the pulse generator case and an axillary subcutaneous lead implanted over the anterior thorax.[199] Although exercise tolerance and cardiac output have been demonstrated to increase to a significantly greater extent with rate-adaptive pacing systems that respond to respiratory rate than with fixed-rate pacemakers,[199–204] the relationship between respiratory rate and oxygen consumption is variable among individuals.[202] In addition, the requirement for an axillary lead has been considered a disadvantage of this pacing system.

Minute ventilation–sensing, rate-adaptive pacing systems have been demonstrated to provide rate modulation that is closely correlated with VO_2 in most patients implanted with these devices.[205–209] Minute ventilation is estimated by frequent measurements of transthoracic impedance between an intracardiac lead and the pulse generator case using a tripolar system.[210] A low-energy pulse of known current amplitude (1 mA with pulse duration 15 μsec) is delivered from the ring electrode of a standard bipolar pacing lead (Figure 2.35). The resultant voltage between the tip electrode and the pulse generator case is measured and the imped-

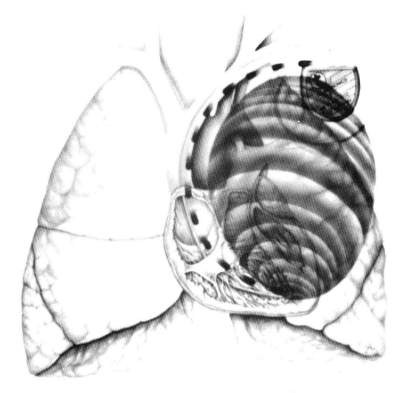

Figure 2.35 Diagrammatic illustration of a Telectronics tripolar transthoracic impedance (minute ventilation) sensing rate-adaptive pacing system. A low-energy pulse is emitted from the ring electrode every 50 msec with measurement of the resultant voltage between the tip electrode and the pulse generator case. (Courtesy of Telectronics Pacing Systems, Inc.)

ance calculated. The impedance pulses are subthreshold and are delivered every 50 msec. Transthoracic impedance increases with inspiration and decreases with expiration. By measuring the frequency of respiration-related fluctuations in impedance (correlated with respiratory rate) and the amplitude of those excursions (correlated with tidal volume), the estimated minute ventilation can be calculated.

The transthoracic impedance signal is a complex parameter that is influenced by several factors. However, the transthoracic impedance is most closely related to the volume and resistivity of blood in the right heart chambers and systemic venous system. The impedance signal fluctuates in response to both respiration and cardiac motion (right ventricular ejection). The impedance signal may also change with thoracic motion due to arm movements.[211] In order to minimize the cardiac-related component of the impedance signal, low-pass filtering of frequencies greater than 48 to 60 Hz is performed. A potential problem of this approach is that respiratory rates greater than 48 to 60 breaths per minute, which may be observed in children, may be inappropriately sensed.

The impedance signal is processed by comparing the average impedance values accumulated over two periods of time (one minute and one hour). When the short-term average (one minute) exceeds the long-term average (one hour), the pacing rate is increased. The slope of the relationship between changes in minute ventilation and pacing rate is a programmable parameter. Because the initial minute-ventilation pacing systems decreased the paced cycle length linearly with respect to the minute ventilation signal, the sensor was characterized by a relatively slow onset of rate modulation. Newer generations of devices offer a linear relationship between pacing rate and minute ventilation, improving the rate-adaptive algorithm and the initial response to exercise. In general, the minute-ventilation sensor is characterized by a highly proportional relationship to metabolic demand over a wide variety of exercise types.

Minute ventilation has been combined with activity sensors in the Medtronic Legend Plus pulse generator. This device modulates pacing rate by allowing the fastest of these sensors to control the pacing rate. An advantage of this combination of sensors is the ability to separately program the upper rate of each sensor. Thus, the activity sensor can be programmed to provide a very rapid increase in pacing rate at the onset of exercise, yet prevent excessive increases in rate by limiting the maximum activity rate. After minute ventilation has increased during more sustained exercise, the rate response can be controlled by the minute-ventilation sensor. The clinical utility of this sensor combination has been demonstrated in a multicenter trial.[212] Minute-ventilation pacemakers require the use of a bipolar pacing lead to measure transthoracic impedance, limiting the use of this sensor in patients with previously implanted pacing leads. A novel DDDR pacing system manufactured by ELA Medical (Chorus RM) uses the atrial lead to sense the minute-ventilation signal. Although a bipolar atrial lead is required for this device, a unipolar ventricular lead may be used. This device offers continuous self-modulation of the rate-adaptive slope based on a rolling trend of minute-ventilation signals.

Temperature

Central venous temperature has received considerable interest as a rate-adaptive sensor.[218–224] The temperature of venous blood in the right ventricle typically falls at the onset of exercise and is followed by a gradual increase at higher workloads.[218,219,225,226] The initial dip in temperature is caused by the return of cool blood from the extremities to the central circulation. The magnitude and duration of the temperature dip are highly variable among individuals but are most prominent in individuals with congestive heart failure or venous pooling. With subsequent muscular activity and heat generation, the temperature of the venous blood rises linearly with the exercise workload to a maximum difference that averages approximately 1.5°C. Temperature is an easily measured parameter, and the sensors are highly reliable. In rate-adaptive pacing systems, central venous temperature is measured with a thermistor that is mounted several centimeters proximal to the distal electrode of a permanent pacing lead. The thermistors have a resolution of 0.004°C to 0.025°C. The function of the thermistor has been shown to be unaffected by encapsulation of the lead by fibrous tissue.

Temperature-sensing, rate-adaptive pacing systems respond to the initial dip in central venous temperature by an increase in pacing rate, usually to a programmable intermediate value. At the onset of an increase in temperature, the pacing rate increases linearly from the intermediate rate to a maximum rate. The slope of the temperature–heart-rate relationship is programmable, with different slopes available over several ranges of the temperature curve. In addition, because there is a normal diurnal variation in temperature, the device may be programmed to a lower pacing rate when a gradual decrease in temperature is detected, such as occurs during sleep. Separate rate-adaptive slopes are programmable for slow changes in temperature, so that diurnal variation or sustained fever will lead to smaller changes in pacing rate. Relative disadvantages of temperature as a rate-adaptive sensor involve the marked variability in temperature curves among individuals and the requirement for a specialized lead. Despite these concerns, improvements in the rate-adaptive algorithm have produced highly satisfactory results in clinical use.

QT interval

The intracardiac QT interval has been demonstrated to shorten with exercise or sympathetic tone and to lengthen at rest.[229–231] The QT interval also shortens with increasing pacing rate and lengthens at slow heart rates. The QT interval is measured from the onset of the pacing stimulus to the apex of the T wave in the intracardiac ventricular electrogram.[231,232] Although the QT interval varies widely among individuals, it is quite consistent in an individual at rest. The QT interval can be markedly influenced by medications or electrolyte concentrations, however. Initial QT-sensing pacing systems suffered from a high incidence of T-wave undersensing and degradation of the ventricular electrogram over time. In addition, electrodes with high polarization properties were associated with large afterpotentials that interfered with accurate measurement of the QT interval.[233] These problems were significantly improved by the addition of a fast-recharge pulse that minimized afterpotentials and by changes in the T-wave filter.

The QT-pacing system includes an absolute refractory period of 250 msec, which is followed by a programmable T-wave sensing window (250–450 msec). A subthreshold marker pulse that is visible on the surface electrocardiogram is useful for confirming appropriate T-wave sensing. Further improvements in this sensor have involved the use of a curvilinear slope that improves the initial rate response to the onset of exercise.[232] Automation of the slope measurement has also improved the function of this sensor and reduced the time required for calibration of the pacemaker.[234] Disadvantages of the QT sensor involve the requirement for a low-polarization electrode, potentially complex programming, and the fact that the T wave can be reliably sensed only with paced beats. The potential advantages of this sensor are its responsiveness to emotional factors and the lack of a specialized lead.[235] It is also clear that the function of the sensor has been significantly improved by refinements in the rate-adaptive algorithm.[232] The disadvantages of the QT sensor have been largely overcome by combining this sensor with an activity sensor (Vitatron Diamond). This dual-sensor pacing system allows a programmable blending of sensor response to modulate pacing rate.

Mixed venous oxygen saturation

The saturation of oxygen in venous blood in the right heart chambers and pulmonary artery is inversely related to the rate of systemic oxygen extraction.[236,237] The mixed venous oxygen saturation declines within seconds of an increase in systemic oxygen consumption, resulting in a widening of the arteriovenous oxygen gradient. The fall in oxygen saturation is rapid in onset and is proportional to the exercise workload, factors that potentially make this parameter an ideal guide for rate modulation.[238] The oxygen saturation of hemoglobin in venous blood can be accurately measured by the optical reflectance technique.[238] As the oxygen saturation declines, red blood cells reflect a smaller proportion of light, thus appearing darker to the eye. The optical reflectance method of measuring oxygen saturation uses a light-emitting diode as a source of light in the blood pool (Figure 2.36). The amount of light reflected from erythrocytes is measured by a light-sensitive phototransistor.[239]

Permanent pacing systems currently in clinical trials utilize a specialized lead that incorporates both a light-emitting diode (660 nm wavelength) and a photosensitive receiver—these are located several centimeters proximal to the distal pacing electrode. The accuracy of the measurement is increased by recording the reflectance of more than one wavelength of light, with the ratio of the two wavelengths used as the rate-responsive control parameter, although some manufacturers utilize a single wavelength of light. The phototransistor transduces the reflected light into an electrical signal that is transmitted to the timing circuit of the pulse generator to modulate pacing rate. Despite the advantages of mixed venous oxygen saturation as a rate-adaptive sensor, there have been con-

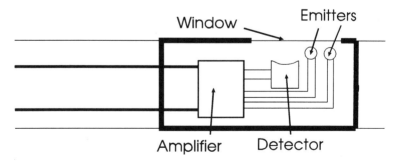

Figure 2.36 Schematic diagram of a Medtronic oxygen-saturation measuring capsule located several centimeters proximal to the tip of the lead. Two light emitters are the source of two different wavelengths of light reflected from erythrocytes in the blood pool and detected by a photosensitive detector. The signal is processed by an amplifier in the lead. (Courtesy of Medtronic, Inc.)

cerns that the sensor might become coated by a fibrous sheath, which would impair the long-term reliability of the specialized lead. Chronic animal implants have shown that coating of the lead reduces the absolute amount of light received by the phototransistor.[181,240] However, relative changes in oxygen saturation continue to be reliably measured. Artifacts in the signal may occur synchronously with the cardiac cycle, suggesting that the sensor may be transiently entrapped in the trabeculae of the right ventricle during systole. This can be reduced by pulsing the light source during end-diastole, a technique that also reduces the current drain of the sensor.

Although initial human implants with this sensor were encouraging, later experience during two years of follow-up has demonstrated that the sensor may deteriorate as a consequence of tissue overgrowth. However, if the problem of tissue overgrowth of the sensor can be solved, mixed venous oxygen consumption will likely become a valuable sensor. It is likely that the first commercial use of this sensor in an implantable device will be to monitor hemodynamics in patients with congestive heart failure.

REFERENCES

1. Hodgkin AL, Huxley AF. A quantitative description of membrane current and its application to conduction and excitation in nerves. *J Physiol* (Lond) 1952;117:500–544.
2. Thomas RC. Electrogenic sodium pump in nerve and muscle cells. *Physiol Rev* 1972;52:563–594.
3. Glitsch HG. Electrogenic Na pumping in the heart. *Ann Rev Physiol* 1982;44:389–400.
4. Gadsky DC. The Na/K pump of cardiac cells. *Ann Rev Biophys Bioeng* 1984;13:373–398.
5. Mullins IJ. The generation of electric currents in cardiac fibers by Na/Ca exchange. *Am J Physiol* 1979;236:C103–110.
6. Hilgemann DW. Numerical approximations of sodium–calcium exchange. *Prog Biophys Mol Biol* 1988;51:1–45.
7. Brown AM, Lee KS, Powell T. Voltage clamp and internal perfusion of single rate heart muscle cells. *J Physiol* (Lond) 1981;318:455–500.
8. Grant AO. Evolving concepts of cardiac sodium channel function. *J Cardiovasc Electrophysiol* 1990;1:53–67.
9. Makielski JC, Sheets MF, Hanck DA, et al. Sodium current

in voltage clamped internally perfused canine cardiac Purkinje cells. *Biophys J* 1987;52:1–11.

10. Cohen CJ, Bean BP, Tsien RW. Maximal upstroke velocity (Vmax) as an index of available sodium conductance: Comparison of Vmax and voltage clamp measurements of I_{Na} in rabbit Purkinje fibers. *Circ Res* 1984;54:636–651.

11. Bodewei R, Hering S, Lemke B, et al. Characteristics of the fast sodium current in isolated rat myocardial cells: Simulation of the clamped membrane potential. *J Physiol* (Lond) 1982;301–315.

12. Kunze DL, Lacerda AE, Wilson DL, et al. Cardiac Na currents and the inactivating, reopening and waiting properties of single cardiac Na channels. *J Gen Physiol* 1985;86:691–719.

13. Fozzard HA, Hanck DA, Makielski JC, et al. Sodium channels in cardiac Purkinje cells. *Experientia* 1987;43:1162–1168.

14. Angelides KJ, Nutter TJ. Mapping the molecular structure of the voltage-dependent sodium channel. *J Biol Chem* 1983; 258:11958–11967.

15. Noda M, Ikeda T, Suzuki H, et al. Expression of functional sodium channels from cloned cDNA. *Nature* 1986;322:826–828.

16. Cohen IS, Datyner NB, Gintant GA, et al. Time-dependent outward currents in the heart. In HA Fozzard et al. (eds.), *The Heart and Cardiovascular System*. New York: Raven Press, 1986.

17. Tsien RW. Calcium channels in excitable cell membranes. *Ann Rev Physiol* 1983;45:341–358.

18. Tsien RW, Hess P, McCleskey EW, et al. Calcium channels: Mechanisms of selectivity permeation and block. *Ann Rev Biophys Biochem* 1987;16:265–290.

19. Rousseau E, Meissner G. Single Cl^- channel from cardiac sarcoplasmic reticulum. *Mol Cell Biochem* 1988;82:155–156.

20. Reuter H. Divalent ions as charge carriers in excitable membranes. *Prog Biophys Mol Biol* 1973;26:1–43.

21. Kline R, Cohen IS. Extracellular $[K^+]$ fluctuations in voltage clamped canine cardiac Purkinje fibers. *Biophys* 1984;J49:663–668.

22. Hume JR, Giles W. Ionic currents in single isolated bullfrog atrial cells. *J Gen Physiol* 1983;81:153–194.

23. Hume JR, Giles W, Robinson K, et al. A time and voltage

dependent K$^+$ current in single cardiac cells from bullfrog atrium. *J Gen Physiol* 1986;88:777–798.

24. Brown HF, DiFrancesco D, Noble SJ. How does adrenalin accelerate the heart? *Nature* 1979;280:235–236.
25. DiFrancesco D, Ferroni A, Mozzanti M, et al. Properties of the hyperpolarizing activated current (if) in cells isolated from the rabbit sinoatrial node. *J Physiol* 1986;377:61–88.
26. Dewey MM, Barr L. A study of the structure and distribution of the nexus. *J Cell Biol* 1964;23:553–585.
27. DeMello WC. Intracellular communication in cardiac muscle. *Circ Res* 1982;51:1–9.
28. Barr L, Dewey MM, Berger W. Propagation of action potentials and the structure of the nexus in cardiac muscle. *J Gen Physiol* 1965;48:797–823.
29. Fozzard HA. Conduction of the action potential. In RM Berne, N Sperelakis, SR Geiger (eds.), *Handbook of Physiology, Section 2: The Cardiovascular System, Volume 1, The Heart.* Washington, DC: American Physiological Society, 1979; pp 335–356.
30. Walton MK, Fozzard HA. Experimental study of the conducted action potential in cardiac Purkinje strands. *Biophys J* 1983;44:1–8.
31. Walton MK, Fozzard HA. The conducted action potential: Models and comparison to experiments. *Biophys J* 1983;44:9–26.
32. Spach MS, Miller WT III, Geselowitz DB, et al. The discontinuous nature of propagation in normal canine cardiac muscle. Evidence for recurrent discontinuities of intracellular resistance that affect the membrane currents. *Circ Res* 1981;48:39–54.
33. Spach MS, Dolber PC, Heidlage JR, et al. Propagating depolarization in anisotropic human and canine cardiac muscle: Apparent directional differences in membrane capacitance. A simplified model for selective directional effects of modifying the sodium conductance on Vmax, τ_{foot}, and the propagation safety factor. *Circ Res* 1987;60:206–219.
34. Inoue H, Zipes DP. Conduction over an isthmus of atrial myocardium in vivo: A possible model of Wolff-Parkinson-White syndrome. *Circulation* 1987;76:637–647.
35. Winfree AT. The electrical thresholds of ventricular myocardium. *J Cardiovasc Electrophysiol* 1990;1:393–410.

36. Irnich W. The fundamental law of electrostimulation and its application to defibrillation. *PACE* 1990;13:1433–1477.
37. Lapicque L. Définition expérimentale de l'excitabilité. *Soc Biol* 1909;77:280–283.
38. Hoorweg L. Über die elektrische nerve merregung. *Pflugers Arch Physiol* 1892;52:87–99.
39. Weiss G. Sur la possibilite de rendre comparable entre eux les apparels servant a l'excitation electrique. *Arch Ital Biol* 1901;35:413–446.
40. Blair HA. On the intensity–time relations for stimulation by electric currents. *J Gen Physiol* 1932;15:709–729.
41. Irnich W. The chronaxie time and its practical importance. *PACE* 1980;3:292.
42. Ripart A, Mugica J. Electrode–heart interface: Definition of the ideal electrode. *PACE* 1983;6:410.
43. Irnich W. Comparison of pacing electrodes of different shape and material—recommendations. *PACE* 1983;6:422–426.
44. Sylven JC, Hellerstedt M, Levander-Lingren M. Pacing threshold interval with decreasing and increasing output. *PACE* 1982;5:646.
45. Timmis GC, Westveer DC, Holland J, et al. Precision of pacemaker thresholds: The Wedensky effect. *PACE* 1983; 6:A-60.
46. Stokes K, Bornzin G. The electrode-biointerface: Stimulation. In SS Barold (ed.), *Modern Cardiac Pacing*. Mount Kisco: Futura, 1985; pp 37–77.
47. Barold SS, Ong LS, Heinle RA. Stimulation and sensing thresholds for cardiac pacing: Electrophysiologic and technical aspects. *Prog Cardiovasc Dis* 1981;24:1–29.
48. Timmis GC, Jordan S, Holland J. Enhanced electrode stability: The endocardial screw. In Y Watanabe (ed.), *Cardiac Pacing: Proceedings of the Fifth International Symposium*. Amsterdam: Excerpta Medica, 1976; pp 516–526.
49. Albert HM, Glass BA, Pittman B, et al. Cardiac stimulation threshold: Chronic study. *Ann NY Acad Sci* 1964;111:889.
50. Zoll PM, Frank HA, Zarsky LR, et al. Long-term electric stimulation of the heart for Stokes-Adams disease. *Ann Surg* 1961;154:330.
51. Contini C, Strata G, Pauletti M, Gerberoglio B. Measurement of the myocardial stimulation threshold in chronic and acute patients with pacemakers implanted. *G Ital Cardiol* 1978;8:273.

52. Luceri RM, Furman S, Hurzeler P, et al. Threshold behavior of electrodes in long-term ventricular pacing. *Am J Cardiol* 1977;40:184.

53. Kay GN, Anderson K, Epstein AE, Plumb VJ. Active fixation atrial leads: Randomized comparison of two lead designs. *PACE* 1989;12:1355–1361.

54. Chaptal AP, Ribot A. Statistical survey of strength–duration threshold curves with endocardial electrodes and long-term behavior of these electrodes. In C Meerg (ed.), *Proceedings of the Fifth World Symposium on Cardiac Pacing.* Montreal: Pacesymp, 1979; pp 21–22.

55. Mond HG. *The Cardiac Pacemaker: Function and Malfunction.* New York: Grune & Stratton, 1983; pp 54–55.

56. Kertes P, Mond H, Sloman G, et al. Comparison of lead complications with polyurethane tined, silicone rubber tined and wedge tip leads: Clinical experience with 822 ventricular endocardial leads. *PACE* 1983;6:957.

57. Williams WG, Hesslein PS, Kormos R. Exit block in children with pacemakers. *Clin Prog Electrophysiol Pacing* 1983;4: 478–489.

58. Furman S, Hurzeler P, Mehra R. Cardiac pacing and pacemakers IV. Threshold of cardiac stimulation. *Am Heart J* 1977;94:115–124.

59. Platia EV, Brinker JA. Time course of transvenous pacemaker stimulation impedance, capture threshold, and electrogram amplitude. *PACE* 1986;9:620–625.

60. Brandt J, Attewell R, Fahraeus T, Schuller H. Atrial and ventricular stimulation threshold development: A comparative study in patients with a DDD pacemaker and two identical carbon-tip leads. *PACE* 1990;13:859–866.

61. de Buitleir M, Kou WH, Schmaltz S, Morady F. Acute changes in pacing threshold and R- or P-wave amplitude during permanent pacemaker implantation. *Am J Cardiol* 1990;65:999–1003.

62. Furman S, Parker B, Escher D. Decreasing electrode size and increasing efficiency of cardiac stimulation. *J Surg Res* 1971;11:105.

63. Smyth NPD, Tarjan PP, Chernoff E, et al. The significance of electrode surface area and stimulation thresholds in permanent cardiac pacing. *J Thorac Cardiovasc Surg* 1976;71: 559.

64. Furman S, Hurzeler P, Parker B. Clinical thresholds of en-

docardial cardiac stimulation: A long-term study. *J Surg Res* 1975;19:149.

65. Irnich W. The electrode myocardial interface. *Clin Prog Electrophysiol Pacing* 1985;3:338–348.

66. Irnich W. Engineering concepts of pacemaker electrodes. In M Schaldach, S Furman (eds.), *Advances in Pacemaker Technology*. New York: Springer-Verlag, 1975; p 241.

67. Parsonnet V, Zucker IR, Kannerstein ML. The fate of permanent intracardiac electrodes. *J Surg Res* 1966;6:285.

68. Thalen HJTh, Van den Berg JW. Threshold measurements and electrodes of the cardiac pacemaker. *Acta Physiol Pharmacol Nederl* 1966;14:227.

69. Beyersdorf F, Schneider M, Kreuzer J, et al. Studies of the tissue reaction induced by transvenous pacemaker electrodes. I. Microscopic examination of the extent of connective tissue around the electrode tip in the human right ventricle. *PACE* 1988;11:1753–1759.

70. Guarda F, Galloni M, Ossone F, et al. Histological reactions of porous tip endocardial electrodes implanted in sheep. *Int J Artif Organs* 1982;5:267.

71. Szabo Z, Solti F. The significance of the tissue reaction around the electrode on the late myocardial threshold. In M Schaldach, S Furman (eds.), *Advances in Pacemaker Technology*. New York: Springer-Verlag, 1975; p 273.

72. Beanlands DS, Akyurekli T, Keon WJ. Prednisone in the management of exit block. In C Meerg (ed.), *Proceedings of the Fifth World Symposium on Cardiac Pacing*. Montreal: Pacesymp, 1979;18–23.

73. Walls JT, Maloney JD, Pluth JR. Clinical evolution of a sutureless cardiac pacing lead: Chronic threshold changes and lead durability. *Ann Thorac Surg* 1983;36(3):328.

74. Thiele G, Lachmann W, Eschemann B, et al. Zur Beeinflussung des Reizschwellenanstieges nach Herzschrellmacherimplantation durch Prednisolon. *Z Gesamte Inn Med* 1980;35:863.

75. Nagatomo Y, Ogawa T, Kumagae H, et al. Pacing failure due to markedly increased stimulation threshold two years after implantation: Successful management with oral prednisolone: A case report. *PACE* 1989;12:1034–1037.

76. Stokes KB, Graf JE, Wiebusch WA. Drug-eluting electrodes improved pacemaker performance. In *Proceedings of the Fourth*

Annual Conference IEEE Engineering in Medicine and Biology Society. New York: IEEE, 1982; p 499.

77. Mond H, Stokes K, Helland J, et al. The porous titanium steroid eluting electrode: A double blind study assessing the stimulation threshold effects of steroid. *PACE* 1988;11:214–219.

78. Benditt DG, Stokes KB, Marrone JM. Long-term canine performance of a porous steroid electrode. *Proceedings of the Symposium on Pacemaker Leads.* Leuven: Belgium, 1984; p 85.

79. Kruse IM, Terpstra B. Acute and long-term atrial and ventricular stimulation thresholds with a steroid eluting electrode. *PACE* 1985;8:45.

80. King DH, Gillette PC, Shannon C, et al. Steroid-eluting endocardial lead for treatment of exit block. *Am Heart J* 1983;106:1438.

81. Timmis GC, Gordon S, Westveer DC, et al. A new steroid-eluting low threshold lead. *Proceedings of the Seventh World Symposium on Cardiac Pacing, Vienna.* Darmstadt: Steinkopff-Verlag, 1983; p 361.

82. Pirzada FA, Moschitto LJ, Diorio D. Clinical experience with steroid-eluting unipolar electrodes. *PACE* 1988;11:1739–1744.

83. Brewer G, Mathivanar R, Skolsky M, Anderson N. Composite electrode tips containing externally placed drug-releasing collars. *PACE* 1988;11:1760–1769.

84. Stokes KB. Preliminary studies on a new steroid eluting epicardial electrode. *PACE* 1988;11:1797–1803.

85. Brooks CMcC, Hoffman BF, Suckling EE, Orias O. *Excitability of the Heart.* New York: Grune & Stratton, 1955; pp 196–197.

86. Orias O, Brooks CMcC, Suckling EE, Gilbert JL, Siebens AA. Excitability of the mammalian ventricle throughout the cardiac cycle. *Am J Physiol* 1950;163:272–279.

87. Buxton AE, Marchlinski FE, Miller JM, et al. The human atrial strength–interval relation. Influence of cycle length and procainamide. *Circulation* 1989;79:271–280.

88. Boyett MR, Jewell BR. A study of the factors responsible for rate-dependent shortening of the action potential in mammalian ventricular muscle. *J Physiol* 1978;285:359–380.

89. Kay GN, Mulholland DH, Epstein AE, Plumb VJ. Effect of pacing rate on the human–strength duration curve. *J Am Coll Cardiol* 1990;15:1618–1623.

90. Plumb VJ, Karp RB, James TN, Waldo AL. Atrial excitability and conduction during rapid atrial pacing. *Circulation* 1981;63:1140–1149.
91. Johnson EA, McKinnon MG. The differential effect of quinidine and pyrilamine on the myocardial action potential at various rates of stimulation. *J Pharmacol Exp Ther* 1957;120:460–468.
92. Refsum H, Landmark K. The effect of nifedipine on the effective refractory period and excitability of the isolated rat atrium at different calcium levels and frequencies of stimulation. *Acta Pharmacol et Toxicol* 1976;39:353–364.
93. Landmark K. The action of promazine and thioridazine in isolated rat atrium. 3. Effects of varying concentrations of calcium and different frequencies and strengths of stimulation on contractile force and excitability. *Eur J Pharmacol* 1972;17:365–374.
94. Preston TA, Fletcher RD, Lucchesi BR, Judge RD. Changes in myocardial threshold. Physiologic and pharmacologic factors in patients with implanted pacemakers. *Am Heart* 1967;74:235.
95. Levick CE, Mizgala HF, Kerr CR. Failure to pace following high dose antiarrhythmic therapy-reversal with isoproterenol. *PACE* 1984;7:252.
96. Westerholm CJ. Threshold studies in transvenous cardiac pacemaker treatment. *Scand J Thorac Cardiovasc Surg* 1971 (Suppl);8:1.
97. Sowton E, Barr I. Physiological changes in threshold. *Ann NY Acad Sci* 1969;167:679.
98. O'Reilly MV, Murnaghan DP, Williams MB. Transvenous pacemaker failure induced by hyperkalemia. *JAMA* 1974;228:336.
99. Surawiez B, Chlebus H, Reeves JT, Gettes LS. Increase of ventricular excitability threshold by hyperpotassemia. *JAMA* 1965;191:71.
100. Gettes LS, Shabetai R, Downs TA, Surawiez B. Effect of changes in potassium and calcium concentrations on diastolic threshold and strength–interval relationships of the human heart. *Ann NY Acad Sci* 1969;167:693.
101. Lee D, Greenspan R, Edmands RE, Fisch C. The effect of electrolyte alteration on stimulus requirement of cardiac pacemakers. *Circulation* 1968;38 (Suppl):VI–124.
102. Hughes HC, Tyers GFO, Forman HA. Effects of acid–base

imbalance on myocardial pacing thresholds. *J Thorac Cardiovasc Surg* 1975;69:743.

103. Haywood J, Wyman MG. Effects of isoproterenol, ephedrine, and potassium on artificial pacemaker failure. *Circulation* 1965;32 (Suppl):II–110.

104. Kubler W, Sowton E. Influence of beta-blockade on myocardial threshold in patients with pacemakers. *Lancet* 1970;2:67.

105. Wallace AG, Cline RE, Sealy WC, et al. Electrophysiologic effects of quinidine. *Circ Res* 1966;19:960–969.

106. Gay RJ, Brown DF. Pacemaker failure due to procainamide toxicity. *Am J Cardiol* 1974;34:728.

107. Hellestrand KF, Burnett PJ, Milne JR, et al. Effect of the antiarrhythmic agent flecainide acetate on acute and chronic pacing thresholds. *PACE* 1983;6:892.

108. Salel AF, Seagren SC, Pool PE. Effects of encainide on the function of implanted pacemakers. *PACE* 1989;12:1439–1444.

109. Nielsen AP, Griffin JC, Herre JM, et al. Effect of amiodarone on acute and chronic pacing thresholds (abstract). New York: North American Society of Pacing and Electrophysiology, May 1984.

110. Irnich W, Gebhardt U. The pacemaker–electrode combination and its relationship to service life. In HJTh Thalen (ed.), *To Pace or Not to Pace, Controversial Subjects in Cardiac Pacing.* The Hague: Martinus Nyhoff, 1978; p 209.

111. Lindemans FW, Denier van der Gon JJ. Current thresholds and luminal size in excitation of heart muscle. *Cardiovasc Res* 1978;12:477.

112. Moore WJ. The electro-chemical cell. In •• *Physical Chemistry.* Englewood Cliffs, NJ: Prentice-Hall, 1972; p 510.

113. Mindt W, Schaldach M. Electrochemical aspects of pacing electrodes. In M Schaldach, S Furman (eds.), *Advances in Pacemaker Technology.* New York: Springer-Verlag, 1975; p 297.

114. Amundson D, McArthur W, MacCarter D, et al. Porous electrode–tissue interface. *PACE* 1979;2:40–50.

115. MacGregor DC, Wilson GJ, Lixfeld W, et al. The porous-surfaced electrode. A new concept in pacemaker lead design. *J Thorac Cardiovasc Surg* 1979;78:281.

116. Timmis GC, Helland J, Westveer, et al. The evolution of low threshold leads. *Clin Prog Electrophysiol Pacing* 1983;1:313–334.

117. Sinnaeve A, Willems R, Backers J, et al. Pacing and sensing: How can one electrode fulfill both requirements? *PACE* 1987;10:546–559.

118. Elmqvist H, Schuller H, Richter G. The carbon tip electrode. *PACE* 1983;6:436.

119. Garberoglio B, Inguaggiato B, Chinaglia B, et al. Initial results with an activated pyrolytic carbon tip electrode. *PACE* 1983;6:440–447.

120. Thuesen L, Jensen PJ, Vejby-Christensen H, et al. Lower chronic stimulation threshold in the carbon-tip than in the platinum-tip endocardial electrode: A randomized study. *PACE* 1989;12:1592–1599.

121. Walton C, Gergely S, Economides AP. Platinum pacemaker electrodes. Origins and effects of the electrode–tissue interface impedance. *PACE* 1987;10:87–99.

122. Bornzin GA, Stokes KB, Wiebush WA. A low threshold, low polarization, platonized endocardial electrode. *PACE* 1983; 6:A–70.

123. Mugica J, Duconge B, Henry L, et al. Clinical experience with new leads. *PACE* 1988;11:1745–1752.

124. Djordjevic M, Stojanov P, Velimirovic D, et al. Target lead-low threshold electrode. *PACE* 1986;9:1206–1210.

125. Sedney MI, Rodrigo FA, Buis B, Koops J. Behavior of stimulation resistance and stimulation theshold of pacemaker leads during and after implantation. In *Cursus Pacemakers.* Nederlandse Werkgroep Hartstimulatie, 1982; p 10.

126. Breivik K, Engedal H, Ohm OJ. Electrophysiological properties of a new permanent endocardial lead for uni- and bipolar pacing. *PACE* 1982;5:268.

127. Lewis T. *The Mechanism and Graphic Registration of the Heartbeat.* London: Shaw and Sons, Ltd, 1925.

128. Furman S, Hurzeler P, DeCaprio V. The ventricular endocardial electrogram and pacemaker sensing. *J Thorac Cardiovasc Surg* 1977;73:258.

129. Kleinert M, Elmqvist H, Strandberg H. Spectral properties of atrial and ventricular signals. *PACE* 1979;2:11.

130. Parsonnt V, Myers GH, Kresh YM. Characteristics of intracardiac electrogram II. Atrial endocardial electrograms. *PACE* 1980;3:406.

131. Breivik K, Ohm OJ. Myopotential inhibition of unipolar QRS-inhibited (VVI) pacemakers, assessed by ambulatory

Holter monitoring of the electrocardiogram. *PACE* 1980;3:470.

132. Watson WS. Myopotential sensing in cardiac pacemakers. In SS Barold (ed.), *Modern Cardiac Pacing*. Mount Kisco, NY: Futura, 1985; pp 813–837.

133. Hurzeler P, DeCaprio V, Furman S. Endocardial electrograms and pacer sensing. In M Schaldach, S Furman (eds.), *Advances in Pacemaker Technology*. New York: Springer-Verlag, 1975; p 307.

134. DeCaprio V, Hurzeler P, Furman S. Comparison of unipolar and bipolar electrograms for cardiac pacemaker sensing. *Circulation* 1977;56:750.

135. Bridges JD, Frazier MJ, Hauser RG. Effects of 60 Hz electrical fields and current on implanted cardiac pacemakers. In *Proceedings of the International Symposium on Electromagnetic Compatibility*. New York: IEEE, Inc., 1978; p 258.

136. Irnich W, deBakker JMT, Bisping HF. Electromagnetic interference in implantable pacemakers. *PACE* 1978;1:52.

137. Sowton E. Environmental hazards for pacemaker patients. *J R Coll Physicians Lond* 1982;16:159.

138. Belott PH, Sands S, Warren J. Resetting of DDD pacemakers due to EMI. *PACE* 1984;7:169.

139. Nathan DA, Center S, Wu CY, Keller W. An implantable synchronous pacemaker for the long-term correction of complete heart block. *Am J Cardiol* 1963;11:362.

140. Goldreyer BN, Oliver AL, Leslie J, et al. A new orthogonal lead for P-synchronous pacing. *PACE* 1981;4:638.

141. Goldreyer BN, Knudson M, Cannom DS, Wyman MG. Orthogonal electrogram sensing. *PACE* 1983;6:464.

142. Aubert AE, Ector H, Denys BG, DeGeest H. Sensing characteristics of unipolar and bipolar orthogonal floating atrial electrodes: Morphology and spectral analysis. *PACE* 1986;9:343–359.

143. Varriale P, Pilla AG, Tekriwal M. Single-lead VDD pacing system. *PACE* 1990;13:757–766.

144. Thull R, Schaldach M. Electrochemistry or after-pacing potentials on electrodes. *PACE* 1986;9:1191–1196.

145. Hauser RG, Susmano A. After potential oversensing by a programmable pulse generator. *PACE* 1981;4:391.

146. Potential cross-talk in early Gemini 415A papers with dual anodal rings. Product Safety Alert, Cordis Corporation, October 19, 1989.

147. Parsonnet V, Bilitch M, Furman S, et al. Early malfunction of transvenous pacemaker electrodes. A three-center study. *Circulation* 1979;60:590.

148. Furman S, Hurzeler P, DeCaprio V. Cardiac pacing and pacemakers. III. Sensing the cardiac electrogram. *Am Heart J* 1977;93:795.

149. Shandling AH, Castellanet MJ, Thomas LA, et al. Variation in P-wave amplitude immediately after pacemaker implantation: Possible mechanism and implications for early programming. *PACE* 1989;12:1797–1805.

150. Shandling AH, Castellanet M, Rylaarsdam A, et al. Screw versus nonscrew transvenous atrial leads: Acute and chronic P-wave amplitudes (abstract). *PACE* 1989;12:689.

151. Platia EV, Brinker JA. Endocardial screw-in versus tined J atrial pacing leads: Lead impedance, capture threshold and sensitivity as a function of time (abstract). *PACE* 1985;8:291.

152. Greatbatch W. Metal electrodes in bioengineering. *CRC Crit Rev Bioeng* 1981;5:1.

153. Greatbatch W, Piersma B, Shannon FD, et al. Polarization phenomena relating to physiological electrodes. *Ann NY Acad Sci* 1969;167:722.

154. Raber MB, Cuddy TE, Israel DA. Pacemaker electrodes act as high-pass filter on the electrogram. In Y Watanabe (ed.), *Cardiac Pacing.* Amsterdam and Oxford: Excerpta Medica, 1977; p 506.

155. Mond H, Holley L, Hirshorn M. The high impedance dish electrode—Clinical experience with a new tined lead. *PACE* 1982;5:529–534.

156. Lagergren H, Edhag O, Wahlberg I. A low threshold nondislocating endocardial electrode. *J Thorac Cardiovasc Surg* 1976;72:259.

157. Gould L, Patel C, Becker W. Long-term threshold stability with porous tip electrodes. *PACE* 1986;9:1202–1205.

158. McCarter DJ, Lundberg KM, Corstjens JPM. Porous electrodes: Concept, technology and results. *PACE* 1983;6:427–435.

159. Bobyn JD, Wilson GJ, Mycyk TR, et al. Comparison of a porous-surfaced with a totally porous ventricular endocardial pacing electrode. *PACE* 1981;4:405–416.

160. Mugica J, Henry L, Attuel P, et al. Clinical experience with 910 carbon tip leads: Comparison with polished platinum leads. *PACE* 1986;9:1230–1238.

161. Brummer SB, Robblee LS, Hambrecht FT. Criteria for selecting electrodes for electrical stimulation: Theoretica and practical considerations. *Ann NY Acad Sci* 1983;405:159–171.

162. Stokes K, Stephenson WL. The implantable cardiac pacing lead—Just a simple wire? In SS Barold, J Mugica (eds.), *The Third Decade of Cardiac Pacing: Advance in Technology and Clinical Applications.* Mount Kisco, NY: Futura, 1982; pp 365–416.

163. Van Heeckeren DW, Hogan JF, Glenn WWL. Engineering analysis of pacemaker electrodes. *Ann NY Acad Sci* 1969; 167:774.

164. Ross AM, Hohler H, Gundersen T. Siemens–Elema tined carbon tip lead: A multicenter study of acute and long-term thresholds as measured by the various functions of the Siemens–Elema 688 pacemaker. *PACE* 1983;6:A–68.

165. Holmes DR, Nissen RG, Maloney JD, et al. Transvenous tined electrode systems: An approach to acute dislodgement. *Mayo Clin Proc* 1979;54:219–222.

166. Furman S, Pannizzo F, Campo I. Comparison of active and passive adhering leads for endocardial pacing. *PACE* 1979; 2:417–427.

167. Bisping HJ, Kreuzer J, Birkenheir H. Three-year clinical experience with a new endocardial screw-in lead with introduction protection for use in the atrium and ventricle. *PACE* 1980;3:424–435.

168. Pehrsson SK, Bergdahl L, Svane B. Early and late efficacy of three types of transvenous atrial leads. *PACE* 1984;7:195–202.

169. Bredikis J, Dumcius A, Stirbys P, et al. Permanent cardiac pacing with electrodes of a new type of fixation in the endocardium. *PACE* 1978;1:25–30.

170. Markewitz A, Wenke K, Weinhold C. Reliability of atrial screw-in leads. *PACE* 1988;11:1777–1783.

171. Ormerod D, Walgren S, Berglund J, Heil R. Design and evaluation of a low threshold porous tip lead with a monitor coated screw-in tip ("sweet tip"). *PACE* 1988;11:1784–1790.

172. Stokes K. The biostability of polyurethane leads. In SS Barold (ed.), *Modern Cardiac Pacing.* Mount Kisco, NY: Futura, 1985; pp 173–198.

173. Hanson JS. Sixteen failures in a single model of bipolar polyurethane-insulated ventricular pacing lead: A 44-month experience. *PACE* 1984;7:389–394.

174. Raymond RD, Nanian KB. Insulation failure with bipolar polyurethane pacing leads. *PACE* 1984;7:378–380.
175. Byrd CL, McArthur W, Stokes K, et al. Implant experience with unipolar polyurethane pacing leads. *PACE* 1983;6:868–882.
176. Stokes KB, Frazer WA, Christopherson RA. Environmental stress cracking in implanted polyurethanes. In *Proceedings of the Second World Congress on Biomaterials, Tenth Annual Meeting of the Society of Biomaterials.* Washington. DC, 1984; p 254.
177. Phillips RE, Thoma RJ. Metal ion complexation of polyurethane. A proposed mechanism of calcification. In H Plank, et al. (eds.), *Polyurethanes in Biomedical Engineering II: Proceedings of the Second International Conference on Polyurethanes in Biomedical Engineering.* Amsterdam: Elsevier, 1987; pp 91–108.
178. Korhonen U, Karkola P, Takkunem J, et al. One turn more; threshold superiority of 3-turn versus 2-turn screw-in myocardial electrodes. *PACE* 1984;7:678–682.
179. Calfee RV, Saulson SH. A voluntary standard for 3.2 mm unipolar and bipolar pacemaker leads and connectors. *PACE* 1986;9:1181–1185.
180. Love JW, Jahnke EJ. The rechargeable cardiac pacemaker. *Arch Surg* 1975;110:1186.
181. Hoover MD, Forino RV, Snell JR. In vivo experience with a hemo-reflective oxygen sensor for rate responsive pacing (abstract). *PACE* 1987;10:1214.
182. Tyers GFO, Brownlee RR. Power pulse generators, electrodes, and longevity. *Prog Cardiovasc Dis* 1981;23:421.
183. Aubert AE, Goldreyer BN, Wyman ME, et al. Filter characteristics of the atrial sensing circuit of a rate responsive pacemaker. To see or not to see. *PACE* 1989;12:525–536.
184. Irnich W. Muscle noise and interference behavior in pacemakers: A comparative study. *PACE* 1987;10:125–132.
185. Bicik V, Kristan L. Sine^2/triangle/square wave generator for pacemaker testing. *PACE* 1985;8:484–493.
186. Anderson KM, Moore AA. Sensors in pacing. *PACE* 1986;9:954.
187. Humen DP, Kostuk WJ, Klein GJ. Activity-sensing rate responsive pacing: Improvement in myocardial performance with exercise. *PACE* 1985;8:52.
188. Benditt DG, Mianulli M, Fetter J, et al. Single chamber cardiac pacing with activity-initiated chronotropic response.

Evaluation by cardiopulmonary exercise testing. *Circulation* 1987;75:184.

189. Lindemans FW, Rankin IR, Murtaugh R, Chevalier PA. Clinical experience with an activity sensing pacemaker. *PACE* 1986;9:978.

190. Humen PP, Anderson K, Brumwell D, et al. A pacemaker which automatically increases its rate with physical activity. In K Steinbach, D Glogar, A Laszkovics, et al. (eds.), *Proceedings of the Seventh World Symposium, Vienna.* Darmstadt: Steinkopff Verlag, 1983; p 259.

191. Alt E, Heinz M, Theres H, et al. A new body motion activity based rate responsive pacing system. *PACE* 1987;10:422.

192. Matula M, Alt E, Theres H, et al. A new mechanical sensor for the detection of body activity and posture suitable for rate responsive pacing (abstract). *PACE* 1987;10:1221.

193. Lau CP, Scott JRR, Toff WD, et al. Selective vibration sensing: A new concept for activity-sensing rate-responsive pacing. *PACE* 1988;11:1299–1309.

194. Kubisch K, Peters W, Chiladakis I, et al. Clinical experience with the rate responsive Sensalog[R] 703. *PACE* 1988; 11:1829–1839.

195. Lau CP, Butrous G, Ward DE, Camm AJ. Comparison of exericse performance of six rate-adaptive right ventricular cardiac pacemakers. *Am J Cardiol* 1989;63:833–838.

196. Toff WD, Leeks C, Joy M, et al. The effect of aircraft vibration on the function of an activity-sensing pacemaker (abstract). *Br Heart J* 1987;57:573.

197. Matula M, Alt E, Fotuhi P, et al. Influence of varied types of exercise on the rate adaptation of activity pacemakers. *PACE* 1992;15:578.

198. Alt E, Millerhagen JO, Heemels J-P. Accelerometers. In KA Ellenbogen, GN Kay, BL Wilkoff (eds.), *Clinical Cardiac Pacing.* Philadelphia: WB Saunders, 1995; p 275.

199. Rossi P, Plicchi G, Canducci G, et al. Respiratory rate as a determinant of optimal pacing rate. *PACE* 1983;6:502.

200. Rossi P, Plicchi G, Canducci G, et al. Respiration as a reliable physiological sensor for controlling cardiac pacing rate. *Br Heart J* 1984;51:7.

201. Alt E, Volker R, Wirtzfeld A. Directly and indirectly measured respiratory parameters compared with oxygen uptake and heart rate (abstract). *PACE* 1985;8:A–21.

202. Rossi P, Rognoni G, Occhetta E, et al. Respiration-dependent ventricular pacing compared with fixed ventricular and atrial-ventricular synchronous pacing aerobic and hemo-dynamic variables. *J Am Coll Cardiol* 1985;6:646.
203. Rossi P, Aina F, Rognoni G, et al. Increasing cardiac rate by tracking the respiratory rate. *PACE* 1984;7:1246.
204. Melissano G, Prezuiso M, Menegazzo G, Cammilli L. Our experience with different rate responsive systems (abstract). *PACE* 1987;10:1221.
205. Kay GN, Bubien RS, Epstein AE, Plumb VJ. Rate-modulated cardiac pacing based on transthoracic impedance measurements of minute ventilation: Correlation with exercise gas exchange. *J Am Coll Cardiol* 1989;14:1283–1289.
206. Alt E, Heinz M, Hirgsletter C, et al. Control of pacemaker rate by impedance-based respiratory minute ventilation. *Chest* 1987;92:247.
207. Lau CP, Antoniou A, Ward DE, Camm AJ. Initial clinical experience with a minute ventilation sensing rate modulated pacemaker: Improvements in exercise capacity and symptomatology. *PACE* 1988;11:1815–1822.
208. Val F, Bonnet JL, Ritter PH, Pioger G. Relationship between heart rate and minute ventilation, tidal volume and respiratory rate during brief and low level exercise. *PACE* 1988;11:1860–1865.
209. Mond H, Strathmore N, Kertes P, et al. Rate responsive pacing using a minute ventilation sensor. *PACE* 1988;11:1866–1874.
210. Nappholz T, Valenta H, Maloney J, Simmons T. Electrode configurations for a respiratory impedance measurement suitable for rate responsive pacing. *PACE* 1986;9:960.
211. Lau CP, Ritchie D, Butrous GS, et al. The effects of arm movement on rate modulation of respiratory dependent rate responsive pacemakers (abstract). *PACE* 1987;10:1217.
212. Alt E, Millerhagen JO, Heemels J-P. Accelerometers. In KA Ellenbogen, GN Kay, BL Wilkoff (eds.), *Clinical Cardiac Pacing*. Philadelphia: WB Saunders. 1995; p 275.
213. McKay RG, Spears JR, Aroesty JM, et al. Instantaneous measurement of left and right ventricular stroke volume and pressure volume relationships with an impedance catheter. *Circ* 1984;69:703.

214. Woodard JC, Bertram CD, Gow BS. Right ventricular volumetry by catheter measurement of conductance. *PACE* 1987;10:862.

215. Salo RW, Pederson BD, Olive AL, et al. Continuous ventricular volume assessment for diagnosis and pacemaker control. *PACE* 1984;7:1267.

216. Chirife R. The pre-ejection period: An ideal physiologic variable for closed loop rate responsive pacing (abstract). *PACE* 1987;10:425.

217. Klein H, Olive A, Pederson B, et al. The pre-ejection interval: A reliable biosensor for rate-responsive pacing (abstract). *PACE* 1987;10:1215.

218. Sellers TD, Fearnot NE, Smith HJ, et al. Right ventricular blood temperature profiles for rate responsive pacing. *PACE* 1987;10:467–479.

219. Alt E, Hirgstetter C, Heinz M, et al. Rate control of physiologic pacemakers by central venous blood temperature. *Circulation* 1986;73:1206–1212.

220. Fearnot NE, Evans ML. Heart rate correlation, response time and effect of previous exercise using an advanced pacing rate algorithm for temperature-based rate modulation. *PACE* 1988;11:1846–1852.

221. Sugiura T, Kimura M, Shizuo M, et al. Cardiac pacemakers regulated by respiratory rate and blood temperature. *PACE* 1989;11:1077–1084.

222. Griffin JC, Jutzy KR, Claude JP, et al. Central body temperature as a guide to optimal heart rate. *PACE* 1983;6: 498.

223. Fearnot NE, Jolgren DL, Tacker WA, et al. Increasing cardiac rate by measurement of right ventricular temperature. *PACE* 1984;7:1240.

224. Alt E, Theres H, Heinz M, et al. A new rate-modulated pacemaker system optimized by combination of two sensors. *PACE* 1988;11:1119.

225. Shellock FG, Rubin SA, Ellrodt AG, et al. Unusual core temperature decrease in exercising heart failure patients. *J Appl Physiol* 1983;54:544.

226. Fearnot NE, Smith HJ, Sellers D, Boal B. Evaluation of the temperature response to exercise testing in patients with single chamber, rate-adaptive pacemakers: A multicenter study. *PACE* 1989;12:1806–1815.

227. Richards AF, Normal J. Relation between QT interval and heart rate. *Br Heart J* 1981;45:56.

228. Milne JR, Ward DE, Spurrell RAJ, Camm AJ. The ventricular paced QT interval—The effects of rate and exercise. *PACE* 1982;5:352.
229. Oda E. Changes in QT interval during exercise testing in patients with VVI pacemakers. *PACE* 1986;9:36.
230. Hedman A, Norlander R, Pehrsson SK. Changes in QT and A-aT intervals at rest and during exercise with different modes of cardiac pacing. *PACE* 1985;8:825.
231. Richards AF, Donaldson RM, Thalen HJTh. The use of the QT interval to determine pacing rate: Early clinical experience. *PACE* 1983;6:346.
232. Heijer PD, Nagelkerke D, Perrins EJ, et al. Improved rate responsive algorithm in QT driven pacemakers—Evaluation of initial response to exercise. *PACE* 1989;12:805–811.
233. Fananapizir L, Rademaker M, Bennett DH. Reliability of the evoked response in determining the paced ventricular rate and performance of the T rate responsive (TX) pacemaker. *PACE* 1985;8:701.
234. Boute W, Gebhardt U, Begemann MJS. Introduction of an automatic QT interval drive rate responsive pacemaker. *PACE* 1988;11:1804–1814.
235. Jordaens L, Backers J, Moerman E, Clement DL. Catecholamine levels and pacing behavior of QT-driven pacemakers during exercise. *PACE* 1990;13:603–607.
236. Eityzgrlf A, Goedel-Meinem L, Bock T, et al. Central venous saturation for the control of automatic rate-responsive pacing. *PACE* 1982;5:829.
237. Wirtzfeld A, Heinze R, Stangl K, et al. Regulation of pacing rate by variations of mixed venous saturation. *PACE* 1984;7:1257.
238. Snell J, Cohen D, Hedberg SE. In vivo performance of a hemo-reflective type oxygen sensor for rate responsive pacing (abstract). *PACE* 1988;11:504.
239. Stangl K, Wirtzfeld A, Heinze R, Laule M. First clinical experience with an oxygen saturation controlled pacemaker in man. *PACE* 1988;11:1882–1887.
240. Bennett T, Bornzing BM, Olson W. Rate responsive pacing using mixed venous oxygen saturation in heart blocked dogs (abstract). *Circulation* 1984;70:II–246.

Hemodynamics of Cardiac Pacing

Dwight W. Reynolds

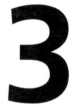

INTRODUCTION

Knowledge, as well as interest, in hemodynamics has evolved substantially since 1960, essentially pari passu with the technology of cardiac pacing. While general knowledge of this subject has played an important role in the evolution of sophisticated pacing capabilities, the technology itself has facilitated the expansion of knowledge of cardiovascular hemodynamics generally and as it relates to pacing.

The vogue in pacing since 1980 has been the accomplishment of "physiologic" pacing. Our concepts of physiologic pacing have evolved in concert with our understanding of pacing-related cardiovascular hemodynamics, as well as with technologic sophistication. Although in 1996 we speak of optimizing and providing for rate-varied atrioventricular (AV) intervals, differentiating between atrial sensed and atrial paced AV intervals, different ventricular pacing sites for improved hemodynamic performance, and fine-tuning rate modulation, in 1960 it was certainly a fact that asynchronous ventricular pacing was more physiologic than the alternative—no pacing—in such ominous maladies as acquired third-degree AV block. And now that we have alluded to progress, it is also important to point out that there continues to be a number of unanswered questions relating to cardiovascular hemodynamics and, perhaps more generally, to cardiovascular physiology, as this in turn relates to cardiac pacing. More is to be learned, especially in the application of pacing to special cardiovascular problems (e.g., hypertrophic and dilated cardiomyopathies and neurocardiogenic syncope) but much of what we strive to learn and accomplish henceforth may be properly described as "fine-tuning," because much has been accomplished to allow approximation of normal physiology with pacing.

The key concepts of physiologic pacing, considered most broadly, include the proper sequencing of atrial and ventricular contraction and physiologic rate modulation. These topics will be discussed in this chapter, as well as a practical guide for selection of a pacing mode as it relates to these physiologic/hemodynamic issues.

AV SYNCHRONY

For semanticists, the term *AV synchrony* can imply simultaneous atrial and ventricular activation and/or contraction. This issue notwithstanding, *AV synchrony* is the term used most commonly to describe the normal physiologic sequencing of atrial and ventricular activation/contraction. *AV sequencing* (or *AV sequential*) may be a better term; due to common usage, however (and the fact that *AV sequential* is a term used specifically for DVI mode), *AV synchrony* is the term used here.

The hemodynamics of AV synchrony have been addressed both qualitatively and quantitatively for centuries.[1] Elegant work was published in the early part of this century.[2,3] The topic has been more extensively examined since 1960, during which time pacemakers have been developed that are capable of providing AV synchrony. The hemodynamics of AV synchrony (and the absence thereof) are discussed in the context of advantages that might accrue from maintaining AV synchrony. In addition, issues relating to optimization of the AV interval, the merit of atrial versus AV pacing, and what has been called "pacemaker syndrome" will be discussed.

Advantages of AV synchrony

Blood pressure and cardiac output: Systemic blood pressure and cardiac output have been the subjects of much of the discussion regarding the importance of maintaining AV synchrony. It has been observed that certain individuals have marked drops in blood pressure when ventricular pacing is instituted.[4,5] Indeed, some individuals have dramatic and symptomatic decreases in systemic blood pressure similar to that shown in Figure 3.1. In the figure, the blood pressure, measured by radial artery line, drops from around 110/70 mmHg during sinus rhythm to around 75/55 mmHg

125

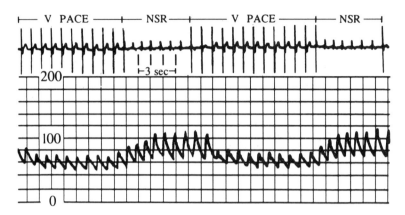

Figure 3.1 Radial artery pressure recording from a patient during right ventricular pacing (V PACE) at 80 ppm and normal sinus rhythm (NSR). The scale is in mmHg.

during ventricular pacing. Several mechanisms may be responsible for this phenomenon. Loss of left ventricular preload volume from mistimed atrial contraction (loss of atrial "kick") and loss of neural cardial reflexes (due also to inappropriately timed atrial contraction) have been the mechanisms most commonly focused on. Whatever the precise mechanisms—and these may vary—it appears that these dramatic changes in occasional patients are related to mistiming of atrial contraction such that the atrial contraction occurs after closure of the mitral (and tricuspid) valve at the onset of ventricular systole. This marked hypotension, although uncommon, can produce dramatic symptoms, including syncope. In a clinical setting, if this problem is suspected but hypotension with symptoms cannot be reproduced in a supine position, upright or semiupright posture may unmask the problem, especially if this is related to left ventricular preload deficiency caused by loss of atrial contribution to ventricular filling.

Although such dramatic examples of hypotension during ventricular pacing do occur, they are relatively uncommon. A more typical example of the blood pressure comparison among atrial, AV, and ventricular pacing is shown in Figure 3.2. Here, as is more typically the case, essentially no differences exist between the blood pressures comparing atrial to AV pacing (left and middle panels). The blood pressure during ventricular pacing (right panel) is slightly, though not dramatically, lower than during either atrial or AV pacing. In a study done at the University of Oklahoma,[6] in a heterogeneous group of pacemaker patients, statistically significant differences were found in femoral artery systolic pressure (Figure 3.3 and Table 3.1) but not in diastolic and mean pressures (see Table 3.1). This study, however, involved measurements made in a supine position, which may have masked the more dramatic differences that may have been found if patients had been evaluated in an upright posture.

An important digression is the issue of ventriculoatrial (VA) conduction. VA conduction, the ability to conduct electrically retrograde from the ventricles through the AV junction (or, in certain situations, an accessory pathway) to the atria, can lead to a fixed, though abnormal, relationship between ventricular and atrial contraction such that the atria contract during ventricular systole

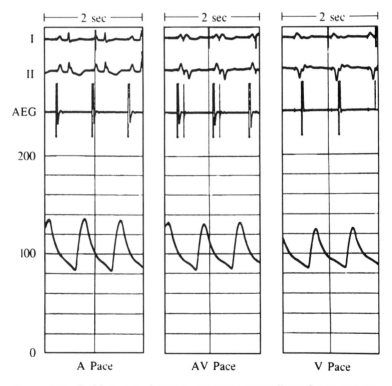

Figure 3.2 (left) Femoral artery pressure recordings from one patient during atrial pacing (A Pace). (center) AV sequential pacing (AV Pace). (right) Ventricular pacing (V Pace). All are at 80 ppm with AV interval of 150 msec during AV pacing. The scale is in mmHg. I = ECG lead I, II = ECG lead II, AEG = atrial electrogram.

(or in cases of long VA conduction, early diastole). This can cause loss of the atrial contribution to ventricular filling as well as other hemodynamic problems, as discussed below. VA conduction has been found in as many as 90 percent of patients with sick sinus syndrome and in 15 to 35 percent of individuals with a variety of forms of AV block.[7-9] This is problematic—once VA conduction is established, there is a propensity for it to continue. This has been a major issue in the use of hysteresis, a feature commonly included in ventricular pacemakers since 1980.

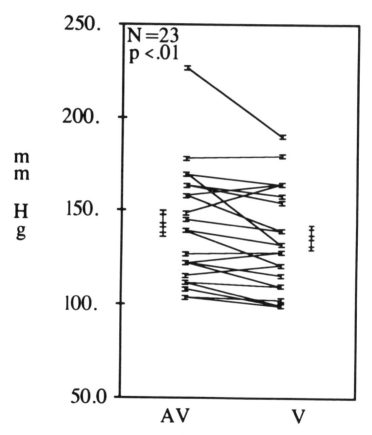

Figure 3.3   A comparison of femoral artery systolic pressures in a group of 23 pacemaker patients during (left) AV sequential pacing and (right) ventricular pacing, both at 80 ppm with AV interval during AV pacing =150 msec. Individual comparisons are inside and connected by solid lines. Group comparison ± SEM is outside. Paired t tests used for statistical comparison.

Table 3.1   Hemodynamic Evaluation of Atrioventricular and Ventricular Pacing

	AV[a]	V[a]	N	P[b]
RA mean (mmHg)	6.0 ± 0.6	8.1 ± 0.6	22	<0.001
PA systolic (mmHg)	24.5 ± 1.6	28.3 ± 1.7	23	<0.001
PA diastolic (mmHg)	12.6 ± 1.0	14.3 ± 1.1	23	<0.02
PA mean (mmHg)	17.1 ± 1.1	20.6 ± 1.2	23	<0.001
PCW mean (mmHg)	7.7 ± 1.0	13.4 ± 1.2	22	<0.001
LV systolic (mmHg)	141.3 ± 5.2	132.0 ± 5.1	23	<0.01
LV end-diastolic (mmHg)	9.8 ± 1.4	10.1 ± 0.8	22	NS
FA systolic (mmHg)	141.4 ± 5.1	133.4 ± 5.1	23	<0.01
FA diastolic (mmHg)	80.3 ± 2.0	80.9 ± 2.4	23	NS
FA mean (mmHg)	105.6 ± 2.8	103.1 ± 3.4	23	NS
CI.TD (L/min/m²)	2.575 ± 0.148	2.073 ± 0.126	23	<0.001
CT.Angio (L/min/m²)	3.337 ± 0.210	2.878 ± 0.157	19	<0.001
LV.EDVI (ml/m²)	85.7 ± 7.4	76.6 ± 6.8	19	<0.001
LV.ESVI (ml/m²)	46.2 ± 5.9	42.2 ± 5.4	19	<0.05
LV.SVI (ml/m²)	39.7 ± 2.6	34.3 ± 2.0	19	<0.001
LV.EF (%)	48.9 ± 2.8	47.6 ± 2.8	19	NS
SVR (dyne · sec · cm⁻⁵)	1856.1 ± 160.3	2178.0 ± 180.6	23	<0.001
PVR (dyne · sec · cm⁻⁵)	169.0 ± 16.3	152.1 ± 15.0	22	NS

[a] Mean ± SEM.
[b] Paired *t* tests.
RA = right atrium, PA = pulmonary artery, PCW = pulmonary capillary wedge, LV = left ventricle, FA = femoral artery, CI = cardiac index, TD = thermodilution, Angio = angiography, EDVI = end-diastolic volume index, ESVI = end-systolic volume index, SVI = stroke volume index, EF = ejection fraction, SVR = systemic vascular resistance, PVR = pulmonary vascular resistance, NS = not statistically significant.

If a patient with intact VA conduction has sinus node dysfunction as the indication for pacing and a ventricular pacemaker is in place with the hysteresis feature employed, the following scenario commonly occurs. If, for example, the pacemaker is programmed to a pacing rate of 70 ppm and a hysteresis rate of 50 ppm, ventricular pacing at 70 ppm will not occur until the patient's intrinsic rate falls below 50 ppm. The ventricular pacing will continue until the patient's own sinus rate increases above 70 ppm rather than being inhibited (as seen with normal AV synchrony) when the sinus rate exceeds 50 ppm. This creates inordinately prolonged periods of ventricular pacing with the potential hemo-dynamic problems (noted above and below) associated with this. Because of this relatively common scenario, the use of the hyster-esis function in *ventricular* pacemakers must be carefully considered and is usually inappropriate. On the other hand, the use of hyster-esis or similar types of features in *dual-chamber* (AV) pacemakers may have a role to play in reducing the symptoms and hypotension of neurocardiogenic syncope.[10]

Although VA conduction is generally (and appropriately) viewed as a negative when considering ventricular pacing, the converse is not true. Specifically, during ventricular pacing, even when VA conduction is not intact, if the ventricular pacing rate is unequal to atrial rate, there will be periods of time when atrial contraction occurs during ventricular systole with the resulting disadvantageous hemodynamics.

Cardiac output, more than any other hemodynamic feature, has been the focus of discussions and investigations relating to AV synchrony.[11–13] Properly timed atrial contraction provides a signifi-cant increase in ventricular end-diastolic volume and is responsible for the so-called atrial kick. Studies have shown a wide range in the actual importance of the atrial contribution to ventricular filling. This variance is likely related to differences in patient populations and study conditions. By increasing the end-diastolic volumes (right and left ventricles), the cardiac output is, in turn, increased. The average increase in cardiac output in a broad-based pacing population, if AV synchrony is maintained, appears to be between 20 and 25 percent in comparison to non–AV-synchronized ven-tricular pacing.

In our study, similar results were found in a broad-based pacing population (Figure 3.4 and Table 3.1). In this study, AV pacing at 80 ppm with an AV interval of 150 msec was compared with ventricular pacing at 80 ppm during which VA conduction was intact or was created by VA pacing. Consistently higher cardiac outputs by maintaining AV synchrony were seen in both thermodilution and angiographic evaluations (the apparent differ-ences in cardiac index measured by thermodilution and angio-graphic techniques in this study relate to variances of measure-ment techniques, different times of measurement, and the absence of angiography in some of the patients in whom thermo-dilution measurements were made). Upright posture might amplify these differences seen in a supine position, because ventricular diastolic filling is more dependent on atrial kick due to loss of

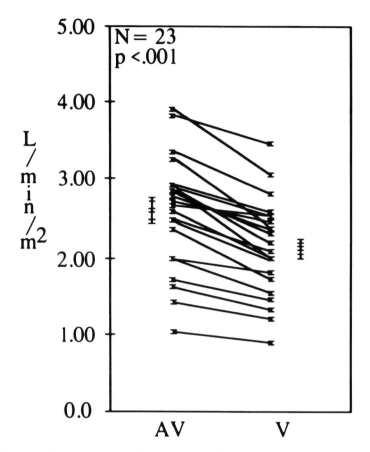

Figure 3.4 A comparison of cardiac index, measured by thermodilution technique, in 23 pacemaker patients during (left) AV sequential pacing and (right) ventricular pacing, both at 80 ppm with AV interval during AV pacing =150 msec. Individual comparisons are inside and connected by solid lines. Group comparison ± SEM is outside. Paired *t* tests used for statistical comparison.

venous return of blood to the heart (lower extremity pooling) in the upright posture.[14]

Similar results have been found in comparisons between AV-synchronized and ventricular pacing in patients after myocardial infarction[15] and after cardiac surgery.[16,17] Patients with reduced cardiac output—especially if such reduced function is due to relative volume depletion or only mild to moderately depressed left ventricular function—frequently benefit significantly from maintenance of AV synchrony; this should be kept in mind when dealing with patients in these and other situations.

There has been a general perception that patients with abnormal cardiac function benefit most from maintenance of AV synchrony. This may be true, but the reasons are frequently not due to better cardiac output.[12,18] In fact, if cardiac output were the only consideration hemodynamically—and, obviously, it is not—it is patients with very poor ventricular function (markedly increased end-diastolic volume and depressed ejection fraction) that benefit least from AV synchrony. This can be best understood by using the concept of ventricular function curves that compare stroke volume or cardiac output to left ventricular (LV) end-diastolic volume or preload.

Figure 3.5 shows hypothetical ventricular function curves for a patient with normal ventricular function (curve 1), one with moderate LV dysfunction (curve 2), one with very poor LV function and a markedly dilated ventricle (curve 3), and a patient with hypertrophic cardiomyopathy (curve 4). These curves describe the performance of the left ventricle in generating stroke volume (or cardiac output) in relationship to the end-diastolic volume (or preload). In patients with normal LV function (curve 1), as end-diastolic volume increases, stroke volume (and cardiac output) increases until the flat (and, perhaps arguably, eventually, the de-

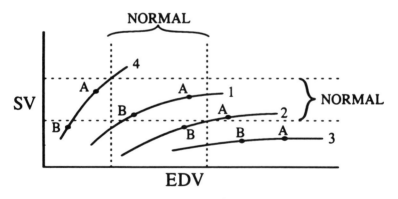

Figure 3.5 Hypothetical ventricular function curves comparing (1) stroke volume (SV) and left ventricular end-diastolic volume (EDV) in patients with normal ventricular function, (2) moderately depressed ventricular function, (3) severely depressed ventricular function, and (4) hyperdynamic ventricular function. Point A = with normal AV sequence. Point B = without normal AV sequence.

scending) portion of the curve is reached. In patients with depressed LV function (curves 2 and 3) there is reduction in the increase in stroke volume that depends on end-diastolic volume to the point that in patients with poor LV function (curve 3) there is negligible improvement in stroke volume with increased end-diastolic volume. On the other hand, patients with hypertrophic cardiomyopathies tend to have small ventricles that are normal (i.e., normal systolic function) or hyperdynamic in function (curve 4). Small increases in end-diastolic volume can significantly increase stroke volume in this situation.

As has been discussed, AV synchrony provides the atrial kick that increases end-diastolic volume. Point A on these curves represents the hypothetical stroke volume and end-diastolic volume during AV pacing. Point B represents stroke volume and end-diastolic volume during ventricular pacing (with associated loss of atrial kick). In the normal situation (curve 1), although end-diastolic volume is greater and hence stroke volume is greater during AV-synchronized pacing, the loss of AV synchrony during ventricular pacing does not drop the end-diastolic volume and the stroke volume to significantly low levels. This, however, might not be the case if filling volume were otherwise reduced by volume depletion due to blood loss, diuresis, and so on. In these situations, even with normal LV function, the higher end-diastolic volumes and stroke volumes provided by properly timed atrial contraction might be important. With depressed LV function of a moderate degree (curve 2), although maintenance of AV synchrony provides for a greater end-diastolic volume, the stroke volume advantage is diminished. It is possible that, due to overall reduction in stroke volume (and cardiac output), even this modest increment in stroke volume would be of important benefit. In patients with more severely depressed LV function and extremely flat LV function curves (curve 3), although end-diastolic volume can be augmented with maintenance of AV synchrony, there is little or no advantage in stroke volume. Other important reasons exist, however, for maintenance of AV synchrony, as will be described later. With regard to patients with hypertrophic cardiomyopathies (curve 4), because of the relatively small end-diastolic volumes, maintenance of AV synchrony may be very important in enhancing stroke volume (and cardiac output). This is because small increments in end-diastolic volume, due to the steep slope of the curve, may substantially increase the stroke volume. This relatively steep-sloped ventricular function curve is also characteristic of patients

with diastolic ventricular dysfunction, a group for whom maintenance of AV synchrony is very important. Figure 3.6 displays this
concept in a relatively small number of patients studied at the
University of Oklahoma[18] (quantitative nuclear techniques were
used). Although only data from the supine position at 80 ppm are
shown (AV interval 15 msec during AV-synchronized pacing), the
same situation hemodynamically was found to be present at a faster
pacing rate (100 ppm) and in an upright posture.

It should be pointed out that movement along single ventricular function curves is probably simplistic in that such variables as
afterload, which could be modulated by a number of factors, might
cause shifting from one curve to another as well as movement
along a given curve. However, for practical understanding, this
conceptual approach is useful.

Although it is beyond the scope of this discussion to examine
in-depth the special situation of patients with hypertrophic *obstructive* cardiomyopathy, a brief discussion is warranted. These patients
have obstruction to LV outflow caused by hypertrophy of the
interventricular septum, typically in the subaortic area, combined
with systolic anterior motion of the mitral valve. Several studies,

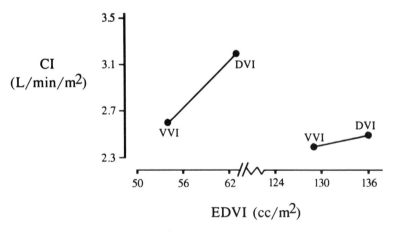

**Figure 3.6 Ventricular function curves comparing cardiac index
(CI) and left ventricular end-diastolic volume index (EDVI) from
(left) a group of nine patients with relatively normal ventricular
function and (right) a group of four patients with markedly depressed ventricular function. VVI = ventricular pacing (no AV
synchrony), DVI = AV sequential pacing (AV synchrony). Patients
studied in supine position at pacing rate = 80 ppm. AV interval
during DVI pacing = 150 msec. Points are group means.**

including several from the National Institutes of Health (NIH),[19] suggest that dual-chamber (AV) pacing, by producing dys-synchrony of LV contraction (modifying the normal way in which the left ventricle contracts) reduces in many patients the degree of outflow obstruction and symptoms (angina, syncope, dyspnea) frequently associated with this obstruction. Confirmatory work is underway and full understanding of mechanism(s) responsible for improvement is lacking; nevertheless, this represents a unique potential indication for pacing, the benefits of which are almost certainly to be on a basis different from that described elsewhere in this section. In this regard, however, it is appropriate to point out that this group of patients also tend to be very dependent on atrial kick for maintenance of cardiac output, similar to those described hypothetically in curve 4 of Figure 3.5.

Even more preliminary data[20,21] have suggested that AV pacing, perhaps involving "multisite" independent pacing of right and left ventricles,[22] may be helpful in improving hemodynamics and/or symptoms in patients with dilated cardiomyopathy. Identification of mechanisms of improvement and subsets of this large population that could be benefited by this therapy is still not adequately elucidated. Further, development of technology that would facilitate this type of special therapy is in its infancy.

Atrial pressures: Cardiac output and blood pressure have been the primary focus of most discussions about the importance of AV synchrony, and the most extreme cases of intolerance to ventricular pacing relate to these factors. It is likely, however, that increase in atrial pressures during ventricular pacing is the most common mechanism by which symptoms are produced when AV synchrony is not maintained.

In Figure 3.7, the left panel shows recordings of pulmonary capillary wedge pressure (also reflecting pulmonary venous and left atrial pressures) in one patient during AV-synchronized pacing (80 ppm/AV interval 150 msec). The right panel shows pulmonary capillary wedge pressure during ventricular pacing (80 ppm) with intact ventriculoatrial conduction. Relatively normal pulmonary capillary wedge pressure tracing is produced during AV pacing with mean pressures between 4 and 8 mmHg and without significant phasic aberration. In contrast, during ventricular pacing, one can see that the mean pressures are elevated to between 8 and 12 mmHg with large A waves (or VA waves) that, at times, exceed 16 mmHg. This elevation in atrial pressures, and specifically the

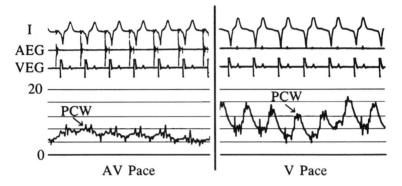

Figure 3.7 Pulmonary capillary wedge (PCW) pressure recordings from a single patient during (left) AV pacing (AV Pace) and (right) ventricular pacing (V Pace) at 80 ppm with AV interval =150 msec. I = ECG lead I, AEG = atrial electrogram, VEG = ventricular electrogram. Scale = mmHg.

production of giant or "cannon" A waves, occurs because of left atrial contraction against a closed mitral valve; the increased pressure wave is present not only in the left atrium but also in the pulmonary veins and pulmonary capillary wedge position.

The same phenomenon occurs on the right side of the heart. Figure 3.8 is a display of simultaneous pulmonary capillary wedge and right atrial recordings during ventricular pacing (80 ppm) in which VA conduction is intact. Typically, the large A waves are present not only in the pulmonary capillary wedge position but also in the right atrium, comparable to those that occur on the left side of the heart. This is due to right atrial contraction against the closed tricuspid valve. The importance of the timing of atrial contraction in producing these giant waves is shown in Figure 3.9. Here, a display of both pulmonary capillary wedge and right atrial pressure recordings made during ventricular pacing (80 ppm) documents the giant A waves with every other ventricular complex due to 2:1 VA conduction that can be seen in the electrical recordings at the top of the tracing.

Figure 3.10 is a display of mean pulmonary capillary wedge pressure measurements made during AV and V pacing (80 ppm) in patients in a supine position studied at the University of Oklahoma. As described above, this study involved a heterogeneous pacing population. During ventricular pacing, ventriculoatrial conduction was intact or reproduced by ventriculoatrial pacing. As shown, quite consistent increases in pulmonary capillary wedge (and, by implication, left atrial) pressure occur when AV synchrony is lost if atrial contraction occurs during ventricular systole, at which time the tricuspid and mitral valves are closed. Although it is not individually shown, the same physiologic phenomenon is seen in the right atrium. Although the actual increase in mean left atrial

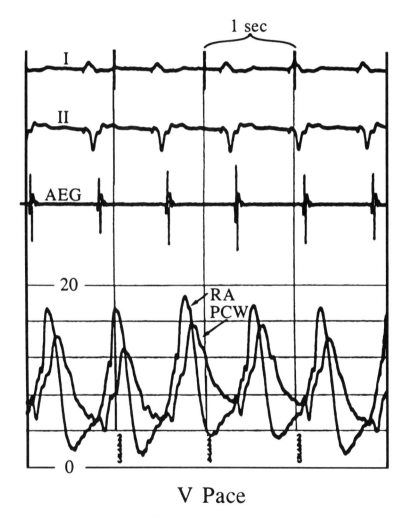

V Pace

Figure 3.8 Right atrial (RA) and pulmonary capillary wedge (PCW) pressure recordings during ventricular pacing (V Pace) at 80 ppm with 1:1 VA conduction. I = ECG lead I, II = ECG lead II, AEG = atrial electrogram. Scale = mmHg.

and right atrial pressures during ventricular pacing may not be dramatic (see Table 3.1), some patients, especially those with already elevated pressures, may become significantly symptomatic due to this mechanism. If one considers the extent of elevation in phasic pressures due to the giant A waves, this potential is magnified. Patients with poor LV function generally also have elevated LV end-diastolic volume and left atrial, pulmonary capillary wedge, and pulmonary artery pressures. Superimposing the giant A waves only worsens the problem and is the most common cause of patient

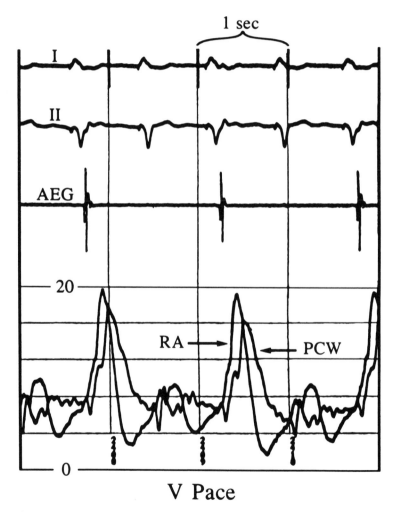

Figure 3.9   Same as Figure 3.8 except 2:1 VA conduction.

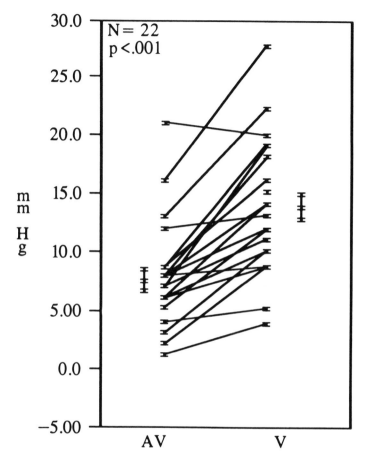

Figure 3.10 A comparison of pulmonary capillary wedge pressures in a group of 22 pacemaker patients during (left) AV sequential pacing and (right) ventricular pacing, both at 80 ppm with AV interval during AV pacing =150 msec. Individual comparisons are inside and connected by solid lines. Group comparison ± SEM is outside. Paired *t* tests used for statistical comparison.

intolerance to ventricular pacing in the population of patients with poor LV function.

Intact VA conduction produces consistent elevations in pressure in the left atrium and right atrium due to the contraction of the atria against closed AV valves, even when VA conduction is not intact. If VA conduction is not intact, because of unequal atrial and ventricular rates, however, there will be frequent periods when atrial contraction occurs during ventricular systole, during which the AV valves are closed; hence the problems of elevated pressures in the atria and approaching veins occur. It has been our experience that some patients are actually more symptomatic when VA conduction is not intact, due to the intermittency of these elevated pressures, thus preventing patients from establishing tolerance for this phenomenon.

The relationship of the phasic changes in the pulmonary capillary wedge (and left atrial) pressures to LV pressures can be seen in Figures 3.11, 3.12, and 3.13. Figure 3.11 is a display of normal LV and pulmonary capillary wedge pressure recordings during AV pacing (80 ppm/AV interval of 150 msec). The appropriately timed A wave can be seen in both the LV and pulmonary capillary wedge pressure recordings. In contrast, as Figure 3.12 shows, during ventricular pacing (80 ppm) with a consistent 1:1 VA relationship, the loss of the A wave contribution to the upstroke of the LV pressure recording and the giant A wave, late in ventricular systole, can be seen consistently in the pulmonary

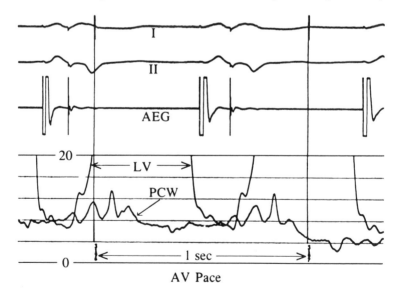

Figure 3.11 Left ventricular (LV) and pulmonary capillary wedge (PCW) pressure recordings during AV pacing at 80 ppm with AV interval = 150 msec. I = ECG lead I, II = ECG lead II, AEG = atrial electrogram. Scale = mmHg.

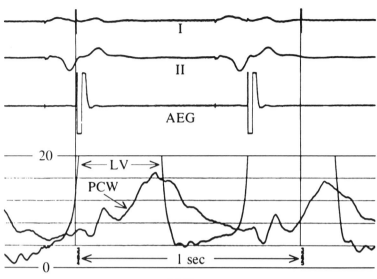

Figure 3.12 Same as Figure 3.11 except ventricular pacing at 80 ppm.

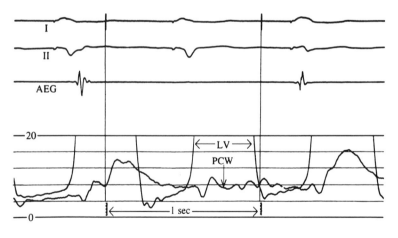

Figure 3.13 Same as Figure 3.11 except ventricular pacing at 80 ppm with VA dissociation.

capillary wedge pressure recording. Figure 3.13 displays this relationship when the atrial contraction is random in relationship to ventricular contraction.

Although it is relatively clear that the mechanism for the giant A waves is the contraction of the atria against closed AV valves, some have speculated that AV valvular regurgitation is responsible for much of the increase in phasic pressure in the atria.[23,24] This appears not to be the case, however, on the basis of the results of a study done at this institution in which pacemaker patients underwent LV cineangiography during both AV and V pacing for assessment of mitral regurgitation.[25] The presence and degree of mitral regurgitation was assessed by two experienced angiographers in a blinded fashion. Conventional definitions of degrees of mitral regurgitation were used. Of the 16 patients who underwent paired LV cineangiograms in this study, five (approximately 30 percent) had slight worsening in the degree of mitral regurgitation during ventricular pacing compared with AV pacing. Of the five that worsened, two who had no mitral regurgitation during AV pacing developed a trace of mitral regurgitation during ventricular pacing and three patients developed what was judged to be 1+ mitral regurgitation during ventricular pacing and only a trace of mitral regurgitation during AV pacing. It is possible that an occasional patient will have substantial worsening or production of mitral (and tricuspid) regurgitation during ventricular pacing (as opposed to AV pacing), but it is unlikely that in a majority of patients this contributes significantly to the problem of atrial pressure elevation and giant A waves seen consistently during ventricular pacing. To reiterate, it appears that the mechanism of these increases in atrial pressure is related to the contraction of the atria against the closed AV valves during ventricular systole.

Other advantages: Additional hemodynamic comparisons between AV and V pacing are presented in Table 3.1. It is likely that the higher pulmonary artery pressures during ventricular pacing are related to the giant A waves produced when atria contract against the closed AV valves. Pulmonary vascular resistance, at least in this study, was not significantly different between AV and V paced patients. Systemic vascular resistance was significantly higher during ventricular pacing. Mechanistically, it is likely that this increase in systemic vascular resistance is related to neural reflexes supportive of blood pressure when cardiac output is diminished.[4,5]

A hemodynamic variable that is not significantly affected in most individuals (AV versus V pacing) is that of ejection fraction (see Table 3.1). Although the components of ejection fraction— both end-diastolic volume and stroke volume—are significantly lower during ventricular pacing, ejection fraction is unaffected because both the numerator (stroke volume) and the denominator (end-diastolic volume) of the ejection fraction vary directly. Ejection fraction is a crude measurement of contractile performance, so it is not surprising that presence or absence of AV synchrony, which primarily affects preload and cardiac output, has no effect on ejection fraction.

It appears that pacing modalities have little effect on most hormonal levels, but atrial natriuretic peptide (ANP), an atrially produced hormone, does appear to be increased during ventricular pacing. This increase is probably related to release of the hormone in response to the stress of higher atrial pressures.[21,22] The importance of the increase is unclear.

Although the issue of mortality rates comparing patients in whom AV synchrony is maintained with those in whom it is not may not be entirely related to hemodynamics, a brief discussion is warranted. Studies by Alpert et al. in groups of pacemaker patients for whom the indication for pacing was AV block or sinus node dysfunction and who had congestive heart failure addressed five-year survival in patients paced ventricularly and patients paced with AV synchrony.[28,29] In the AV block group, the five-year survival in V paced patients was 47 percent, whereas in the AV paced group it was 69 percent—a difference that is statistically significant. In the group of patients with sinus node dysfunction, the V paced patients had a five-year survival of 57 percent, whereas the AV paced patients had a 75 percent survival—also statistically significant.

In another study, done by Rosenqvist et al., the four-year survival, development of congestive heart failure, development of atrial fibrillation, and occurrence of stroke were compared in two populations of patients with sinus node dysfunction, comparing atrial and ventricular paced groups.[30] The incidence of stroke was not different, but statistically significant differences occurred in the other parameters. At four years, the occurrence of congestive heart failure, defined by clinical parameters, was 15 percent in the A paced group but 37 percent in the V paced group. Atrial fibrillation had developed in 6.7 percent of the A paced group and 47 percent of the V paced group. Finally, mortality in the A paced group was 8 percent and was 23 percent in the V paced group.

Hesselson et al.,[31] in a review of previous studies and in a report of the experience at their hospital, described their experience with 950 patients who underwent pacing. Of these, 581 (61%) were paced DDD, 84 (9%) DVI, and 285 (30%) VVI. The incidence of previous atrial fibrillation in each group was 18 to 19 percent. Mean age at implant was 70, 69, and 71 years for the DDD, DVI, and VVI groups, respectively. Atrial fibrillation developed within seven years of implantation in 7 percent, 12 percent, and 38 percent, respectively, of all patients, in 9 percent, 12 percent, and 45 percent, respectively, of patients with sinus node dysfunction, and in 11 percent, 47 percent, and 63 percent, respectively, of patients with both sinus node dysfunction and prior atrial tachyarrhythmias. Survival at seven years after implantation was, respectively, 55 percent, 53 percent, and 36 percent for all patients, 60 percent, 66 percent, and 37 percent, respectively, for patients with sinus node dysfunction. For patients with non–sinus node dysfunction (patients mainly with AV block) the survival rates were 54 percent, 47 percent, and 33 percent in DDD, DVI, and VVI groups, respectively. Although mortality in these and other studies could reflect differences in hemodynamics, it is also likely that differences in atrial arrhythmias and their complications are participatory.

AV interval

Rate-adaptive optimization: The preceding section dealt with the importance of maintaining AV synchrony, but did not address the appropriate AV interval. This issue has been the focus of a number of investigations since 1985. It appears that, at rest, 125 to 200 msec is generally the optimal range if both atria and ventricles are paced.[32,33] On the other hand, more precise optimization may be possible, although it may vary from patient to patient and from time to time in a specific patient. Capacity for fine-tuning the AV interval based on hemodynamic measurements is somewhat limited by accuracy of the measurement technology. Noninvasive measurements may be helpful, although methodologic limitations (including intra- and intertechnician and interpreter variations) are substantial.

There is some predictability in certain aspects of AV interval optimization. Specifically, with exercise there is a relatively linear decrease in the normal PR interval as exercise increases from the resting state to near maximal exertion.[34] The total reduction in spontaneous PR interval in normal subjects appears to be about 20 to 50 msec and about 4 msec for each 10-beat increment in heart rate. Pacing systems have already been developed that incorporate this concept and are substantially sophisticated in this regard. It appears that cardiac output can be more effectively increased and pulmonary capillary wedge pressures (and presumably atrial pressures) can be effectively maintained at lower levels using rate-variable AV intervals rather than preselected fixed AV intervals.

Atrial sensed versus atrial paced AV intervals: Another issue relating to hemodynamics involves the appreciation of the difference in the appropriate AV intervals, depending on whether the atrium is sensed or paced. If atrial activity is sensed and this serves as the basis for initiation of the pacemaker AV interval, atrial activation is already underway and the AV interval based on this sensed atrial activity ideally should be shorter than when the atrium is paced at the initiation of the AV interval. This concept is shown in Figure 3.14. The appropriate difference in the atrial sensed AV interval setting and the atrial paced AV interval setting is probably variable in different patients; the most appropriate values for these parameters are somewhat empirically determined.[35] Generally, a difference of 20 to 50 msec (atrial sensed AV interval < atrial paced

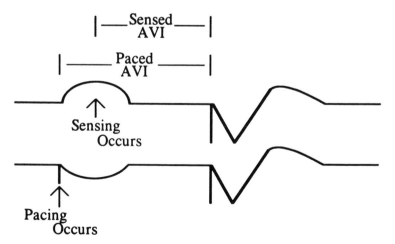

Figure 3.14 Hypothetical relationship of appropriate AV intervals (AVI) during atrial sensing versus atrial pacing at initiation of the AVI.

145

AV interval) has been used at our institution. As noted in the previous section, this represents fine-tuning and is somewhat difficult to quantify in many situations because of technologic shortcomings. Keeping AV intervals as short as is appropriate has benefits other than in hemodynamics. In particular, maintenance of shorter AV intervals—both rate-adaptively and in atrial sensed ventricular paced situations—facilitates shorter total atrial refractory periods. These shorter refractory periods, in turn, maintain greater time for sensing atrial activity. The downside of keeping AV intervals short, however, is that in patients without AV block, short AV intervals may commit the patient to ventricular pacing unnecessarily. This is discussed further in Chapter 6.

Atrial versus AV pacing

Both atrial and AV pacing have the advantage of providing AV synchrony. The choice of atrial versus AV pacing is usually made on the basis of considerations other than hemodynamics. We compared hemodynamics of atrial and AV pacing in a group of pacemaker patients unselected for hemodynamic status.[36] The results of the comparison are shown in Table 3.2. The pacing rate in this study was 80 ppm, and the AV interval during AV pacing was 150 msec (with ventricular activation by pacing confirmed electrocardiographically). The study was done with patients in the supine position. Except for pulmonary artery and pulmonary capillary wedge pressures, there were no statistically significant differences comparing atrial to AV pacing. For example, significantly, cardiac index for the group as a whole, showed no significant difference between atrial and AV pacing, although small differences were seen in some patients.

It is likely that the small but statistically significant differences in pulmonary artery and pulmonary capillary wedge pressures are related to nonoptimization of the AV interval during AV pacing. This has not been fully ascertained, however. Whether mean pulmonary capillary wedge pressure was normal or elevated did not seem to affect whether AV pacing would be associated with larger A waves than would atrial pacing. Figure 3.15 shows simultaneous pulmonary capillary wedge and right atrial pressure tracings in both phasic and mean displays during atrial pacing, on the left, and AV pacing (AV interval 150 msec), on the right. Although it is not entirely obvious in the figure, some patients have slightly larger A waves, especially in the pulmonary capillary wedge position during

Table 3.2 Hemodynamic Evaluation of Atrial and Atrioventricular Pacing

	A[a]	AV[a]	N	P[b]
RA mean (mmHg)	5.8 ± 0.7	6.7 ± 0.6	19	NS
PA systolic (mmHg)	24.1 ± 1.5	25.4 ± 1.7	20	0.05
PA diastolic (mmHg)	12.1 ± 0.9	13.4 ± 1.0	20	0.01
PA mean (mmHg)	16.5 ± 1.0	18.0 ± 1.2	20	0.02
PCW mean (mmHg)	6.7 ± 0.9	8.3 ± 1.0	20	0.01
LV systolic (mmHg)	143.8 ± 7.1	145.7 ± 7.2	20	NS
LV end-diastolic (mmHg)	8.8 ± 0.9	10.7 ± 1.4	20	NS
AO systolic (mmHg)	145.0 ± 7.0	146.2 ± 7.1	20	NS
AO diastolic (mmHg)	81.8 ± 2.0	82.1 ± 2.4	20	NS
AO mean (mmHg)	107.2 ± 3.2	108.1 ± 3.5	20	NS
CI (L/min/m^2)	2.66 ± 0.15	2.62 ± 0.15	20	NS
PVR (dyne · sec · cm^{-5})	168 ± 17	174 ± 20	20	NS
SVR (dyne · sec · cm^{-5})	1769 ± 148	1816 ± 166	20	NS

[a] Mean ± SEM.
[b] Paired t tests.
RA = right atrium, PA = pulmonary artery, PCW = pulmonary capillary wedge, AO = aortic, LV = left ventricle, CI = cardiac index, SVR = systemic vascular resistance, PVR = pulmonary vascular resistance, NS = not statistically significant.

AV pacing. We believe these A waves are related to suboptimal AV sequencing. The relationship between pulmonary capillary wedge pressure and left ventricular pressure during atrial pacing can be seen in Figure 3.16 and can be compared, in the same patient, with recordings made during AV pacing (see Figure 3.11) and ventricular pacing (see Figures 3.12 and 3.13). When we compare the recordings during atrial pacing (see Figure 3.16) and AV pacing (see Figure 3.11), both at 80 ppm (AV interval during AV pacing 150 msec), it appears that during AV pacing there is a greater (though only slightly so) phasic perturbation in the pulmonary capillary wedge pressure and a slightly higher post–A wave LV pressure that may be related to the obviously shorter AV interval during AV pacing than during atrial pacing.

Certain patients, especially those with diastolic dysfunction of the left ventricle, tolerate less well the abnormal activation of the ventricles that occurs with AV pacing. More profoundly negative hemodynamic effects can occur in these patients. This should be taken into consideration when choosing pacing modes in the situations in which either atrial or AV pacing is electrically appropriate.

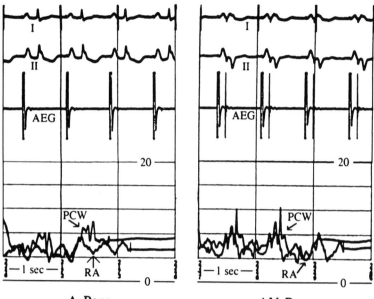

Figure 3.15 Phasic and electronically mean pulmonary capillary wedge (PCW) and right atrial (RA) pressure recordings during atrial (A Pace) and AV (AV Pace) pacing at 80 ppm with AV interval = 150 msec during AV pacing. I = ECG lead I, II = ECG lead II, AEG = atrial electrogram. Scale = mmHg.

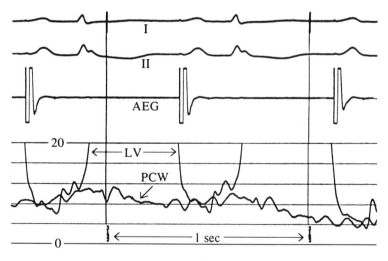

A Pace

Figure 3.16 Same as Figure 3.11 except atrial pacing at 80 ppm.

Generally, then, it appears that although occasional patients may benefit significantly from atrial rather than AV pacing, due to the more normal activation sequence of the ventricles in atrial pacing, most patients do equally well with atrial and AV pacing, especially if AV interval optimization is accomplished. Typically, as noted earlier, the selection of atrial or AV pacing modes is most appropriately determined by electrical considerations (e.g., the presence of abnormal AV conduction) or logistics (e.g., the preference to implant both atrial and ventricular leads during the initial procedure rather than taking the chance of needing to implant the ventricular lead subsequently, especially if cardioactive drugs or dynamic disease processes are involved) than by hemodynamic preference between the two.

Pacemaker syndrome

Pacemaker syndrome is a term proposed in 1974 to describe a condition or conditions composed of a variety of symptoms and signs produced by ventricular pacing.[37] This is particularly relevant in the discussion of AV synchrony in that it appears that most of the symptoms and signs of this syndrome are related to the hemodynamic abberations that are related to loss of AV synchrony. The symptoms frequently associated with pacemaker syndrome include, at the extreme, syncope. Syncope is very uncommon and is most likely related to profound hypotension and, in some, a decrease in cardiac output, associated with loss of AV synchrony. Additional symptoms related to blood pressure and cardiac output include malaise, easy fatigability, a sense of weakness, lightheadedness, and dizziness. Symptoms related to higher atrial and venous pressures include dyspnea (frequently at rest), orthopnea, paroxysmal nocturnal dyspnea, fullness and/or pulsations in the neck and chest, and palpitations or forceful heartbeats. Experience has shown that careful questioning is frequently necessary to elucidate these symptoms. It is not uncommon for patients who have had a pacemaker implanted for some time to deny symptoms but, on specific questioning, to admit to symptoms that can be directly related to ventricular pacing with loss of AV synchrony.

Similarly, careful examination is necessary to find physical signs related to ventricular pacing. Some of these signs include relative or absolute hypotension that can be continuous or fluctuating, neck vein distension with prominent ("cannon") A waves, pulmonary rales, and, rarely, peripheral edema.

Two difficulties in ascribing symptoms and signs specifically to pacemaker syndrome are commonly encountered. First, patients who have pacemakers implanted are frequently patients with other cardiovascular problems that produce the symptoms and signs described. Second, unfortunately, many pacemaker patients have the belief that having the pacemaker, de facto, forces them to accept a less than normal sense of well-being. The following example is illustrative. A 70-year-old man who had been a hard-working farmer/rancher for most of his life began to have syncopal episodes that occurred one or two times per month for three months before he sought medical evaluation. The syncopal episodes markedly compromised his ability to do his work, and he had to hire others to help him. On finally seeking medical attention, he was found to have, by Holter monitoring, periods of third-degree AV block with a wide complex escape rate at 20 ppm, some associated with dizziness comparable to the prodrome he had experienced with his syncopal episodes. A ventricular pacemaker was implanted and the patient was told that he would be "just fine." Six months later, on the insistence of a family member who felt that the patient had not "bounced back" from the pacemaker implantation and had not resumed his normal work and leisure activities, he was seen in our pacemaker clinic. On questioning, he had several of the symptoms noted above, including malaise and easy fatiguability, resting dyspnea, and episodic fullness in his neck and chest. Examination revealed intermittent giant pulsations in his neck that appeared to be cannon A waves, bibasilar pulmonary rales, and normal, nonfluctuating blood pressure. His electrocardiogram revealed third-degree AV block with a ventricular paced rhythm at 70 ppm with an apparently normal underlying atrial rhythm. On questioning the patient as to why he had waited so long and had been reluctant to seek medical attention and further evaluation, the patient, an intelligent individual, said he was so relieved that his syncopal episodes had resolved that he was willing to tolerate (albeit with a significantly modified lifestyle) the symptoms that he had experienced. This patient, like many, believed that simply because he had a pacemaker, he must tolerate feeling less than well. This patient underwent revision of his pacing system to a dual-chamber (DDD) system and began "feeling normal" almost immediately thereafter. One week after the revision, he returned to his more vigorous lifestyle, which he continues now, years later.

Pacemaker syndrome has been defined differently by different authors, but the broadest definition is probably most appropriate. It is best thought of as any combination of the variety of symptoms and signs occurring with ventricular pacing that are relieved by restoration of AV synchrony.

Although uncommon today, since the culprit modes are not frequently utilized because of more sophisticated options, DDI and DVI, both AV pacing modes, can result in pacemaker syndrome if atrial rates exceed the programmed pacing rate and if AV block is present. The pacemaker syndrome in this situation occurs because these are nonatrial tracking modes; when the atrial rates are greater than the programmed rate, AV dissociation occurs if AV block is also present.

RATE MODULATION

As with AV synchrony, terminology here can be confusing. The earliest term used to describe the physiologic property of pacing systems was *rate responsive*. Significant objection to this term (for grammatical reasons) has led to the more acceptable use of the terms *rate adaptive* and *rate modulating*. All these terms are used to describe the capacity of a pacing system to respond to physiologic need by increasing and decreasing pacing rate. The capability of a pacing system depends on the presence of one of a variety of physiologic sensors that monitor need or indication for rate variability.

The predominant need for rate modulation derives from physical activity or exertion. There are other physiologic situations in which normally there are modulations of heart rate, for example, fever and emotional stress. These, however, are substantially less important, especially in the context of pacing systems. A comprehensive discussion of exercise physiology is beyond the scope of this book, although the more important and relevant concepts will be addressed. Further, because the technology of physiologic sensors has been discussed in Chapter 2, a detailed discussion of these sensors will not be repeated.

Exercise physiology

The importance of rate modulation in pacing systems is related directly and specifically to the importance of matching cardiac output with body need. To understand this, a brief discussion of exercise physiology is warranted.[14]

During exercise, or "work," as it is frequently referred to by physiologists, there is an increase in demand for oxygen by body

151

tissues. In addition, there is increased need for removal of metabolic by-products, such as CO_2, from the tissues. The body has a number of mechanisms in place to provide for these increased needs during exercise. Redistribution of blood flow to working tissues, increased ability of working tissues to extract oxygen from the blood, and, most important, increased cardiac output are these mechanisms. This discussion will focus on the last of these—specifically, the body's ability to increase cardiac output with exercise, as this is what rate modulation provides.

The importance of cardiac output during work must be appreciated. A direct, relatively linear relationship exists between amount of work accomplished and oxygen consumption. Maximal work capacity, therefore, is specifically related to maximum oxygen consumption. The hypothetical relationship between work and oxygen consumption is shown in Figure 3.17. Further, consistent with the Fick principle, cardiac output = O_2 consumption/AV O_2 difference, where AV means arterial–venous. Also, cardiac output = stroke volume × heart rate. By substitution in these equations, O_2 consumption = stroke volume × heart rate × AV O_2 difference. Because oxygen consumption is directly, linearly proportional to work (see Figure 3.17), work ≈ stroke volume × heart rate × AV O_2 difference. Maximum work, in normal individuals, is accomplished by an increase in stroke volume to approximately 150 percent of the resting value, an increase in heart rate to approximately 300 percent of the resting value, and an increase in AV O_2 difference by about 250 percent of the resting value. These changes allow an increase in work to over 10 times resting levels.

In normal individuals cardiac output during maximum exercise is approximately 4.5 times greater than the resting value. As above, stroke volume is increased to approximately 150 percent of resting value during peak exercise. This increase in stroke volume, depicted in Figure 3.18, is not linear and is achieved at approximately the halfway point between the rest and maximal exercise levels. The increased stroke volume is accomplished by an increase in ventricular filling. This increase, in turn, is due to greater muscular "pumping" of blood from working muscles and to a general increase in venous tone. In addition, there is augmentation of ventricular emptying due to the increased end-diastolic volume as well as to both increased myocardial contractility and decreased vascular resistance. Loss of AV synchrony can compromise stroke volume, even with exercise, although it appears that AV synchrony is usually less important during exercise in providing ventricular

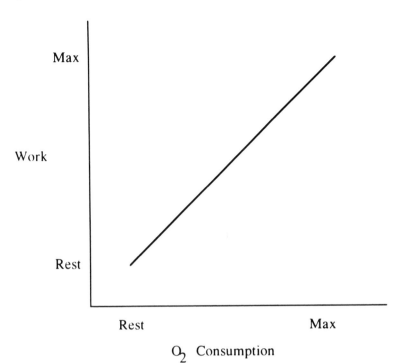

Figure 3.17 Relationship between work and O₂ consumption at rest and exercise.

filling than it is at rest. It is ideal, however, to optimize stroke volume because this is a more energy-efficient way of accomplishing cardiac output (ml of cardiac output/ml of O_2 consumption) than by increase in heart rate.

Clearly, the most important mechanism by which cardiac output is increased during exercise is by increasing heart rate. Increase in heart rate with exercise, in normal individuals, is accomplished by both neural and neurohumoral mechanisms. There is a rapid withdrawal of parasympathetic (vagal) tone and a slightly slower increase in sympathetic tone. There is a still slower rise in circulating catecholamine levels. As depicted in Figure 3.18, there is a direct and relatively linear relationship between heart rate and exercise level and, in turn, between heart rate and cardiac output during exercise. In normal individuals, peak cardiac output can be increased to 300 percent of resting values simply by an increase in heart rate.

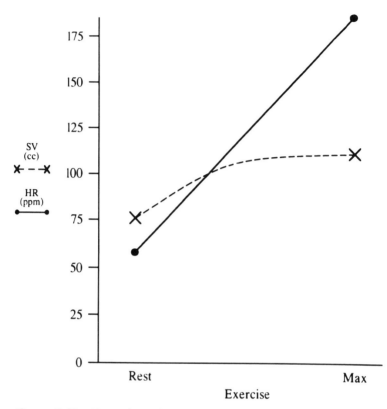

Figure 3.18 Normal stroke volume (SV) and heart-rate (HR) response to exercise.

An additional point relating to rate-modulation capabilities in pacing systems is that, in normal individuals, there is a relatively rapid achievement of the appropriate heart rate for a given level of exercise. This is depicted in Figure 3.19. As shown, the appropriate heart rate for the exercise level is achieved within 1 to 1.5 minutes after the beginning of the particular level of exercise. To recapitulate normal physiology, therefore, it is important for pacing systems to respond rather quickly to exercise.

Advantage of rate modulation

As is obvious by the foregoing discussion of exercise physiology, the ability of patients to increase heart rate with exercise—and to a lesser extent, other metabolic stress—is important in attaining and maintaining optimal physiologic status. Exertional intolerance, manifested by a number of clinical symptoms, can be very limiting, but it is almost obligatory if heart rate cannot be increased.

In pacemaker patients, compromised ability to increase heart rate due to the underlying cardiac electrical problem and/or super-imposed drug therapy is common. The inability to increase and maintain heart rate appropriately with exercise has been called chronotropic incompetence.[38] Some individuals are totally chronotropically incompetent in that they have essentially no or markedly blunted chronotropic response to exercise. Others have a more modestly blunted chronotropic response to exercise such that, although their heart rate increases somewhat with exercise, the increase is inappropriate for age or other factors. Some patients are able to achieve the appropriate heart rate for level of exercise but do so more slowly than is normal. Patients with any of these forms of chronotropic incompetence are candidates for pacing systems with rate-modulation capabilities.

Diagnosis of chronotropic incompetence is relatively easy at times. Patients with third-degree and, frequently, lesser degrees of

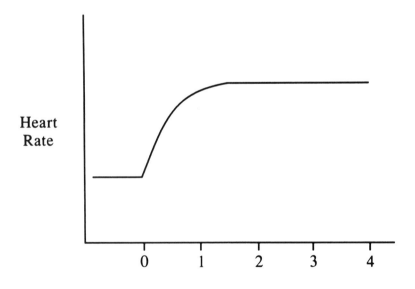

Figure 3.19   Normal heart-rate equilibration time requirement at a constant exercise level.

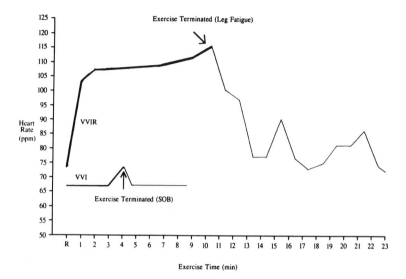

Figure 3.20 Heart rate and exercise time in a patient with normal left ventricular function during rate-modulated (VVIR) and non–rate-modulated (VVI) ventricular pacing. The exercise testing method used was the modified Naughton protocol. Exercise was terminated due to leg fatigue during VVIR pacing and shortness of breath during VVI pacing.

AV block are typically chronotropically incompetent. The neural and, to a lesser extent, neurohumoral reasons for rate increase with exercise have less of an effect on the ventricles than the atria. The diagnosis of chronotropic incompetence in patients with sinus node dysfunction is frequently more difficult. A number of different criteria have been proposed, including the inability to increase heart rate with exercise to at least 70 to 85 percent of the maximum predicted heart rate (maximum predicted heart rate = 220 − age in years). This is a useful criterion for diagnosing chronotropic incompetence, but it is likely that this criterion cannot be used in many individuals due to limitations of exercise function unrelated to cardiopulmonary status. Further, there are patients with delayed chronotropic responses that could benefit from rate-modulating pacing systems that might be missed by this criterion. More complicated formulas have been developed to allow determination of the presence of chronotropic incompetence by exercise testing with assessments made by stage.[39] The Wilkoff chronotropic assessment exercise protocol (CAEP) is an easily accomplished test and has become widely utilized for chronotropic competency evaluation.

Rate-modulating pacing systems have been shown not only to improve the heart-rate response with exercise but also to increase work capacity (by criteria such as exercise time). Figures 3.20 and 3.21 are graphic presentations of heart rates during exercise testing (modified Naughton treadmill protocol) in two patients comparing their exercise performance during VVI (non–rate-modulating ventricular pacing) to VVIR (rate-modulating ventricular pacing). Both these patients have atrial fibrillation with third-degree AV block. The patient whose data are displayed in Figure 3.20 has normal cardiac function; the one whose data are displayed in Figure 3.21 has poor LV function. From a clinical perspective, it is

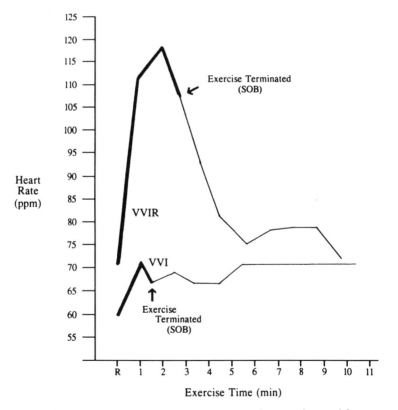

Figure 3.21 **Same as in Figure 3.20 except in a patient with poor left ventricular function. Exercise was terminated due to shortness of breath during both VVIR and VVI pacing.**

interesting that the patient with poor LV function, although his exercise time was not dramatically different between the two modes of pacing, felt dramatically better in the rate-modulating mode of pacing. Quantification of the improvement in work capacity in pacemaker populations comparing non–rate-modulating with rate-modulating modes has consistently shown advantages for the rate-modulating systems. This is dependent to a large extent, however, on the presence of chronotropic incompetence. Nordlander et al., in review of studies addressing work capacity in rate-modulating versus non–rate-modulating systems, noted that for every 40 percent increase in paced rate during rate-modulated pacing compared with non–rate-modulated pacing, there is a 10 percent increase in work capacity.[40]

Exercise testing and assessment of improvement in maximal work capacity represent quantifiable parameters for assessing improvement in patients with pacemakers; but most pacemaker patients, like most normal individuals, function at submaximal levels of exertion most of the time. Optimization of heart rate at these submaximal levels of exertion by providing rate modulation is the principal gain of enfranchising this physiologic concept. Protocols such as CAEP can be helpful. In Figure 3.22, the heart rate, all paced, during a 24-hour period is displayed. The Holter monitor data are taken from the same individual for whom the exercise test is Figure 3.21 was performed. The low rate of the pacemaker was 50 ppm during the test. As can be seen, the patient was at submaximal exercise levels, based on a comparison of the Holter and exercise test data, during the entire 24-hour Holter monitoring period. This heart-rate graph is fairly typical of many patients with rate-modulating pacing systems, whether the rate modulation is accomplished by tracking of normal P waves or using some other physiologic sensor, especially if the patients are com-

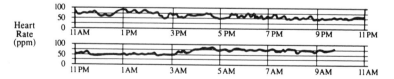

Figure 3.22 Heart-rate trend during 24-hour ambulatory ECG recording in same patient as in Figure 3.21 in 100 percent paced, rate-modulated ventricular pacing mode (low rate = 50 ppm).

promised by underlying cardiovascular or other problems that limit exertion.

Relationship of rate modulation to AV synchrony

An unfortunate competition developed a number of years ago between rate modulation and AV synchrony for preeminence as the most important physiologic pacing concept. This competition was caused by technological limitations that forced a choice between either rate-modulation capabilities or AV synchrony. For example, patients with sinus node dysfunction and chronotropic incompetence as well as AV conduction abnormalities could pose such a problem. Specifically, although a dual-chamber pacemaker can provide AV synchrony in this situation, if a physiologic sensor-driven rate-modulating capability was not present in this pacemaker, the problem of chronotropic incompetence would not be treated. On the other hand, if a physiologic sensor-driven rate-modulating ventricular pacemaker was implanted in this patient, AV synchrony would be lost. Frequently the less-than-ideal decision enfranchising one of the physiologic concepts but not the other had to be made on the basis of whether the patient was more likely to need AV synchrony or rate modulation. This was frequently a difficult decision. Understanding the physiology involved could help direct the decision. If a patient was predominantly sedentary, had LV dysfunction with some elevation in atrial pressures, and had intact ventriculoatrial conduction, maintenance of normal AV synchrony would likely be preferred. On the other hand, if the patient was totally chronotropically incompetent, was very active (including vigorous physical exertion), and had no ventriculoatrial conduction, rate modulation might be of greater importance.

In Figure 3.23 the relative hemodynamic benefit, for a general population, of rate modulation and AV synchrony scaled from rest to maximum exertion can be seen. At rest, AV synchrony is of preeminent benefit, whereas this benefit is diminished as one approaches maximal exercise, especially in relationship to rate modulation. Rate modulation is of very little value at rest, but it becomes quite important early in exercise and increases in relative benefit approaching maximal exercise. Rate modulation and AV synchrony are complementary, not competitive, physiologic concepts. In the past, choices had to be made between these concepts for particular patients in particular situations. Technology today,

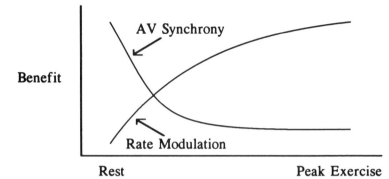

Figure 3.23 Hypothetical, general relationship between AV synchrony and rate modulation with respect to hemodynamic benefit, both at rest and during exercise.

Table 3.3 Sensors in Use or Proposed for Use in Pacemaker Rate Modulation

Atrial rate (P wave)	Body activity/motion
Blood pH	QT/ST interval
Mixed venous O_2 saturation	Respiratory rate
Mixed venous blood temperature	Minute ventilation
Right ventricular stroke volume	Evoked response
Right ventricular pressure (dP/dt)	Systolic time intervals

however, allows us to accomplish both AV synchrony and rate modulation in virtually all patients for whom cardiac pacing is indicated. Physiologic sensors coupled with dual-chamber pacing systems have made this possible.

Sensors

A chronotropically competent sinus node unaffected by disease, drugs, or procedures is the ideal physiologic sensor to accomplish rate modulation. Unfortunately, chronotropic incompetence of the sinus node is not uncommon, and alternative physiologic sensors are sometimes needed. A number of physiologic sensors have been incorporated into implantable pacing systems or have been proposed for incorporation. A listing of a number of these sensors is included in Table 3.3. As the technology and mechanisms of the most important of these are discussed in Chapter 2, a detailed discussion of this will not be provided here.

Choice of sensors for pacing systems is dependent on a number of factors. Ideally, physiologic sensors and their implementation are inexpensive, require no modification in implantation technique, are chronically stable and free of interference, consume little energy, and allow for recapitulation of normal physiology. In regard to the last of these, the ideal sensor-driven rate-modulating system is appropriately responsive to varying levels of physical (and, arguably, other) stress, has a rapid response time, has negative as well as positive feedback capability, and is eminently flexible both manually and automatically. To date, no single sensor or combination of sensors has been proven to have all of these desirable characteristics. On the other hand, even with the early iterations of many of these sensors, acceptable (although perhaps not ideal) rate modulation for most situations has been provided. It is appropriate to continue to search for and develop sensor-driven rate-modulating systems that are closer to the ideals described above, but the caveat is that the ideals of simplicity and ease of use must be heavily weighted in trying to strike a balance with the ideal of physiologic optimization.

The rate-modulation functions in some, if not most, of these systems can be mainly self-initiated and periodically "self-evaluated." Some systems presently have a number of manually programmable features that allow for optimization. Exercise testing, formal or informal, of a variety of types and ambulatory ECG monitoring have been the tools that this institution has used most frequently to optimize the rate-modulation functions. Many currently available models have rate memory functions that preclude the need for external monitoring for this process.

MODE SELECTION

Selection of the appropriate pacing mode to fit the patient's electrical and hemodynamic status is usually not difficult. Striving to provide both AV synchrony and rate modulation, whenever possible, assists in this decision-making process. Mode-selection decisions related to electrical considerations take into account three principal issues. These are atrial rhythm status, status of AV conduction, and presence of chronotropic competence. A mode-selection flow chart is shown in Figure 3.24. Difficulties arise principally in the assessment of atrial rhythm status. It is not uncommon for patients who are predominantly in sinus rhythm to have episodes of atrial tachyarrhythmias. Historically, the decision whether to use atrial or AV pacing systems rather than ventricular pacing systems in these individuals has been difficult. The advent of AV pacemakers capable of functioning in atrial tracking modes (DDD, DDDR, VDD, VDDR) during sinus rhythm but switching to non-tracking modes (DDI, DDIR, VVI, VVIR) if atrial tachyarrhythmias occur (and back to atrial tracking modes when they resolve) has simplified this decision and has been referred to as "mode switching." At present, at this institution, preservation of AV synchrony using atrial or AV pacing is typically chosen if there are any periods of significant sinus rhythm.

A lesser difficulty in mode selection is related to the determination of AV conduction status. Careful evaluation of AV conduction status dramatically reduces the likelihood that subsequent AV conduction problems will develop, but a small risk remains. This risk is about 2 to 6 percent in five years.[41,42] For this reason, although we may program an atrial pacing mode, a dual-chamber pacing system is usually implanted.

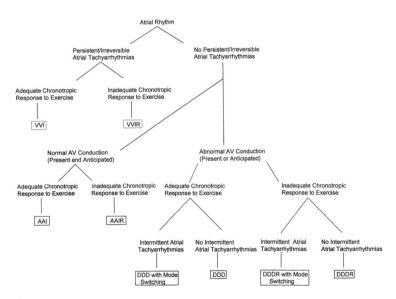

Figure 3.24 Mode choice algorithm based on the presence and persistance of atrial tachyarrhythmias, status of AV conduction, and adequacy of chronotropic response to exercise. VVI = ventricular demand pacing, VVIR = rate-modulated ventricular demand pacing, DDD = AV universal pacing, DDDR = rate-modulated AV universal pacing, AAI = atrial demand pacing, AAIR = rate-modulated atrial demand pacing. The pacemaker code is discussed in detail in Chapter 6.

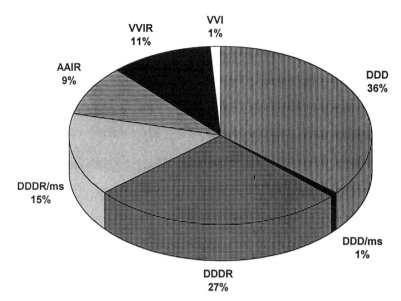

Figure 3.25   Mode selected at implant in a recent series of 100 consecutive patients at the University of Oklahoma. Modes are the same as in Figure 3.24 (ms = mode switching).

The mode of pacing selected in the last 100 implants performed at the University of Oklahoma is shown in Figure 3.25. Notably, all of these implants occurred early in the mode-switching DDDR (sensor-driven rate-modulating dual-chamber) era.

In summary, a reasonable approach—or at least the one used at the University of Oklahoma in selection of pacing mode—is to preserve AV synchrony with atrial or, most commonly, AV pacing in all but the most extenuating circumstances. Further, we judge the patient's chronotropic response capabilities and provide this as well, when it is intrinsically blunted or absent, using devices with as simple and automatic but appropriate physiologic sensors as are available.

REFERENCES

1. Harvey W. *Exercitatio Anatomica de Motu Cordis et Sanguinis in Animalibus* (1628). R Willis, translator. England: Barnes Survey, 1874.
2. Lewis T. Fibrillation of the auricles: Its effects upon the circulation. *J Exp Med* 1912;16:395–398.

3. Gesel RA. Auricular systole and its relation to ventricular output. *Am J Physiol* 1911;29:32–63.
4. Alicandri C, Fouad FM, Tarazi RC, et al. Three cases of hypotension and syncope with ventricular pacing: Possible role of atrial reflexes. *Am J Cardiol* 1978;42:137–142.
5. Erlebacher JA, Danner RL, Stelzer PE. Hypotension with ventricular pacing: An atrial vasodepressor reflex in human beings. *J Am Coll Cardiol* 1984;4:550–555.
6. Reynolds DW, Olson EG, Burow RD, et al. Hemodynamic evaluation of atrioventricular and ventriculoatrial pacing. *PACE* 1984;7:463.
7. Goldreyer B, Bigger T. Ventriculoatrial conduction in man. *Circulation* 1970;41:935–946.
8. Klementowicz P, Ausubel K, Furman S. The dynamic nature of ventriculoatrial conduction. *PACE* 1986;9:1050–1054.
9. Levy S, Corbelli JL, Labrunie P. Retrograde (ventriculoatrial) conduction. *PACE* 1983;6:364–371.
10. Petersen MEV, Chamberlain-Webber R, Fitzpatrick AP, et al. Permanent pacing for cardioinhibitory malignant vasovagal syndrome. *Br Heart J* 1994;71:274–281.
11. Karloff I. Hemodynamic effect of atrial triggered vs. fixed rate pacing at rest and during exercise in complete heart block. *Acta Med Scand* 1975;197:195–210.
12. Greenberg B, Chatterjee K, Parmley WW, et al. The influence of left ventricular filling pressure on atrial contribution to cardiac output. *Am Heart J* 1979;98:742–751.
13. Kruse I, Arnman K, Conradson TB, Ryden L. A comparison of the acute and long-term hemodynamic effects of ventricular inhibited and atrial synchronous ventricular inhibited pacing. *Circulation* 1982;675:846–855.
14. Astrand PO, Rodahl K. *Textbook of Work Physiology.* 2nd ed. New York: McGraw-Hill, 1977.
15. Topol E, Goldschlager N, Ports TA, et al. Hemodynamic benefit of atrial pacing in right ventricular myocardial infarction. *Ann Intern Med* 1982;96:594–597.
16. Hartzler GO, Maloney JD, Curtis JJ, Barnhorst DA. Hemodynamic benefits of atrioventricular sequential pacing after surgery. *Am J Cardiol* 1977;40:232–236.
17. Chamberlain DA, Leinbach RC, Vassaux CE, et al. Sequential atrioventricular pacing in heart block complicating acute myocardial infarction. *N Engl J Med* 1970;282:577–582.

18. Reynolds DW, Wilson MF, Burow RD, et al. Hemodynamic evaluation of atrioventricular sequential vs. ventricular pacing in patients with normal and poor ventricular function at variable heart rates and posture. *J Am Coll Cardiol* 1983;1: 636.
19. Epstein ND, Curiel RV, Panza JA, et al. Long-term results of dual-chamber (DDD) pacing in obstructive hypertrophic cardiomyopathy. Evidence for progressive symptomatic and hemodynamic improvement and reduction of left ventricular hypertrophy. *Circulation* 1994;90:2731–2742.
20. Hochleitner M, Hortnagl H, Fridrich L, et al. Long-term efficacy of dual-chamber pacing in treatment of end-stage idiopathic dilated cardiomyopathy. *Am J Cardiol* 1992; 70:1320–1325.
21. Nishimura RA, Hayes DL, Holmes DR, Tajik AJ. Mechanism of hemodynamic improvement by dual-chamber pacing for severe left ventricular dysfunction: An acute Doppler and catheterization hemodynamic study. *J Am Coll Cardiol* 1995;25:281–288.
22. Cazeau S, Ritter P, Bakdach S, et al. Four chamber pacing in dilated cardiomyopathy. *PACE* 1994;17:1974–1979.
23. Ogawa S, Dreifus LS, Shenoy PN, et al. Hemodynamic consequences of atrioventricular and ventriculoatrial pacing. *PACE* 1978;1:8–15.
24. Morgan DE, Norman R, West RO, Burggraf G. Echocardiographic assessment of tricuspid regurgitation during ventricular demand pacing. *Am J Cardiol* 1986;58:1025–1029.
25. Reynolds DW, Olson EG, Burrow RD, et al. Mitral regurgitation during atrioventricular and ventriculoatrial pacing. *PACE* 1984;7:476.
26. Nakaoka H, Kitahara Y, Imataka K, et al. Atrial natriuretic peptide with artificial pacemakers. *Am J Cardiol* 1987;60:384–385.
27. Stangl K, Weil J, Seitz K, et al. Influence of AV synchrony on the plasma level of atrial natriuretic peptide (ANP) in patients with total AV block. *PACE* 1988;11:1176–1181.
28. Alpert M, Curtis J, Sanfelippo J, et al. Comparative survival after permanent ventricular and dual-chamber pacing for patients with chronic high degree atrioventricular block with and without preexistent congestive heart failure. *J Am Coll Cardiol* 1986;7:925–932.

29. Alpert M, Curtis J, Sanfelippo J, et al. Comparative survival following permanent ventricular and dual-chamber pacing for patients with chronic symptomatic sinus node dysfunction with and without congestive heart failure. *Am Heart J* 1987;113:958–965.

30. Rosenqvist M, Brandt J, Schuller H. Long-term pacing in sinus node disease: Effects of stimulation mode on cardiovascular morbidity and mortality. *Am Heart J* 1988;116:16–22.

31. Hesselson AB, Parsonnet V, Burnstein AD, Bonavita GJ. Deleterious effects of long-term single-chamber ventricular pacing in patients with sick sinus syndrome: The hidden benefits of dual-chamber pacing. *J Am Coll Cardiol* 1992;19:1542–1549.

32. Haskell RJ, French WJ. Optimum AV interval in dual-chamber pacemakers. *PACE* 1986;9:670–675.

33. Janosik DL, Pearson AC, Buckingham TA, et al. The hemodynamic benefit of differential atrioventricular delay intervals for sensed and paced atrial events during physiologic pacing. *J Am Coll Cardiol* 1989;14:499–507.

34. Luceri RM, Brownstein SL, Vardeman L, Goldstein S. PR interval behavior during exercise: Implications for physiological pacemakers. *PACE* 1990;13:1719–1723.

35. Alt E, von Bibra H, Blomer H. Different beneficial AV intervals with DDD pacing after sensed or paced atrial events. *J Electrophysiol* 1987;1:250–256.

36. Reynolds DW, Olson EG, Burow RD, et al. Atrial vs. atrioventricular pacing: A hemodynamic comparison. *PACE* 1985;8:148.

37. Hass JM, Strait GB. Pacemaker induced cardiovascular failure: Hemodynamic and angiographic observations. *Am J Cardiol* 1974;33:295–299.

38. Ellestad MH, Wan MKC. Predictive implications of stress testing: Follow-up of 2700 subjects after maximum treadmill testing. *Circulation* 1975;51:363–369.

39. Wilkoff BL, Corey J, Blackburn G. A mathematical model of the cardiac chronotropic response to exercise. *J Electrophysiol* 1989;3:176–180.

40. Nordlander R, Hedman A, Pehrsson SK. Rate responsive pacing and exercise capacity—A comment. *PACE* 1989;12:749–751.

41. Rosenqvist M, Obel IWP. Atrial pacing and the risk for AV block: Is there time for a change in attitude? *PACE* 1989;12:97–101.

42. Santini M, Aexidou G, Ansalone G, et al. Relation of prognosis in sick sinus syndrome to age, conduction defects, and modes of permanent cardiac pacing. *Am J Cardiol* 1990;65:729–735.

Temporary Cardiac Pacing

Mark Wood and Kenneth A. Ellenbogen

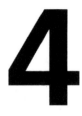

INTRODUCTION

Temporary cardiac pacing serves as the definitive and frequently lifesaving therapy in the acute management of medically refractory bradyarrhythmias. In recent years the field of temporary cardiac pacing has expanded considerably in terms of the diversity and sophistication of pacing techniques. In addition, the applications of temporary pacing have expanded to include management of certain tachyarrhythmias and use in provocative diagnostic cardiac procedures. Therefore, as the need for a thorough understanding of these techniques has become more widespread, the techniques themselves have become more numerous and complex. The purpose of this chapter is to describe in detail the salient clinical aspects of the temporary pacing techniques currently in use. The final section of this chapter summarizes the rationale for selection among these techniques in the clinical setting.

MECHANICAL CARDIAC PACING

Mechanical cardiac pacing techniques involve stimulation of excitable myocardial tissue by direct or transmitted physical forces. Clinically, these techniques include percussion pacing (single or serial "chest thumps") administered by a medical attendant and cough-induced cardiac resuscitation performed by the patient himself or herself. Although lacking in technical sophistication, these techniques persist as useful clinical maneuvers by virtue of their sheer simplicity and immediacy of application.

Percussion pacing for bradyarrhythmias involves the administration of sharp blows with the ulnar aspect of the fist to the mid to lower two-thirds of the patient's sternum. The blows are delivered from a height of 15 to 20 cm above the sternum with a recommended force estimated to be $\frac{1}{4}$ to $\frac{1}{3}$ of that routinely applied for attempted conversion of ventricular tachyarrhythmias.[1] The blows may be repeated serially at a rate of approximately 60 to 90 per minute depending on the duration of bradycardia and the resultant cardiac response (Figure 4.1). True ventricular depolarization and mechanical response must be documented by palpatation of a pulse because percussion artifacts may convincingly simulate QRS complexes (even in corpses with the heart explanted).[2] A true cardiac pulse must be differentiated from the transmitted percussion wave.

The mechanism by which chest wall percussion stimulates myocardial depolarization is not fully understood but is assumed to involve mechanical–electrical transduction properties of the cardiac tissue. The actual threshold for cardiac stimulation by percussion of the chest was 0.04 to 1.5 J as determined by Zoll et al. in 10 human subjects using a calibrated external mechanical stimulator.[3] The ventricles are routinely activated by external mechanical pacing. It is unclear whether the atria are directly stimu-

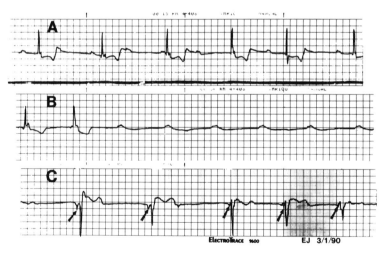

Figure 4.1 Percussion pacing during asystolic cardiac arrest. (A) High-degree atrioventricular block with slow ventricular escape rhythm. (B) Onset of ventricular asystole with continued atrial activity. (C) Percussion pacing artifacts (arrows) each followed by ventricular depolarization.

169

lated by this technique. Experimentally, the percussion pacing technique demonstrates absolute and relative refractory periods and supernormal response periods when applied as coupled or synchronized stimuli.[3] A constant delay of 40 msec between the mechanical stimulus and the electrical ventricular response has been noted in dogs.[3]

The myocardial response to external mechanical pacing appears to depend on the duration of bradyasystolic arrest and the metabolic state of the myocardium. Percussion pacing is most successful very early in the course of witnessed arrests; in this setting it usually elicits a single myocardial depolarization for each blow delivered. As myocardial hypoxia and ischemia intervene, the evoked QRS complexes widen and occur in salvos or extended runs. Further metabolic compromise appears to be associated with loss of QRS voltage, appearance of injury patterns, induction of ventricular fibrillation, and, eventually, failure of response.[4] If percussion pacing initially fails, repeated attempts after the administration of chest compressions and inotropic agents may be successful.[5]

In canines, percussion pacing has maintained cardiac output and blood pressure at levels twice those achieved by conventional chest compressions.[5] Systematic studies on the hemodynamic responses to percussion pacing in humans are lacking. When effective in bradyasystolic arrests, percussion pacing has sustained patients for up to 60 minutes as the sole mechanism of cardiac stimulation.[4] Conscious patients receiving percussion pacing have described the experience as "unpleasant" but tolerable. Single and serial chest blows have also been used to terminate ventricular tachycardia in humans.[6,7]

The true incidence of myocardial "capture" during percussion pacing in bradyasystolic situations is uncertain. Reports from advocates of the technique are encouraging; however, the patient numbers cited are small, and the reports are largely anecdotal.[1,4,6] In addition to undocumented reliability, percussion pacing has precipitated ventricular fibrillation according to several reports.[7,8] The technique is otherwise free of reported complications. Unstable chest wall lesions and recent sternotomy are potential contraindications to the technique.

Cough-induced ventricular depolarization has been suggested and would presumably share a mechanical–electrical transduction mechanism with percussion pacing.[9,10] A forceful cough can generate up to 25 J of kinetic energy within the chest cavity.[10] It is more probable, however, that coughing sustains cardiac output by compression of intrathoracic structures with up to 250 to 450 mmHg of pressure generated by the cough.[10]

To perform this maneuver, the conscious patient is instructed to cough *forcefully* every one to three seconds until either an effective native rhythm returns or definitive treatment is administered. Paroxysms of coughing are ineffective. Clinically, cough-induced resuscitation has maintained mean aortic systolic blood pressures above 130 mmHg during ventricular fibrillation as opposed to only 60 mmHg during conventional external chest compressions in the same patients.[9] Patients performing cough-induced resuscitation during ventricular fibrillation have remained conscious for up to 92 seconds.[9] The technique has the disadvantage of requiring a conscious patient able to immediately generate effective coughs very early (5–11 sec) into the course of a witnessed arrest. Although it is not strictly a cardiac pacing technique, the maneuver is extremely useful in certain situations.

TRANSCUTANEOUS CARDIAC PACING

Due largely to advances in electronic technology and dissatisfaction with other emergency pacing modalities, transcutaneous cardiac pacing has reemerged as a valuable, if not preeminent, initial mode of cardiac pacing for bradyasystolic arrest situations and prophylactic pacing applications. The technique can be quickly, safely, and easily initiated by minimally trained personnel and may be effective when endocardial pacing fails or is contraindicated.[11] A variable incidence of cardiac capture and patient intolerance represent the only significant disadvantages to transcutaneous pacing.

Transcutaneous cardiac pacing is based on the depolarization of excitable myocardial tissue by pulsed electrical current conducted through the chest between electrodes adherent to the skin. The self-adhesive surface patch electrodes are large in area—typically 8 cm in diameter—nonmetallic, and impregnated with a high-impedance conductive gel at the electrical interface with the skin. Currently available transcutaneous pacing generators vary in size and complexity, but ideally one should feature asynchronous and demand pacing modes, a built-in oscilloscope display that electronically filters the large pacing artifact, widely adjustable settings for pacing rate and current output, and extended battery life (Figure 4.2). Available units provide up to 200 mA of current per pulse and utilize a rectangular or truncated exponential pulse waveform of 20 or 40 msec duration. The long pulse widths permit the lowest

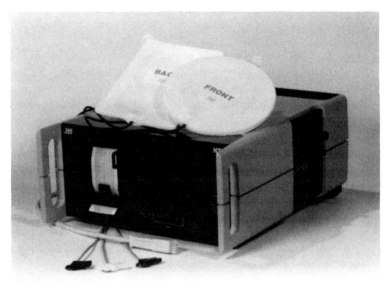

Figure 4.2 Commercially available transcutaneous cardiac pacing generator and surface patch electrodes.

pacing thresholds while minimizing skeletal muscle and cutaneous nerve stimulation.

To initiate transcutaneous pacing, the patch electrodes are secured anteriorly and posteriorly to the chest wall. Several electrode configurations have been recommended and appear to be equally effective in healthy subjects.[12] For effective capture, it is essential that the anterior chest electrode be of negative polarity. Thresholds may be unobtainable or intolerably painful if the negative electrode is placed posteriorly. The anterior (negative) electrode is routinely centered over the palpable cardiac apex, or over the chest lead V_3 position along the left sternal border if pectoral muscle stimulation is to be minimized (Figure 4.3). In animal studies, placement of the negative electrode over the point of maximal cardiac impulse provides the lowest thresholds.[13] The posterior (positive) electrode is centered at the level of the inferior aspect of the scapula between the thoracic spinous processes and either the right or left scapula, but it is equally effective when positioned on the anterior right chest in healthy subjects.[12] Placement directly over the scapula or spine may increase the pacing threshold, however. Before electrode placement, the skin should be thoroughly cleaned with alcohol to remove salt deposits and skin

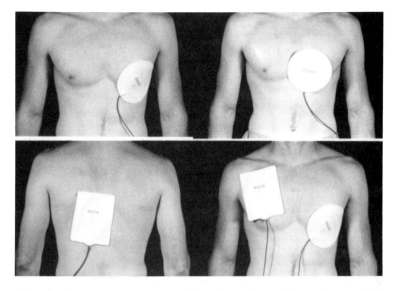

Figure 4.3 Transcutaneous pacing electrode positions. (upper left) Anterior cathodal patch placement over cardiac apex. (upper right) Alternate anterior cathodal patch position over position of electrocardiographic chest lead V_3. (lower left) Posterior anodal patch centered between lower aspect of the left scapula and the spine. (lower right) Placement of anterior anodal patch on the right chest. Note that cathodal (negative) electrode must be positioned anteriorly.

debris, which contribute to patient discomfort and elevate pacing thresholds, respectively. Abrading the skin by shaving directly beneath the electrode interface may worsen discomfort and is not recommended.

In emergent bradyasystolic situations or with unconscious patients, transcutaneous pacing should be initiated in the asynchronous mode and at maximal current output to ensure ventricular capture. Chest compressions may be performed directly over the electrodes without disruption of pacing or conduction of significant electrical current to medical personnel. The large pacing stimulus artifact typically obscures ancillary ECG monitors; thus the electronically filtered display on the generator itself must be followed. Cardiac capture is suggested by the appearance of depolarization artifacts following the pacing stimuli, but capture must be confirmed by palpation of a pulse or by Doppler auscultation if prominent muscle contractions interfere with palpation (Figure 4.4).

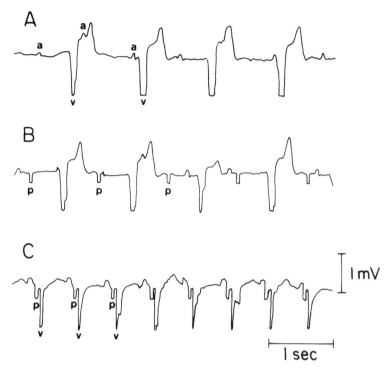

Figure 4.4 **Successful transcutaneous cardiac pacing during complete heart block. (A) Complete heart block with wide complex ventricular escape rhythm (a = atrial depolarization, v = ventricular depolarization). (B) Subthreshold transcutaneous pacing stimuli (p) at 20 mA fail to capture the ventricle. (C) A 1:1 ventricular capture achieved with increased generator current output to 60 mA. Ventricular capture was confirmed by palpation of femoral pulses.**

Once capture is documented, the current may be decreased gradually until loss of capture defines the pacing current threshold. In conscious bradycardic patients or when used prophylactically, transcutaneous pacing is begun in the demand mode at rates slightly faster than the native rhythm and at minimal current output. The current is gradually increased until cardiac capture is documented (threshold) or until intolerable discomfort develops. The final current output is left at or slightly above (5–10 mA) threshold if patient tolerance permits.

Transcutaneous pacing thresholds tend to be lowest in healthy subjects and in patients with minimal hemodynamic compromise.

In these settings, thresholds generally range from 40 to 80 mA but may be slightly higher when stimuli of shorter pulse width are used.[14–17] In clinical use, thresholds of 20 to 140 mA are encountered.[16] No clear correlation has been defined between transcutaneous pacing threshold and age, body weight, body surface area, chest diameter, cardiac drug therapy, or etiology of underlying heart disease.[15,16,18] However, thresholds are elevated for 24 hours following intrathoracic surgery, possibly due to entrapped pericardial and mediastinal air, incomplete rewarming, or transient myocardial ischemia.[18] Elevated thresholds are also suggested in the presence of emphysema, pericardial effusion, positive pressure ventilation, and when used to pace terminate ventricular tachycardias.[16,19,20] As with other forms of cardiac pacing, thresholds tend to be higher and incidence of capture lower as myocardial hypoxia and ischemia worsen during prolonged or delayed rescuscitation efforts. Thresholds may decrease after adequate myocardial perfusion is restored, however. In one study, thresholds tended to fall in the same patients after serial pacing attempts.[12]

The current output that produces unbearable pain is highly variable among individuals; however, it appears that the majority of patients can be paced at tolerable levels of discomfort.[15,16] Patient tolerance has reportedly been enhanced using a three-electrode system with two positive electrodes over the sacrogluteal area.[21] The perception of discomfort may abate somewhat with continued pacing due to accommodation or diminished apprehension. The pain results from stimulation of cutaneous afferent nerves and intense pacing-induced skeletal muscle contraction.

Electrophysiologically, transcutaneous pacing affects ventricular pacing in humans. Simultaneous atrial and ventricular stimulation is common in canine studies but rarely has been reported in humans.[22] Retrograde activation of the atria may occur, depending on the integrity of ventriculoatrial conduction. Intracardiac electrocardiographic and pressure monitoring during transcutaneous pacing have shown the right ventricle to be the site of earliest myocardial activation.[19,23] Theoretically, this follows from the close proximity of the right ventricle to the anterior (cathodal) electrode and from the fact that the stimulating current density declines proportionally to the square of distance from the electrode. Despite initial right ventricular activation, echocardiographic studies in healthy subjects undergoing transcutaneous pacing have shown normal synchronous left ventricular contraction without alterations in ventricular end-diastolic dimension or fractional shortening when compared to sinus rhythm.[14] This pattern suggests near-simultaneous activation of the entire left ventricle. When measured at or near the transcutaneous pacing threshold, ventricular effective refractory periods may be significantly longer than values obtained during right ventricular endocardial stimulation.[15] At 20 mA or more above threshold, ventricular refractory periods are similar for the two techniques.

The hemodynamic responses to transcutaneous pacing are similar to those of right ventricular endocardial pacing.[16] Experimentally, transcutaneous pacing increases cardiac output to a similar or greater degree than right ventricular endocardial pacing in bradycardic dogs.[24,25] In these studies, systemic vascular resistance was reduced by both pacing modalities, and the hemodynamic responses were stable during one hour of continuous pacing.[25] Respiratory alkalosis was induced by transcutaneous pacing in these animals due to stimulation of the chest wall and diaphragm.[25]

In humans, modest reductions in left ventricular systolic pressure and stroke index may occur during transcutaneous pacing when compared to sinus rhythm or atrioventricular (AV) sequential pacing as a result of AV dyssynchrony.[26] The alterations in systemic pressures are similar to those induced by endocardial VVI pacing. Right heart pressures may rise due to loss of AV synchrony. Compared with rapid atrial or ventricular endocardial pacing, transcutaneous pacing reportedly provides greater cardiac output and systolic indices.[23] This phenomenon has been associated with an increased O_2 consumption during transcutaneous pacing and is believed to result from enhanced skeletal muscle metabolism secondary to electrical stimulation. Measured systemic vascular resistance appears to be unaltered, however. Alternatively, the enhanced cardiac output from transcutaneous pacing may result from chest, diaphragmatic, and abdominal muscle contractions simulating cough-induced resuscitation synchronized to cardiac activation.[27]

The reported incidence of ventricular capture with transcutaneous pacing is highly variable and is greatly influenced by the setting in which it is used. In healthy subjects, the reported ability to capture and tolerate transcutaneous pacing is high, ranging from 50 to 100 percent.[15,20,28] Clinically, success rates appear to be highest when transcutaneous pacing is used prophylactically or early (within 5 min) in the course of bradycardic arrests.[16] In these situations, success rates may exceed 90 percent.[16] Successful nonemergent pacing has been reported in 98 percent of patients using a three-electrode configuration, compared with only 72 percent capture with the conventional two-lead system in the same patients.[21] In emergent situations, the success of transcutaneous pacing appears to be much lower, but recent literature shows that it ranges from 10 to 93 percent.[11,16,22] In the largest study, Zoll reports ventricular capture in 105 of 134 patients (78 percent) in diverse clinical situations.[16] Electrical capture was obtained in only 58 percent of cardiac arrests but in 95 percent of cases of expected arrest or standby use. As with any cardiac pacing technique employed during cardiac arrest, time to onset of pacing largely determines the rate of success. Transcutaneous pacing has been used continuously in humans for up to 108 hours and intermittently for 17 days without apparent complications or sequelae.[16,29] This pacing mode has been used to terminate both ventricular and supraventricular tachycardia.[30]

A variety of causes may contribute to failure of transcutaneous pacing. These are outlined with possible solutions in Table 4.1. Efficacy of the technique depends on both the ability to obtain ventricular capture and patient tolerance of the stimulus (Table 4.2).

Complications arising from the use of transcutaneous pacing are extraordinarily rare despite almost 40 years of experience. Although limited areas of focal myofibrillar coagulation necrosis and perivascular microinfarcts have been demonstrated in dogs undergoing transcutaneous pacing, no such lesions have been de-

Table 4.1 Failure to Capture During Transcutaneous Pacing

Cause	Solution
Suboptimal lead position	Reposition leads avoiding scapula, sternum, and spine
Negative electrode placed posteriorly	Place negative electrode anteriorly over apex or V_3
Poor skin–electrode contact	Clean skin of sweat and debris; dry thoroughly
Faulty electrical contacts	Check electrical connections
Generator battery depletion	Charge battery or plug-in generator
Increased intrathoracic air	Reduce positive pressure ventilation, relieve pneumothorax
Pericardial effusion	Drain
Myocardial ischemia/metabolic derangements	CPR, ventilation, correct acidosis/hypoxia/electrolyte abnormalities
High threshold	Use stimuli of longer pulse width

Table 4.2 Painful Transcutaneous Pacing

Cause	Solution
Conductive foreign body beneath electrode	Remove foreign body
Electrode over skin abrasions (shaved)	Reposition, avoid shaving beneath electrodes
Apprehension or low pain tolerance	Administer narcotics or benzodiazepines
Sweat or salt deposits on skin (increased local current density)	Clean skin
High threshold	Use longer pulse width stimuli

scribed in humans.[20] Transcutaneous pacing produces no measurable release of myoglobin, myocardial creatine kinase, or myocardial lactate dehydrogenase in normal subjects.[14] There are no reports of damage to skeletal muscle, lungs, myocardium, or skin (other than mild erythema and irritation) associated with transcutaneous pacing in humans. Caution has been suggested in using this technique within three days of sternotomy; however, actual wound dehiscence from pacing-induced muscle contractions appears to be more a theoretical concern than a practical one. Coughing and discomfort from cutaneous nerve and skeletal muscle stimulation are the most frequent problems. The technique poses no electrical danger to personnel attending the patient. Transcutaneous pacing appears remarkably free from arrhythmic complications despite its use in acute myocardial infarction, digitalis toxicity, during anesthesia, and in cases of endocardial pacing-induced ventricular arrhythmias.[16] There is only one reported case of ventricular tachycardia induced by therapeutic transcutaneous pacing.[31] In dogs, ventricular fibrillation thresholds during the ventricular vulnerable period average 12.6 times the pacing threshold and exceed the current capacity of clinically available generators.[32] In addition, the noninvasive nature and ability to prolong ventricular refractoriness may also contribute to its safety.

TRANSVENOUS PACING

Transvenous endocardial pacing provides the most consistent and reliable means of temporary cardiac pacing in clinical practice. The technique is adaptable to permit atrial and/or ventricular pacing, a feature currently unique to this modality. Once initiated, pacing is generally stable and extremely well tolerated. Considerable cognitive and technical skills are required to implement transvenous pacing safely and effectively, however.[33] Even so, a variety of complications may attend its use. The procedure may also require significant time to implement even under optimal conditions, making it less than ideal for emergent situations.

Transvenous cardiac pacing utilizes intravenous catheter electrodes to stimulate atrial or ventricular myocardial tissue directly with electrical current pulses provided by an external generator. Stimulation may be accomplished by bipolar electrode configurations—in which both anode and cathode are intracardiac in location—or by unipolar pacing—in which one pole, preferably the anode, is extracardiac in location. The bipolar configuration is most commonly employed for temporary pacing, and a variety of pacing leads are available (Figure 4.5). These catheters are typically 3- to 6-Fr in diameter, utilize platinum–coated electrodes (the distal most electrode comprising the tip of the catheter), and are constructed of relatively rigid woven polyester fabric or flexible plastic. The rigid polyester catheters readily transmit thrust and torque for responsive

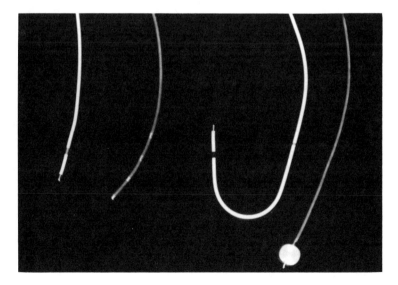

Figure 4.5 Transvenous single-chamber pacing catheters. From left to right: 5-Fr plastic semifloating bipolar catheter; 6-Fr woven polyester fabric quadripolar catheter; preformed 5-Fr semifloating J bipolar catheter; 5-Fr floating bipolar catheter with distal inflatable balloon.

handling but require fluoroscopic guidance to position safely and accurately. Flexible plastic catheters may be flaccid and flow-directed (floating) by means of an inflatable balloon ($1.5 \, cm^3$ volume) between the electrodes, or they may be semirigid (semifloating) without balloons for more responsive yet safer manipulation without fluoroscopy. Rigid and semirigid catheters may be straight or possess preformed distal curvatures (J configurations) to facilitate manipulation and stable atrial positioning.

Other specialized electrode designs include winged atrial J electrodes for atrial pacing without fluoroscopy,[34] single-pass dual-chamber pacing leads (Figure 4.6), and pulmonary artery catheters with proximal atrial and/or distal ventricular electrodes. Lead stability is problematic with pacing pulmonary artery catheters, however. Unipolar cardiac pacing has been described using standard coronary angioplasty guidewires and 0.035-mm catheter guidewires (tips uninsulated) positioned in the coronary arteries and left ventricle, respectively.[35]

Commonly available temporary pacing generators are typically constant-current output devices that are capable of a variety of

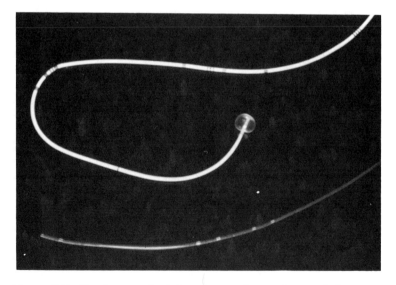

Figure 4.6   Single-pass dual-chamber pacing catheters. Pulmonary artery pressure monitoring catheter with three proximal atrial ring electrodes and two distal ventricular ring electrodes. (top) Woven polyester hexipolar catheter with two distal ventricular electrodes and four proximal atrial electrodes (bottom).

pacing modes (e.g., VVI, DVI, DDD). These devices are powered by disposable commercial batteries and generate output voltages up to 12 to 15 V (Figure 4.7). These generators typically function best against loads of 300 to 1000 ohms. The stimulus pulse width is usually 1 to 2 msec. Temporary pacing generators typically feature adjustable rates (30–180 ppm), sensitivity (0.1 mV-asynchronous), and current output (0.1–20 mA). Specialized rapid atrial pacing generators provide output rates up to 800 ppm. Temporary AV sequential pacing can be accomplished using DVI pulse generators or temporary DDD pacemakers. Temporary DDD generators provide a wide variety of programmability and are capable of most common single- and dual-chamber pacing modes as well as high-rate pacing (Figure 4.8).

Techniques for obtaining central and peripheral venous access are described in detail elsewhere.[36] Decisions regarding the site of venous access for pacing should take into consideration the urgency

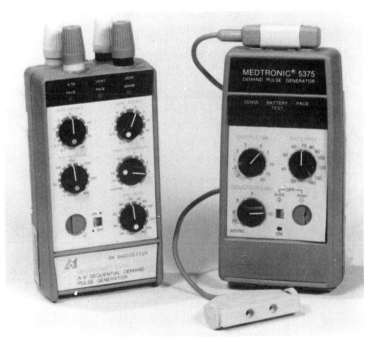

Figure 4.7 Temporary external transvenous pacing generators. (left) Single-chamber generator with adjustable heart rate, current output, and sensitivity. (right) Dual-chamber (DVI) generator with adjustable AV delay and atrial current output.

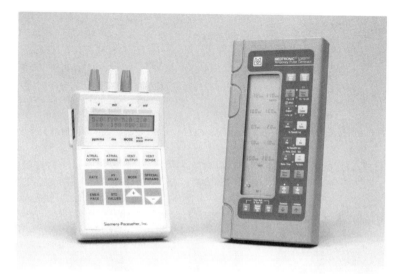

Figure 4.8 Temporary external transvenous DDD pacing generators. Both units are capable of multiple single- and dual-chamber modes as well as high-rate pacing.

to initiate pacing, desired lead stability, need to avoid specific complications, and anticipated duration of pacing. Proper catheter position is most easily and rapidly obtained from the right internal jugular approach.[37] This site and the left subclavian route are the sites of choice during emergent situations. The external jugular and brachial routes are most circuitous and difficult to negotiate without fluoroscopy. The cephalic vein is frequently impassable even with fluoroscopy due to its acute junction with the axillary vein. Catheter stability is maximized by use of the internal jugular or subclavian routes; it is most problematic with peripheral sites, especially brachial, due to movement of the extremities. The peripheral routes do, however, permit greatest control of bleeding complications and avoid inadvertent puncture of the carotid or subclavian artery and pneumothorax. Femoral venous pacing appears to carry the greatest risks of thrombosis, phlebitis, and infection, thus necessitating site changes every 24 hours. Temporary pacing for extended periods is best tolerated and least complicated by using the internal jugular or subclavian routes; however, subclavian access may preclude future use of this vein for permanent pacing if it is needed.

Once venous access is obtained, the catheter may be directed to the desired intracardiac position by electrocardiographic or, ideally, fluoroscopic guidance. Optimal pacing thresholds and lead stability are usually achieved in the right ventricular apex and right atrial appendage. A functional defibrillator should *always* be present during catheter manipulation. For placement in the right ventricular apex, rigid catheters usually require formation and rotation of a loop or bend in the atrium under fluoroscopy but may advance directly across the tricuspid valve by deflecting off the tricuspid annulus (Figures 4.9 and 4.10).

Once in the ventricle, catheters coursing the superior vena cava tend to orient superiorly and require clockwise torque and gentle advancement to reach the right ventricular apex (Figure 4.9). The inferior vena caval approach more favorably orients the catheter tip inferiorly toward the ventricular apex but still requires counterclockwise torque during advancement to avoid lodging against the interventricular septum (Figure 4.10). Under fluoroscopy, the atrial appendage is accessed from the superior vena cava by orienting preformed J catheters anteriorly and slightly medially in the low right atrium. The catheter is withdrawn slowly until the tip demonstrates the typical "to and fro" motion of the atrial appendage. Following cardiac surgery, the atrial appendage may be deformed or absent, requiring approximation of curved atrial catheters against the atrial wall or interatrial septum (see Figures 4.9 and 4.10).

When fluoroscopy is unavailable or impractical, electrocardiographic guidance is possible using flow-directed balloon-tipped catheters or semirigid catheters. While advancing these leads, the distalmost electrode is connected to lead V_1 of a standard ECG recorder. Balloon-tipped catheters are gently inflated in the central circulation. The catheter location is known from the characteristic unipolar electrograms recorded from each chamber (Figure 4.11). Balloon-tipped catheters are deflated upon entry into the ventricle to avoid displacement into the pulmonary artery. Large ventricular electrograms ($\geq 6\,mV$) with ST segment elevation (injury pattern) signal contact with ventricular endocardium. There appears to be no correlation between the magnitude of ST (or PR) segment elevation and pacing threshold, however.[38] In asystole, the catheter is advanced during asynchronous pacing at maximal output until ventricular capture is documented by ECG monitoring or palpation of a pulse. Flow-directed catheters appear to provide the shortest insertion times.[39]

Once positioned, the electrodes are connected to the pacing

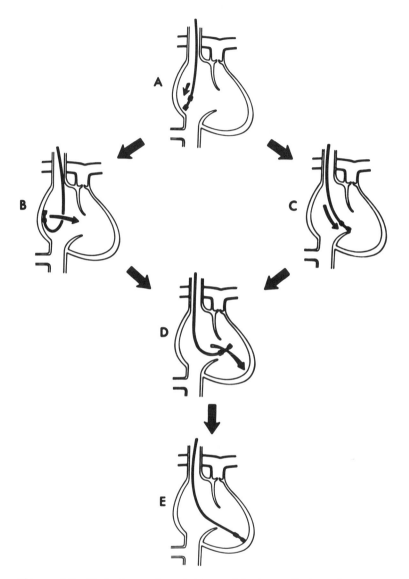

Figure 4.9 Techniques for right ventricular catheter placement from the superior vena cava under fluoroscopic guidance. (A) Catheter advanced to the low right atrium. (B) Further advancement produces a loop or bend in the distal catheter, which is then rotated medially. (C) Alternatively, catheter in low right atrium deflects off tricuspid annulus directly into the right ventricle. (D) Superior orientation of the catheter tip in the ventricle requires clockwise torque during advancement to avoid the interventricular septum. (E) Final catheter position in the right ventricular apex. Catheter position in (B) may be suitable for atrial pacing.

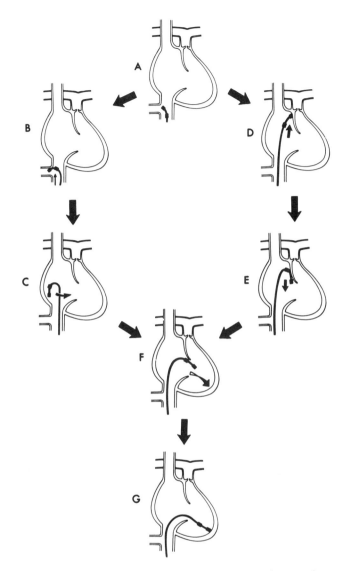

Figure 4.10 Technique for right ventricular catheter placement from the inferior vena cava under fluoroscopic guidance. (A) Catheter is advanced to the hepatic vein. (B) Catheter tip engages proximal hepatic vein and is advanced further, forming a bend in the catheter. (C) The bend in the distal catheter is then rotated medially. (D) Alternatively, the catheter is advanced to the high medial right atrium. (E) With advancement, a bend is formed in the catheter, which is then quickly withdrawn or "snapped" back to the level of the tricuspid orifice. (F) After crossing the tricuspid valve, the catheter is advanced with counterclockwise torque to avoid the interventricular septum. (G) Final catheter position in the right ventricular apex. Catheter positions in (C) and (D) can be used for atrial pacing.

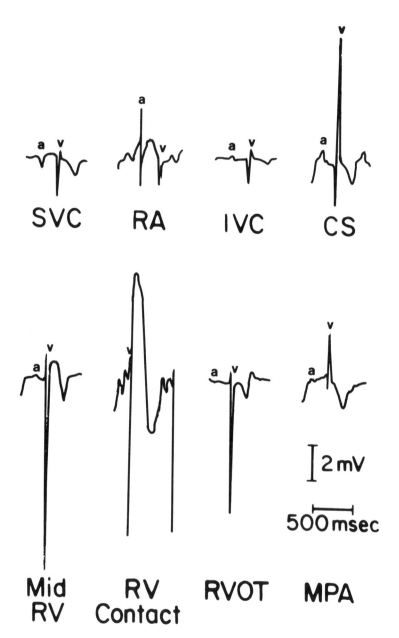

generator; for bipolar pacing, the distal pole serves as the cathode (negative pole), and the proximal pole serves as the anode (positive pole). During unipolar pacing, *cathodal* intracardiac stimulation reduces thresholds and pacing-related arrhythmic complications.[40] The anodal (positive) pole of the generator is secured to a subcutaneous wire electrode or surface patch electrode with surface area $\geq 50\,mm^2$ to reduce threshold (Figure 4.12). During emergent situations, pacing is initiated asynchronously, at maximal outputs, and at rates of 80 to 100 ppm. Following capture, current output is reduced until loss of capture defines the pacing current threshold. During nonemergent situations, pacing is begun at low outputs in the demand mode at rates slightly above (10 ppm) the intrinsic heart rate. Current is increased until capture is achieved. Optimal ventricular and atrial pacing thresholds are less than 1.0 mA (or less than 1.0 V). Pacemaker output is maintained at three to five times threshold current to compensate for subsequent threshold elevations due to inflammation and edema at the electrode–tissue interface, physiologic alterations, and pharmacologic interventions.

Sensing threshold in the demand mode is determined by setting the pacemaker rate below the intrinsic heart rate, then reducing sensitivity (increasing the mV scale) until pacing output occurs. Sensing thresholds should be greater than 6 mV and 1 mV for the ventricle and atrium, respectively. Sensitivity is maintained at 25 to 50 percent of the sensing threshold. AV intervals between 100 and 200 msec are usually optimal during AV sequential pacing. Small changes in the AV interval can significantly influence hemodynamics in some patients.

After initiation of ventricular pacing, the position of the catheter should be confirmed by anteroposterior and lateral chest x-ray *and* electrocardiography. On chest x-ray, a catheter tip in the right ventricular apex should cross to the left of the spine near the lateral

---

Figure 4.11   Unipolar electrograms obtained from the distal electrode of a temporary pacing catheter. a = atrial electrogram, v = ventricular electrogram, SVC = superior vena cava, RA = right atrium, IVC = inferior vena cava, CS = coronary sinus, Mid RV = mid-right ventricular cavity, RV Contact = contact with right ventricular endocardium, RVOT = right ventricular outflow tract, MPA = main pulmonary artery. Note marked ST-segment elevation with right ventricular endocardial contact and predominantly positive ventricular electrogram morphologies with the pulmonary artery and coronary sinus electrograms.

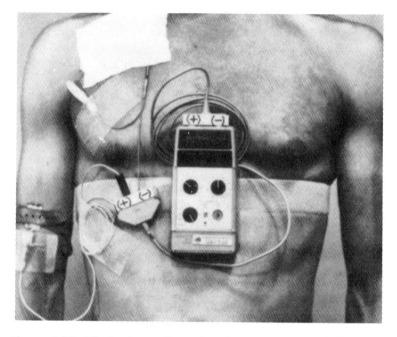

Figure 4.12 Electrode configuration for temporary unipolar cardiac pacing. The negative (cathodal) terminal of the pulse generator connects to the distal pole of a bipolar pacing catheter. The positive (anodal) terminal of the generator connects to a surface plate electrode on the patient's right arm. Note that the second lead of the bipolar temporary pacing catheter is electrically insulated to prevent conduction of extraneous electrical current. Reproduced with permission from Patros RJ, Heart Lung 1983;12:277–280.

cardiac border and point inferiorly and anteriorly. On lateral projections, the catheter tip should be only a few centimeters posterior to the sternum and greater than 3 mm posterior to the epicardial fat pad (Figure 4.13).[41] Even so, the chest x-ray cannot completely exclude malposition of the catheter into the coronary veins, left ventricle, or pericardial space.[42]

Electrocardiographically, paced QRS complexes originating from the right ventricular apex should demonstrate left bundle branch block morphology with a superior axis. A right bundle branch block pattern during temporary ventricular pacing usually indicates coronary sinus pacing or lead perforation into the left ventricle or pericardial space. Rarely, apical pacing can produce a pattern of right bundle branch block due to preferential activation

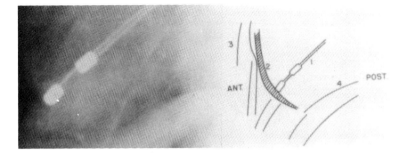

Figure 4.13   Cardiac epicardial "fat-pad" sign. (left) Lateral chest x-ray demonstrates a wide lucent strip corresponding to the anterior epicardial fat pad. The catheter tip is immediately adjacent (within 3 mm) to the fat pad, indicating myocardial perforation. (right) Artist's reproduction of x-ray for clarity. 1 = pacing catheter, 2 = epicardial fat pad, 3 = sternum, 4 = diaphragm. Reproduced with permission from Rubenfire M, *Chest* 1973;63:185–188.

of the interventricular septum or delayed activation of the right ventricle.[43] In this situation, the QRS axis maintains a superior orientation. Various paced QRS morphologies may localize the catheter tip to other locations (Table 4.3).

Unipolar electrograms of intrinsic depolarizations recorded from the right ventricular apex (through lead V_1 of a standard ECG recorder) should demonstrate ST-segment elevation acutely and a predominantly negative QRS morphology (S wave) (Figure 4.14). The absence of acute ST elevation and predominantly positive (R waves) or biphasic electrogram morphology strongly suggests coronary sinus or extracardiac location of the electrode. Coronary sinus pacing is also suggested by high pacing thresholds, atrial or simultaneous atrial and ventricular pacing, posterior orientation of the catheter on chest x-ray, and recording both atrial and ventricular electrograms from the electrode. Although associated with unreliable pacing and early pacing failure, coronary sinus pacing may allow ventricular capture in the presence of impassible tricuspid valve anatomy.

Once in satisfactory position, the lead is sutured securely to the skin, covered with a protective dressing, and examined daily for infection. The generator is affixed to the patient or bed with its controls shielded from inadvertent manipulation. Threshold testing and paced 12-lead ECGs should be performed daily.

For most emergent and prophylactic pacing situations, single-

Table 4.3   Paced QRS Morphology from Various Electrode Positions

Lead Position	QRS Morphology	QRS Axis
Right ventricular apex	LBBB	Superior
Right ventricular inflow tract	LBBB	Normal
Right ventricular outflow tract	LBBB	Inferior or right
Mid or high left ventricle	RBBB	Inferior or right
Inferior left ventricle	RBBB	Superior
Coronary sinus	RBBB	Inferior
Cardiac veins	RBBB	Superior

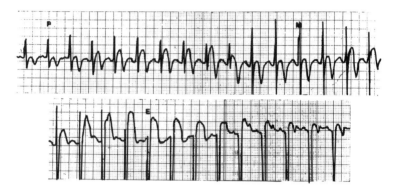

Figure 4.14 Continuous unipolar recording from the distal electrode of a perforated pacing catheter. The catheter is withdrawn from the pericardial space (P), intramyocardially (M) to the right ventricular cavity (E). The characteristic electrocardiographic changes are transition from biphasic QRS morphology at P to negative QRS morphology with ST elevation at E. Reproduced with permission from Van Durme JP, Diagnosis of myocardial perforation by intracardiac electrograms recorded from the indwelling catheter. *J Electrocardiog* 1973;6:97–102. Copyright © Churchill Livingstone, Inc., New York.

chamber ventricular pacing is preferred. Temporary atrial pacing is restricted to those patients with primarily sinus node dysfunction, absence of atrial dysrhythmias, and intact AV nodal function, as documented by 1:1 AV conduction at rates of 125 ppm. The instability of atrial leads and unpredictable effects of autonomic tone and ischemia on AV nodal conduction frequently preclude its use.

Although patients without underlying cardiac disease usually demonstrate similar hemodynamic responses to atrial and ventricular pacing, the maintenance of AV synchrony through atrial or dual-chamber pacing is beneficial in patients with left ventricular systolic and/or diastolic dysfunction.[44,45] In these patients, AV sequential pacing may augment cardiac output by 20 to 30 percent over ventricular pacing alone, while also maintaining higher systemic arterial pressures, lower mean left atrial pressures, lower pulmonary artery pressures, and enhanced ventricular end-diastolic filling. Patients with acute myocardial infarction—especially right ventricular infarction—hypertensive heart disease, hypertrophic or dilated cardiomyopathies, aortic stenosis, or recent cardiac surgery are known to benefit from AV sequential pacing.[46] AV sequential pacing should also be considered in any patient with inadequate hemodynamic responses to ventricular pacing alone (for example, retrograde VA conduction producing pacemaker syndrome).

Initiating and sustaining myocardial capture is dependent on obtaining a stable catheter position, the viability of the paced myocardial tissue, and the electrical integrity of the pacing system. With fluoroscopy, satisfactory catheter position should be obtainable in virtually all patients. The reported incidence of ventricular capture without fluoroscopy using flow-directed or semirigid catheters is variable and ranges from 30 to 90 percent.[34,47,48] Capture is least likely during emergent situations, especially during asystole without fluoroscopy.[47] Catheter coiling in the right atrium poses the most frequent obstacle to ventricular access and may be minimized by using the right internal jugular vein approach, using flow-directed catheters, or by advancing preformed J catheters from subclavian approaches.[49]

Ventricular capture is adversely affected by the setting of hypoxia, myocardial ischemia, acidosis, alkalosis, marked hyperglycemia, and hypercapnia. In emergency situations, electrical capture is least likely in the setting of medically refractory ventricular asystole, probably as a reflection of profound underlying myocardial dysfunction and/or severe metabolic derangement.[47] Electrode contact with previously infarcted or fibrotic myocardium may also prevent capture. Pharmacologic interventions such as administration of propranolol, verapamil, type Ia antiarrhythmics, hypertonic saline, glucose and insulin (by raising intracellular K^+), and mineralocorticoids may also increase ventricular capture thresholds by up to 60 percent.[50] Conversely, threshold may be decreased by epinephrine, ephedrine, glucocorticoids, and hyperkalemia.[50] Isoproterenol may initially decrease and subsequently increase threshold by 20 to 80 percent.[50] Electrolyte effects tend to be transient. Digitalis, calcium gluconate, morphine sulfate, lidocaine, and atropine have minimal effects on ventricular thresholds. Ventricular thresholds may rise by 40 percent during sleep and, conversely, may decrease with activity.[51]

Electronically, cathodal cardiac stimulation provides lower thresholds and greater safety during unipolar pacing than does anodal stimulation.[40] Current thresholds are similar for unipolar and

Table 4.4   Loss of Capture During Transvenous Cardiac Pacing

Cause	Evaluation	Solution
Catheter dislodgment/ perforation	Check position on chest x-ray, paced QRS morphology, or electrograms	Reposition catheter under fluoroscopy, increase output
Poor endocardial contact	Check position on chest x-ray, check electrograms	Reposition catheter, increase output
Local myocardial necrosis/fibrosis	Check electrograms, evaluate for previous infarction	Reposition catheter, possibly increase output
Local myocardial inflammation/edema	Document adequate catheter position (chest x-ray and electrograms)	Increase output, possibly reposition
Hypoxia/acidosis/ electrolyte disturbance/drug effect (type Ia and Ic)	Check appropriate lab values/drug levels	Correct disturbance, reduce drug levels, increase output
Electrocautery/DC cardioversion damaging electrodes and/or tissue interface	Recent exposure to current source	Increase output, replace or reposition catheter, possibly replace generator
Lead fracture	Check unipolar pacing thresholds	Unipolarize functional electrode or replace catheter
Generator malfunction/ battery depletion	Document adequate catheter position, check battery reserve	Replace batteries and/or generator
Unstable electrical connections	Document adequate catheter position, check connections	Secure connections

bipolar pacing, but voltage thresholds tend to be higher with the bipolar configuration.[40] Lead fractures, unstable electrical connections, generator failure, and battery depletion may also preclude myocardial capture.

After successful initiation, malfunction of the pacing system manifesting as inconsistent pacing or sensing may occur in 14 to 43 percent of patients.[52–54] The possible etiologies are numerous and are tabulated with recommended solutions in Tables 4.4, 4.5, and

Table 4.5   Loss of Sensing During Transvenous Cardiac Pacing

Cause	Evaluation	Solution
Lead dislodgment or perforation	Check position on chest x-ray, check unipolar or bipolar electrograms★	Reposition lead under fluoroscopy, increase sensitivity
Local tissue necrosis/ fibrosis	Check unipolar or bipolar electrograms	Reposition lead, increase sensitivity
Electrodes perpendicular to depolarization wavefront, low amplitude electrograms and/or low dV/dt	Check unipolar or bipolar electrograms	Unipolarize lead or reposition
Lead fracture	Check unipolar electrograms from each electrode	Unipolarize functional electrode or replace lead
Electrocautery/DC current damaging electrode or tissue interface	Exposure to current source, check electrograms	Replace or reposition lead, increase sensitivity
Spontaneous QRS during refractory period of generator	Analyze appropriate ECG tracings	No intervention, or replace with generator having shorter refractory period
Generator malfunction	Confirm adequate electrograms and generator sensitivity settings	Replace generator or reset sensitivity
Unstable electrical connections	Confirm adequate electrograms	Secure connections

★Connect bipolar intracardiac leads to right and left arm leads of ECG and monitor lead I.

Table 4.6 Oversensing During Transvenous Cardiac Pacing

Cause	Evaluation	Solution
P-wave sensing	Catheter tip near tricuspid valve on chest x-ray, check electrograms	Reposition further into right ventricular apex, reduce sensitivity
T-wave sensing	Check electrograms	Reduce generator sensitivity, possibly reposition catheter
Myopotential sensing	Check electrograms during precipitating maneuvers	If unipolar, replace with bipolar system or reduce sensitivity
Electromagnetic interference	Check proper electrical grounding and isolation of patient and pacer system, possibly check electrograms	Properly ground equipment, electrically isolate patient, turn off unnecessary equipment, reduce sensitivity
Intermittent electrical contacts, unstable connections, or lead fracture	Monitor sensing during manipulation connections/lead	Secure connections, replace lead

4.6. By far the most common cause of loss of capture is catheter dislodgment or poor initial catheter position. Dislodgment is most common with brachial pacing sites and bears inconsistent relationship to catheter size and stiffness.[52] Most failures occur within the first 48 hours of pacing and are usually corrected by adjusting generator output or sensitivity. Up to 38 percent of malfunctions require catheter replacement or repositioning, however.[53] Lead fractures in bipolar catheters may be overcome by converting the functional electrode to a unipolar configuration (see Figure 4.12) or by replacing the lead. As mentioned, numerous physiologic variables and pharmacologic interventions can also affect pacing threshold.[50,51] Local inflammatory response at the electrode–tissue interface commonly elevates pacing thresholds within hours to days after lead insertion. Similarly, loss of sensing is most frequently related to catheter dislodgment or poor myocardial contact (see Table 4.5). Oversensing is a relatively uncommon problem with temporary pacing systems (Table 4.6).

The complications of transvenous pacing are related to acquisition of venous access, intravascular catheter manipulation, and maintenance of an intravascular foreign body. In large series, the reported incidence of clinical complications ranges from virtually 0 for prophylactic pacemaker insertion in the catheterization laboratory[55] to 20 percent of cases in coronary intensive care units.[53] Complications tend to be more common with brachial or femoral pacing sites. Arterial trauma, air embolism, or pneumothorax may complicate 1 to 2 percent of insertions.[56] Significant bleeding may be seen in 4 percent of patients.[53]

One of the most common complications of temporary pacing is the induction of ventricular tachycardia or fibrillation (up to 20 percent incidence).[57] Ventricular tachycardia is most common during catheter manipulation (3–10 percent incidence) and is usually terminated by withdrawal of the catheter.[58,59] Ventricular tachyarrhythmias are more common in the setting of myocardial ischemia, acute infarction, hypoxia, general anesthesia, vagal stimulation, drug toxicity, and catecholamine administration and during coronary artery catheterization.[60,61] Ventricular fibrillation may complicate up to 14 percent of acute myocardial infarctions requiring temporary pacemaker insertion.[61] Ventricular fibrillation during pacemaker placement is more common within 24 hours of infarction and with inferior infarctions.[61] Supraventricular tachycardias may result from catheter manipulation within the atrium.

Myocardial perforation may complicate temporary pacing in 2 to 20 percent of cases and is probably underdiagnosed clinically.[62,63] Perforation is more common with brachial or femoral catheters and may be more likely with rigid catheters. Immobilization of the extremities is recommended to prevent excessive motion of the catheter. Diagnostic signs and symptoms of myocardial perforation are listed in Table 4.7. Loss of pacing or sensing, changes in paced QRS morphology, and diaphragmatic or skeletal muscle pacing are the most common manifestations; however, perforation to intra- and extracardiac locations can be clinically silent.[63] Penetration *into* the myocardium may occur in up to 30 percent of patients and is suggested by ventricular arrhythmias with the same morphology as paced complexes.[56] Perforation of the interventricular septum is usually hemodynamically inconsequential; however, extracardiac migration of the catheter can produce pericardial tamponade in approximately 1 percent of perforations.[56] Pericarditis may be seen in 5 percent of patients with perforated temporary pacing catheters.[56] In the absence of hemodynamically significant pericardial effusion, myocardial perforation is managed by catheter withdrawal

195

Table 4.7   Diagnostic Features of Myocardial Perforation by Temporary Pacing Catheter

Symptom	Pericardial chest pain, dyspnea (if pericardial tamponade present), skeletal muscle pacing, shoulder pain
Signs	Pericardial rub, intercostal muscle or diaphragmatic pacing, presystolic pacemaker "click" with bipolar systems, failure to pace and/or sense, pericardial tamponade
Chest x-ray	Change in lead position, extracadiac location of tip,[a] "fat-pad" sign,[b] new pericardial effusion
Surface ECG	Change in paced QRS morphology and/or axis, pericarditis pattern
Echocardiography	Extracardiac position of catheter tip,[a] pericardial effusion, loss of paradoxical anterior septal motion or rapid initial left posterior septal motion characteristic of right ventricular apical stimulation
Intracardiac Electrogram	Change in morphology of unipolar electrograms; biphasic or predominantly positive (R wave) unipolar QRS morphology recorded from tip; change in QRS morphology from biphasic, R, or Rs morphology to rS or S configuration with ST elevation and T-wave inversion during catheter withdrawal[a]

[a] Pathognomonic of perforation.
[b] See Figure 4.13 for description.

until effective capture is restored. Careful patient monitoring follows. Unipolar electrograms recorded from the catheter tip will demonstrate a pathognomonic transition from R-wave to S-wave morphology with ST elevation upon withdrawal from extracardiac to intracardiac locations (see Figure 4.14), thereby confirming the diagnosis in cases of uncertainty.[64]

Thromboembolic events from temporary pacing appear to be more frequent than are clinically recognized. Venograms in 29 patients with femoral pacing catheters revealed evidence of femoral venous thrombosis in ten (34 percent) of the subjects despite their receiving subcutaneous heparin prophylaxis.[65] Of these 10 patients, 60 percent had evidence of pulmonary emboli on ventilation perfusion scans. In only one subject was thrombosis suspected by clinical evaluation. The incidence of thrombosis with other pacing sites has not been systematically studied. Systemic anticoagulation with femoral pacing has been recommended by some authors.[66]

Clinical infection or phlebitis complicates 3 to 5 percent of patients paced and is most common with femoral sites.[53] Bacteremia has been demonstrated in 50 percent of patients by the third day of temporary pacing.[56] Sepsis is much less frequent, however. In general, pacing sites should be changed every 72 hours.

Other reported complications include knotting of catheters, induction of right bundle branch block (1 percent), and phrenic nerve or diaphragmatic pacing in the absence of myocardial perforation (10 percent).[41,56]

TRANSTHORACIC PACING

Transthoracic cardiac pacing by direct percutaneous introduction of wire electrodes into the ventricular chambers remains a controversial technique despite more than 30 years of clinical experience. This technique is faster and simpler to implement than transvenous pacing and requires no venous access, blood flow, fluoroscopy, or electrocardiography for guidance. Anecdotally, transthoracic pacing has been effective despite failure of transcutaneous and transvenous pacing.[67] The technique suffers from the high potential for complications and from the absence of controlled, prospective evaluations to dispute the extremely low efficacy pervading the existing anecdotal and retrospective studies.[68,69,70] The advent of effective noninvasive transcutaneous pacing will likely preclude initiation of such prospective trials. Given undocumented efficacy and complication rates, the indications for emergent transthoracic pacing are equally obscure. The technique may be considered in situations of bradyasystolic arrest unresponsive to medical management and in which transcutaneous and transvenous pacing are ineffective, unavailable, or prohibitively time-consuming to initiate.

Percutaneous transthoracic pacing requires a long introducing needle or cannula to access the ventricular cavity, a suitable bipolar or unipolar wire electrode capable of passage through the introducer, a standard temporary (transvenous) pacing generator, and appropriate electrical adapters. Convenient transthoracic pacing kits are highly recommended. A typical commercially available pacing kit provides a 15-cm, 18-gauge steel cannula and trocar, 32-cm bipolar J pacing wire (10-cm electrode spacing), and an electrical connector for adaptation to external pacing generators. Similar components are also available in a single assembled unit.

The right ventricular cavity is the preferred transthoracic wire position; however, left ventricular puncture will also yield successful pacing.[70] Atrial capture with percutaneous transthoracic pacing has not been documented. The right ventricle may be accessed from subxiphoid or left parasternal approaches (Figure 4.15). Studies using human cadavers suggest that left parasternal approaches may provide the greatest accuracy of placement with the fewest "injuries."[71] However, these results have not been validated in actual arrest patients undergoing cardiopulmonary resuscitation. Clinically, the subxiphoid approach is favored. To initiate pacing from this location, the introducing cannula with trocar is advanced to approximately 75 percent of its length from the left xiphochondral notch while being directed toward the left shoulder or sternal notch at an angle of 30 to 45 degrees to the skin (Figure 4.16). Free blood return should occur with removal of the trocar. Needles without trocars are introduced while aspirating until free blood return appears. Chest compressions should be discontinued during the introduction of needles or cannulas until the ventricle is entered. Full ventilation of the lungs is recommended during subxiphoid cannula placement to depress the diaphragm, thus minimizing the risk of liver or stomach injury. Severe kyphosis, scoliosis, or emphysema may complicate ventricular access. Once free blood return is obtained, the pacing wire is advanced through the cannula as far as possible. The cannula is removed from over

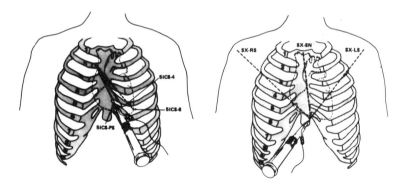

Figure 4.15   Approaches to the right ventricular cavity for percutaneous transthoracic cardiac pacing. (left) Parasternal approaches. 5ICS-PS = fifth intercostal space parasternally, 5ICS-4 and 5ICS-6 = fifth intercostal space 4 and 6 cm lateral to the sternum, respectively. (right) Subxiphoid approaches. SX-RS = subxiphoid directed toward right shoulder, SX-SN and SX-LS = subxiphoid directed toward sternal notch and left shoulder, respectively. All approaches are needle angles of approximately 30° to the skin. Clinically, the SX-SN or SX-LS approaches are recommended. Reproduced with permission from Brown CG, *Am J Emerg Med* 1985;3:193–198.

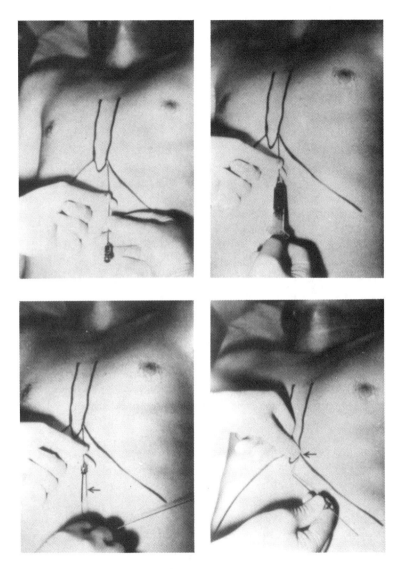

Figure 4.16 Transthoracic pacing wire insertion from the subxiphoid approach. (upper left) Cannula and trochar are advanced from the left xiphochondral notch toward the sternal notch at 30° to the skin. (upper right) After introduction to ¾ its length, the trochar is removed and free blood return is confirmed. (lower left) The pacing wire is straightened with a removable sleeve, then advanced to its full extent through the cannula. (lower right) The wire is secured to the skin as the cannula is withdrawn from over the wire. Reproduced with permission from Robert JR, *Ann Emerg Med* 1981;10:600–612.

the wire, and the electrodes are secured to a pacing generator set asynchronously at 80 to 100 ppm and at maximal output. In skilled hands, the wire can be positioned in as little as 10 to 60 seconds.[72] Failure to achieve capture necessitates manipulation and/or gradual withdrawal of the wire. Ideally, the distal electrode (cathode) should be intraventricular, and the proximal electrode (anode) should be intramyocardial or epicardial in location. The distal electrode need not contact endocardium for capture.[70] During unipolar transthoracic pacing, the intraventricular electrode serves as the cathode, and a subcutaneous wire lead serves as the anode. Capture thresholds range from 1 to 16 mA in animal studies[73] and from 1 to 6 mA in one study of humans.[71]

For left parasternal access, the cannula is advanced at 30° to the skin toward the right second costochondral junction from a site in the left fifth intercostal space immediately adjacent to or 6 cm lateral to the sternum (see Figure 4.15). If the parasternal approach is used, cannula manipulation during full expiration is recommended to minimize the risk of pneumothorax.

Following ventricular capture, the electrode is sutured securely to the skin. A chest x-ray is obtained to document the electrode location and to rule out pneumothorax. The morphology of paced QRS complexes may also localize the lead position (see Table 4.3). Replacement with a transvenous pacing system is recommended as soon as possible, given the undocumented stability of transthoracic leads.

The reported incidence of electrical capture by emergent transthoracic pacing varies from 4 to 100 percent in cardiac arrest patients.[68,72–74] Survival rates are invariably dismal (often 0) in large series;[68,74] however, small series have reported successful transthoracic pacing for up to three weeks in individual patients.[73] Although it is frequently successful in animal models and (from early literature) in nonarresting human subjects,[73] contemporary failure of the technique may stem from delayed application during cardiac arrest (up to 45 min in some studies), traditionally after the failure of medical therapy and conventional pacing techniques.[68] As mentioned, no controlled prospective studies exist that compare early utilization of transthoracic pacing with other modalities.

The analysis of complications of transthoracic pacing is greatly limited by the paucity of even short-term survivors and absence of radiographic or pathologic evaluation of nonsurvivors in most studies. Potential complications are those of vascular and visceral trauma from malpositioned leads, including laceration of the right atrium, ventricles, coronary arteries, great vessels, venae cavae, stomach, liver, and lung. Hemopericardium (up to 100 ml) is a ubiquitous finding in some autopsy studies,[69] and cardiac tamponade has been reported.[68] The development of tension pneumothorax is a particular concern in patients receiving positive pressure ventilation. Theoretically, puncture of ventricular aneurysms may result in elevated thresholds, extensive bleeding, or mobilization of mural thrombi. Nevertheless, a recent review found no evidence of death *directly* attributable to transthoracic pacing.[70] A study utilizing human cadavers suggests the left parasternal approach to minimize internal injury;[75] however, verification on arresting human subjects is lacking.

EPICARDIAL PACING

Transthoracic pacing is also possible using temporary pacing wires passively fixed to the atrial and ventricular epicardium at the time of cardiac surgery or thoracotomy. The wires, usually paired to each chamber with or without a third subcutaneous lead for unipolar pacing, are exposed through the skin in the subxiphoid region. Bipolar leads are also vailable. The wires should be appropriately marked as atrial or ventricular leads. If uncertain, the origin of the lead may be confirmed by pacing, timing unipolar electrograms from the lead with surface ECG signals, or chest x-ray examination. These leads are utilized in a similar fashion to transvenous leads; however, pacing and sensing thresholds tend to deteriorate progressively with time. The use of bipolar electrodes may minimize sensing and pacing failures, especially for atrial pacing.[76] Reversal of bipolar lead polarity or unipolarization of the leads may circumvent high thresholds.

TRANSESOPHAGEAL PACING

The close anatomic proximity of the esophagus to the posterior left atrium makes transesophageal *atrial* pacing possible in nearly all patients. The technique is relatively noninvasive, well tolerated, and virtually free of reported serious complications. Furthermore, the technique requires minimal training to perform successfully. *Ventricular* capture is inconsistent or often intolerably painful, however, thus seriously limiting the therapeutic and emergent applications of the technique.

201

Transesophageal pacing utilizes an intraesophageal electrode positioned in proximity to the heart to deliver stimulating electrical current to the myocardial tissue. The necessary equipment includes a suitable unipolar or bipolar electrode, a specialized transesophageal pulse generator with unique output characteristics, and an ECG recorder. A variety of leads are suitable for transesophageal pacing. Gelatin-encapsulated bipolar "pill" electrodes are convenient and well tolerated in patients capable of swallowing on command (Figure 4.17). Dedicated transesophageal pacing catheters have been introduced and are highly recommended (see Figure 4.17). Alternatively, flexible permanent or temporary transvenous pacing catheters may be used. Specially designed steerable or balloon electrode catheters, while possibly enhancing myocardial capture, are not commercially available.

Theoretically, the optimal interelectrode spacing for bipolar transesophageal pacing is directly proportional to 1.4 times the distance separating the excitable tissue from the midpoint between the pacing electrodes.[77] Fluoroscopic and anatomic studies reveal that the minimum distance from the esophagus to the left atrium in

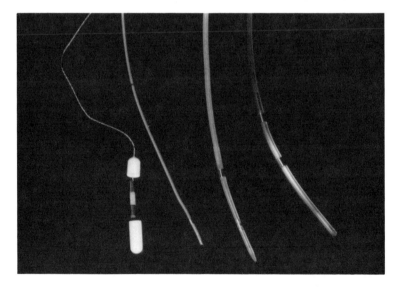

Figure 4.17 Transesophageal pacing catheters and electrodes. From left to right: pill electrode (8 mm spacing) and gelatin capsule; 5-Fr flexible plastic bipolar transvenous pacing catheter (10 mm spacing); implantable coronary sinus electrode (30 mm spacing); 10-Fr flexible transesophageal pacing catheter (30 mm spacing).

humans is 0.5 to 1.5 cm regardless of left atrial size.[78] Therefore, electrode spacings of 0.7 to 2.1 cm would appear optimal. Clinically, spacings of 1.0 to 3.0 cm yield comparable atrial pacing thresholds.[79–81] Interelectrode spacing greater than 30 mm offers the theoretical disadvantages of higher threshold currents and greater extracardiac tissue stimulation.

Transesophageal pacing generators must provide up to 25 to 30 mA of current output into transesophageal impedances of 700 to 2600 ohms.[79] High-voltage outputs of 40 to 75 V are thereby mandatory for these devices. Stimulation pulse width should be 10 to 20 msec in order to minimize pacing thresholds.[77,82] Demand pacing modes are not available. High output rates (>400 ppm) are useful for pacing termination of atrial dysrhythmias—a common application of transesophageal pacing. The short pulse width (1 to 2 msec) and low voltages (12 to 15 V) provided by temporary transvenous pacing generators are rarely adequate for transesophageal myocardial capture.

To initiate transesophageal pacing, the electrode is introduced orally (pill electrodes) or nasally (catheter electrodes), then advanced distally through the esophagus into proximity with the left atrium. Aspiration precautions should be observed during esophageal intubation, and other esophageal catheters (e.g., nasogastric tubes) should be removed if possible. Topical anesthesia to the nares and pharynx is recommended. Gelatin capsules dissolve in 2 to 3 minutes to fully expose the electrodes. The optimal esophageal site for atrial pacing is then identified by one of several methods. This site is best defined by the esophageal electrode position recording the largest peak-to-peak atrial electrogram (Figure 4.18).[82] Unipolar or bipolar electrograms may be used by connecting an electrode pole to lead V_1 (unipolar) or to each arm lead (bipolar) of a standard ECG recorder. Ideally, use of a commercially available preamplifier/filter unit enhances and clarifies the atrial electrograms by limiting respiratory, cardiac motion, and peristalsis artifacts. After introduction to 30 to 40 cm from the teeth or nares, the lead is moved proximally and distally until the largest atrial electrogram is recorded. Both unipolar and bipolar atrial electrograms are typically 0.8 to 0.9 mV in amplitude; however, bipolar recordings enhance the ratio of atrial to ventricular electrogram amplitudes to 3:1 compared with 0.8:1 for unipolar recordings.[83] The optimal site for atrial pacing generally lies at or within 3 cm proximally or distally of this point of maximally recorded atrial activity.[82] This site averages 35 to 40 cm from the teeth or nares in most adult studies.[81,82]

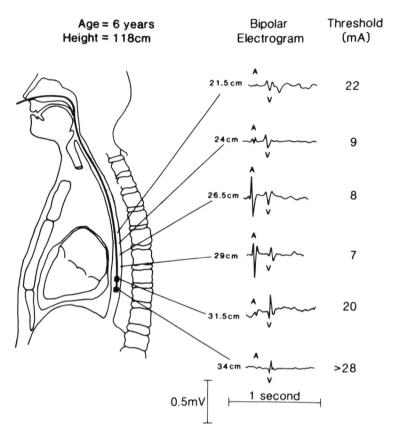

Age = 6 years   Bipolar   Threshold
Height = 118cm   Electrogram   (mA)

21.5cm   22

24cm   9

26.5cm   8

29cm   7

31.5cm   20

34cm   >28

0.5mV   1 second

Figure 4.18   Illustration depicting transesophageal cardiac electrograms obtained from various catheter insertion depths in a 6-year-old child. A = atrial electrogram, V = ventricular electrogram. Minimal transesophageal atrial pacing thresholds correspond to electrode positions recording the atrial electrograms of largest amplitude. Reproduced with permission of the American Heart Association from Benson DW, Transesophageal electrocardiography and cardiac pacing: State of the art. *Circulation* **1987;75 (Suppl III):III-86–III-90.**

The best esophageal site for atrial pacing may also be estimated from the patient's height;[82] however, this correlation is not universally accepted.[84] Empiric introduction of the lead to a depth of 35 to 40 cm from the teeth or nares may provide an adequate pacing location. The lead may be advanced or withdrawn during pacing until myocardial capture is documented. The optimal intraesophageal position for atrial pacing may vary with changes in the patient's posture and position.

The most favorable electrode position for transesophageal ventricular pacing is less well defined but appears to lie 2 to 4 cm distal to the best site for atrial pacing.[84] A ventricular electrogram should be recorded from sites of attempted ventricular pacing; otherwise, the ventricular electrogram amplitude is not helpful. Optimal atrial and ventricular pacing positions have been described at sites consistently 7 to 11 cm and 2 to 4 cm above the gastro-esophageal junction, respectively.[84] Clinically, rapid and accurate utilization of these positions is practical only with the use of specially designed balloon electrode catheters.

Once positioned, the electrodes are connected to the transesophageal pacing generator. Capture thresholds are reduced by cathodal (negative) stimulation through the proximal electrode in bipolar systems.[81] For unipolar systems, the esophageal pole should be cathodal, and the anode (positive) should be a large surface electrode affixed to the thorax or extremity.[81] Generally, pacing is begun at rates slightly above intrinsic heart rates to determine whether atrial and/or ventricular capture is present. Ventricular capture must be excluded before attempting rapid atrial pacing. In conscious subjects, current is begun at low settings, then increased until myocardial capture or intolerable discomfort is achieved. Virtually all patients experience at least a mild thoracic "burning" sensation with effective current outputs. In unconscious or hemodynamically compromised patients, pacing is started at high current outputs to ensure capture. Once capture is achieved, the lead is taped securely to the patient's nose or chin.

In most large series, the incidence of atrial capture with transesophageal pacing equals or approaches 100 percent with mean current thresholds of 8 to 14 mA.[77,79,85,86] Atrial capture thresholds are not influenced by age, height, weight, body surface area, left atrial size, previous coronary bypass surgery, presence of structural heart disease, or size of recorded atrial electrograms in most studies.[87,88] Thresholds greater than 15 mA are frequently associated with increased patient discomfort, but thresholds may be reduced by utilizing stimuli of longer pulse width.[82] Bipolar stimulation appears to provide lower atrial capture thresholds than does unipolar pacing.[81] Optimal lead position is paramount to effective atrial capture. Transesophageal atrial pacing is useful in heart-rate support of sinus bradycardia, in diagnosing or terminating a variety of reentrant supraventricular tachycardias, and diagnostically to induce myocardial ischemia and evaluate sinus node recovery times.[77,89,90]

Ventricular capture using transesophageal pacing is much less reliable. Using conventional transesophageal electrodes and pacing generators, ventricular capture is successful only in 3 to 60 percent of patients.[86,91] Ventricular capture has been reported in 89 percent of patients during arrest using high-voltage pacing generators,[92] however, and in 100 percent of patients using steerable or balloon electrodes.[84,93] Because stimulating current density declines exponentially with distance from the bipolar current source, the ventricle, typically about 3 cm from the esophagus, receives only 20 percent of the current density achieved at the left atrium during transesophageal pacing.[77,87] Therefore, ventricular capture generally requires significantly higher current outputs, of up to 80 mA. Ventricular capture is enhanced by more distal electrode positions (2 to 4 cm above the gastroesophageal junction) and possibly with unipolar pacing or wide-spaced bipolar leads due to more dispersion of current density. Rarely, ventricular pacing thresholds are below those for atrial pacing.[94] Stable transesophageal ventricular pacing has been maintained for up to 60 hours.[91]

To date, the reported serious complications of transesophageal pacing are limited to induction of ventricular tachyarrhythmias during rapid atrial pacing in two patients with prior history of ventricular tachycardia[86] and in one patient with hypertrophic cardiomyopathy.[95] No long-term pacing complications have been reported. Virtually all patients experience tolerable, mild chest or back pain, or burning or "indigestion" during pacing at outputs less than 15 mA.[77] Significant or intolerable discomfort becomes more likely at outputs above 15 to 20 mA and is almost universal above 30 to 50 mA.[81] Animal studies demonstrate visible esophageal lesions with submucosal inflammation following transesophageal pacing with 100 mA output for 10 to 20 minutes.[77] The lesions healed spontaneously within three days, and no esophageal perforation occurred. In humans, endoscopy following transesophageal pacing may reveal focal pressure necrosis typical of any indwelling esophageal catheter in up to 11 percent of patients.[77] Currents used for clinical applications are well below those producing esophageal lesions in animal studies, and no significant esophageal trauma had been reported in humans despite pacing up to 60 hours.[96] Aspiration is a potential complication of any esophageal intubation procedure. Diaphragmatic or phrenic nerve pacing may occur in 1 to 8 percent of patients, especially with distal esophageal catheter positions.[86,89] Coughing may be induced with proximal catheter positions due to tracheal stimulation, and brachial plexus stimulation has been reported in infants.[94]

SELECTION OF THE OPTIMAL TEMPORARY PACING TECHNIQUE

The urgency to initiate temporary cardiac pacing is the foremost consideration in selecting among the available techniques. For prophylactic and nonemergent applications, the duration of pacing, comfort of the patient, and desire to avoid specific complications also become significant. In emergent situations of bradyasystolic arrest, delayed recovery of an effective cardiac rhythm beyond five minutes virtually precludes successful resuscitation.[96] In these situations, *rapid* initiation of *ventricular* pacing is paramount to other considerations. Although transvenous pacing has traditionally served as the mainstay of emergent temporary pacing, the significant time and operator skill needed to implement the technique are less than ideal. As a result, renewed interest in transcutaneous pacing has provided an extremely rapid, simple, and noninvasive alternative to emergent transvenous pacing. The reported incidence of ventricular capture during arrests is quite variable for both techniques. This fact and the lack of prospective studies comparing efficacy of the various emergent pacing techniques prevent endorsement of one technique as superior to others in these settings. Given the narrow therapeutic time constraints in bradyasystolic arrest, it would appear most prudent to proceed with the mode of pacing that will effect ventricular pacing *most rapidly*. Attempts at transcutaneous pacing neither significantly interrupt nor impede performance of cardiopulmonary resuscitation (CPR), and it is usually feasible to attempt transcutaneous pacing while preparations are made for more invasive techniques. Successful transcutaneous pacing is rapid and may obviate the need for invasive procedures. Transvenous or possibly transthoracic pacing would follow failure of transcutaneous pacing and initial medical therapy. The incidence of complications and sequelae of transthoracic pacing is currently undefined—the gravity of the situation should outweigh this concern. Currently, transesophageal pacing, although potentially rapid, cannot be recommended as initial therapy given unreliable ventricular capture.

Of the available techniques, only transthoracic pacing is *inappropriate* for prophylactic or nonemergent use. Transcutaneous pac-

Table 4.8 Comparison of Temporary Pacing Techniques

Method	Time to Initiate	Chambers Paced	Advantages	Disadvantages	Uses
Percussion	Instantaneous	Ventricle	Simple, extremely rapid	Limited capture, short-term use only, dysrhythmias	Transient asystole or bradycardia
Cough resuscitation	Instantaneous	Neither	Simple, extremely rapid	Requires conscious, cooperative patient; short-term use only	Transient asystole or bradycardia
Transcutaneous	<1 min	Ventricle	Simple, rapid, safe	Variable capture, patient tolerance	Arrest, prophylactic
Transvenous	3–10 min	Atrium ventricle	Most reliable, well-	Invasive, time-consuming,	Arrest, prophylactic
Transthoracic	10–60 sec	Ventricle	Extremely rapid, relatively simple	Complications, efficacy unproven	Arrest only
Transesophageal	Minutes	Atrium	Reliable atrial capture, simple, safe	Poor ventricular capture, patient tolerance	Prophylactic atrial pacing, diagnostics, termination SVT

ing is extremely attractive in these settings, given its high efficacy combined with virtual absence of complications. Patient discomfort during pacing represents the only disadvantage. Temporary transvenous pacing, although invasive, provides well tolerated and generally reliable atrial and/or ventricular pacing for extended periods of time. Transesophageal pacing is suitable for most *atrial* pacing applications and finds greatest therapeutic utility in pace termination of atrial flutter and reentrant supraventricular dysrhythmias. Patient discomfort is sometimes a problem, but complications are exceptionally rare. Ventricular capture requires painfully high current outputs, but intraoperative use appears feasible. Mechanical and cough-induced resuscitation techniques are limited to very brief applications. Nevertheless, cough-induced resuscitation is an effective and standard maneuver during asystole induced by coronary angiography. A comparison of the available temporary pacing techniques is shown in Table 4.8.

REFERENCES

1. Chester WL. Spinal anesthesia, complete heart block and the precordial thump: An unusual complication and a unique resuscitation. *Anesth Analg* 1988;69:600–602.
2. Skaaland K. Effect of chest pounding: Electrocardiographic pattern. *Lancet* 1972;1:1121–1122.
3. Zoll PM, Belgard AH, Weintraub MJ, Frank HA. External mechanical cardiac stimulation. *N Engl J Med* 1976;294:1274–1275.
4. Scherf D, Bornemann C. Thumping of the precordium in ventricular standstill. *Am J Cardiol* 1960;5:30–40.
5. Iseri LT, Allen BJ, Baron K, Brodsky MA. Fist pacing, a forgotten procedure in bradysystolic cardiac arrest. *Am Heart J* 1987;113:1545–1550.
6. Caldwell G, Millar G, Quinn E, et al. Simple mechanical methods for cardioversion: Defences of the precordial thump and cough version. *Br Med J* 1985;291:627–630.
7. Margera T, Baldi N, Chersevani D, et al. Chest thump and ventricular tachycardia. *PACE* 1979;2:69–75.
8. Miller J, Tresch D, Horwitz L, et al. The precordial thump. *Ann Emerg Med* 1984;13:791–794.
9. Criley JM, Blaufuss AH, Kissel GL. Cough-induced cardiac compression: Self-administered form of cardiopulmonary resuscitation. *JAMA* 1976;236:1246–1250.

10. Wei JY, Greene HL, Weisfeldt ML. Cough-facilitated conversion of ventricular tachycardia. *Am J Cardiol* 1980;45:174–176.
11. Kelly JS, Royster RL. Noninvasive transcutaneous cardiac pacing. *Anesth Analg* 1989;69:229–238.
12. Falk RH, Ngai STA. External cardiac pacing: Influence of electrode placement on pacing threshold. *Crit Care Med* 1986;14(11):931–932.
13. Geddes LA, Voorhees WD III, Babbs CF, et al. Precordial pacing windows. *PACE* 1984;7:806–812.
14. Madsen JK, Pedersen F, Grande P, Meiborn J. Normal myocardial enzymes and normal echocardiographic findings during noninvasive transcutaneous pacing. *PACE* 1988;11:1188–1193.
15. Klein LS, Miles WM, Heger JJ, Zipes DP. Transcutaneous pacing: Patient tolerance, strength–interval relations and feasibility for programmed electrical stimulation. *Am J Cardiol* 1988;62:1126–1129.
16. Zoll PM, Zoll RH, Falk RH, et al. External noninvasive temporary cardiac pacing: Clinical trials. *Circulation* 1985; 71:937–944.
17. Falk RH, Ngai STA, Kumanki DJ, Rubinstein JA. Cardiac activation during external cardiac pacing. *PACE* 1987;10:503–506.
18. Kelly JS, Royster RL, Angert KC, Case LD. Efficacy of noninvasive transcutaneous cardiac pacing in patients undergoing cardiac surgery. *Anesth Analg* 1989;70:747–751.
19. Luck JC, Grubb BP, Artman SE, et al. Termination of sustained ventricular tachycardia by external noninvasive pacing. *Am J Cardiol* 1988;61:574–577.
20. Hedges JR, Syverud SA, Dalsey WC, et al. Threshold, enzymatic, and pathologic changes associated with prolonged transcutaneous pacing in a chronic heart block model. *J Emerg Med* 1989;7:1–4.
21. Prochaczek F, Birkui PJ, Galecka J, Jarczok K. Is the new electrode configuration a break point in transcutaneous cardiac tolerance? *Rev Eur Technol Biomed* 1994;16:98–101.
22. Altamura G, Bianconi L, Boccadamo R, Pistalese M. Treatment of ventricular and supraventricular tachyarrhythmias by transcutaneous cardiac pacing. *PACE* 1989;12:331–338.
23. Feldman MD, Zoll PM, Aroesty JM, et al. Hemodynamic responses to noninvasive external cardiac pacing. *Am J Med* 1988;84:395–400.

24. Niemann JT, Rosborough JP, Garner D, et al. External noninvasive cardiac pacing: A comparative hemodynamic study of two techniques with conventional endocardial pacing. *PACE* 1984;7:230–236.

25. Syverud SA, Hedges JR, Dalsey WC, et al. Hemodynamics of transcutaneous cardiac pacing. *Am J Emerg Med* 1986;4:17–20.

26. Trigano JA, Remond JM, Mourot F, et al. Left ventricular pressure measurement during noninvasive transcutaneous cardiac pacing. *PACE* 1989;12:1717–1719.

27. Murdock DK, Moran JF, Speranza D, et al. Augmentation of cardiac output by external cardiac pacing: Pacemaker-induced CPR. *PACE* 1986;9 (Part I):127–129.

28. Falk RH, Zoll PM, Zoll RH. Safety and efficacy of noninvasive cardiac pacing: A preliminary report. *N Engl J Med* 1983;309:1166–1168.

29. Zoll PM. Resuscitation of the heart in ventricular standstill by external electrical stimulation. *N Engl J Med* 1952;247:768–771.

30. Estes M, Deering TF, Manolis AS, et al. External cardiac programmed stimulation for noninvasive termination of sustained supraventricular and ventricular tachycardia. *Am J Cardiol* 1989;63:177–183.

31. Béland MJ, Hesslein PS, Rowe RD. Ventricular tachycardia related to transcutaneous pacing. *Ann Emerg Med* 1988;17:279–281.

32. Voorhees WD III, Foster KS, Geddes LA, Babbs CF. Safety factor for precordial pacing: Minimum current thresholds for pacing and for ventricular fibrillation by vulnerable-period stimulation. *PACE* 1984;7 (Part I):356–360.

33. Francis GS, Williams SV, Achord JL, et al. Clinical competence in insertion of a temporary transvenous ventricular pacemaker. *J Am Coll Cardiol* 1994;23:1254–1257.

34. Littleford PO, Pepine CJ. A new temporary atrial pacing catheter inserted percutaneously into the subclavian vein without fluoroscopy: A pereliminary report. *PACE* 1981;4:458–464.

35. Meier B, Rutishauser W. Coronary pacing during percutaneous transluminal coronary angioplasty. *Circulation* 1985;71:557–561.

36. Dailey EK, Tilkian AG. Venous access. In *Cardiovascular Procedures, Diagnostic Techniques and Therapeutic Procedures.* St. Louis: Mosby, 1986.

37. Syverud SA, Dalsey WC, Hedges JR, Hanseits ML. Radio-

logic assessment of transvenous pacemaker placement during CPR. *Ann Emerg Med* 1986;15:131–137.

38. Goldberger J, Kruse J, Ehlert FA, Kadish A. Temporary transvenous pacemaker placement: What criteria constitute an adequate pacing site? *Am Heart J* 1993;126:488–493.

39. Lang R, David D, Klein HO, et al. The use of the balloon-tipped floating catheter in temporary transvenous cardiac pacing. *PACE* 1981;4:491–496.

40. Furman S, Hurzeler P, Mehra R. Cardiac pacing and pacemakers. IV. Threshold of cardiac stimulation. *Am Heart J* 1977;94:115–124.

41. Rubenfire M, Anbe DT, Drake EH, Ormond RS. Clinical evaluation of myocardial perforation as a complication of permanent transvenous pacemakers. *Chest* 1973;63:185–188.

42. Gulotta SJ. Transvenous cardiac pacing: Techniques for optimal electrode positioning and prevention of coronary sinus placement. *Circulation* 1970;42:701–718.

43. Castellanos A, Maytin O, Lemberg L, Castillo C. Unusual QRS complexes produced by pacemaker stimuli with special reference to myocardial tunneling and coronary sinus stimulation. *Am Heart J* 1969;77:732–742.

44. Befeler B, Hildner FJ, Javier RP, et al. Cardiovascular dynamics during coronary sinus, right atrial, and right ventricular pacing. *Am Heart J* 1971;81:372–380.

45. Benchimol A, Ellis JG, Dimond EG. Hemodynamic consequences of atrial and ventricular pacing in patients with normal and abnormal hearts. *Am J Med* 1965;39:911–922.

46. Hartzler GO, Maloney JD, Curtis JJ, Barnhorst DA. Hemodynamic benefits of atrioventricular sequential pacing after cardiac surgery. *Am J Cardiol* 1977;40:232–236.

47. Hazard PB, Benton C, Milnor JP. Transvenous cardiac pacing in cardiopulmonary resuscitation. *Crit Care Med* 1981;9:666–668.

48. Phillips SJ, Butner AN. Percutaneous transvenous cardiac pacing initiated at bedside: Results in 40 cases. *J Thorac Cardiovasc Surg* 1970;59:855–858.

49. Davis MJE. Emergency ventricular pacing using a J-electrode without fluoroscopy. *Med J Aust* 1990;152:194.

50. Preston TA, Fletcher RD, Luccesi BR, Judge RD. Changes in myocardial threshold. Physiologic and pharmacologic factors in patients with implanted pacemakers. *Am Heart J* 1967;74:235–242.

51. Sowton E, Barr I. Physiologic changes in threshold. *Ann NY Acad Sci* 1969;167:678–685.
52. Krueger SK, Rakes S, Wilkerson J, et al. Temporary pacemaking by general internists. *Arch Intern Med* 1983;143:1531–1533.
53. Austin JL, Preis LK, Crampton RS, et al. Analysis of pacemaker malfunction and complications of temporary pacing in the coronary care unit. *Am J Cardiol* 1982;49:301–306.
54. Lumia FJ, Rios JC. Temporary transvenous pacemaker therapy. An analysis of complications. *Chest* 1973;64:604–608.
55. Harvey JR, Wyman RM, McKay RG, Baim DS. Use of balloon flotation pacing catheters for prophylactic temporary pacing during diagnostic and therapeutic catheterization procedures. *Am J Cardiol* 1988;62:941–944.
56. Silver MD, Goldschlager N. Temporary transvenous cardiac pacing in the critical care setting. *Chest* 1988;93:607–613.
57. Paulk EA, Hurst JW. Complete heart block in acute myocardial infarction. *Am J Cardiol* 1966;17:695–706.
58. Hynes JK, Holmes DR Jr, Harrison CE. Five-year experience with temporary pacemaker therapy in the coronary care unit. *Mayo Clin Proc* 1983;58:122–126.
59. Jowett NI, Thompson DR, Pohl JEF. Temporary transvenous cardiac pacing: A year's experience in one coronary care unit. *Postgrad Med J* 1989;65:211–215.
60. Lehmann MH, Cameron A, Kemp HG Jr. Increased risk of ventricular fibrillation associated with temporary pacemaker use during coronary arteriography. *PACE* 1983;6 (Part I):923–928.
61. Mooss AN, Ross WB, Esterbrooks DJ, et al. Ventricular fibrillation complicating pacemaker insertion in acute myocardial infarction. *Cath Cardiovasc Diag* 1982;8:253–259.
62. Weinstein J, Gnoj J, Mazzara JT, et al. Temporary transvenous pacing via the percutaneous femoral vein approach. *Am Heart J* 1973;85:695–705.
63. Nathan DA, Center S, Pina RE, et al. Perforation during indwelling catheter pacing. *Circulation* 1966;33:128–130.
64. Van Durme JP, Heyndrickx G, Snoeck J, et al. Diagnosis of myocardial perforation by intracardiac electrograms recorded from the indwelling catheter. *J Electrocard* 1973;6:97–102.
65. Nolewajka AJ, Goddard MD, Broun TC. Temporary transvenous pacing and femoral vein thrombosis. *Circulation* 1980;62:646–650.
66. Cohen SI, Smith KL. Transfemoral cardiac pacing and phlebitis. *Circulation* 1974;49:1018–1019.

67. Roe BB, Katz HJ. Complete heart block with intractable asystole and recurrent ventricular fibrillation with survival. *Am J Cardiol* 1965;15:401–403.
68. Tintinalli JE, White BC. Transthoracic pacing during CPR. *Ann Emerg Med* 1981;10:113–116.
69. Roberts JR, Greenburg MI, Crisant JW, Gayle SW. Successful use of emergency transthoracic pacing in bradyasystolic cardiac arrest. *Ann Emerg Med* 1984;13:277–283.
70. Roberts JR, Greenburg MI. Emergency transthoracic pacemaker. *Ann Emerg Med* 1981;10:600–612.
71. Brown CG, Hutchins GM, Gurley HT, et al. Placement accuracy of percutaneous transthoracic pacemakers. *Am J Emerg Med* 1985;3:193–198.
72. Gessman LJ, Wertheimer JH, Davison J, et al. A new device and method for rapid emergency pacing: Clinical use in 10 patients. *PACE* 1982;5:929–933.
73. Kodjababian GH, Gray RE, Keenan RL, Iseri LT. Percutaneous implantation of cardiac pacemaker electrodes. *Am J Cardiol* 1967;19:372–376.
74. White JD. Transthoracic pacing in cardiac asystole. *Am J Emerg Med* 1983;3:264–266.
75. Brown CG, Gurley HT, Hutchins GM, et al. Injuries associated with percutaneous placement of transthoracic pacemakers. *Ann Emerg Med* 1985;14:223–228.
76. Scherhag A, Gulbins H, Lange R, Saggaw W. Improved reliability of postoperative cardiac pacing by use of bipolar temporary pacing leads. *Eur J.C.P.E.* 1995;5:101–108.
77. Jenkins JM, Dick M, Collins S, et al. Use of the pill electrode for transesophageal atrial pacing. *PACE* 1985;8:512–527.
78. Binkley PF, Bush CA, Kolibash AJ, et al. The anatomic relationship of the esophageal lead to the left atrium. *PACE* 1982;5:853–859.
79. Kerr CR, Chung DC, Wickham G, et al. Impedence to transesophageal atrial pacing: Significance regarding power sources. *PACE* 1989;12:930–935.
80. Benson DW. Transesophageal electrocardiography and cardiac pacing: State of the art. *Circulation* 1987;75 (Suppl III):III-86–III-92.
81. Nishimura M, Katoh T, Hanai S, Watanabe Y. Optimal mode of transesophageal atrial pacing. *Am J Cardiol* 1986;57:791–796.
82. Benson DW, Sanford M, Dunnigan A, Benditt DG. Transesophageal atrial pacing threshold: Role of interelectrode

spacing, pulse width, and catheter insertion depth. *Am J Cardiol* 1984;53:63–67.

83. Hammill SC, Pritchett ELC. Simplified esophageal electrocardiography using bipolar recording leads. *Ann Intern Med* 1981;95:14–18.

84. Andersen HR, Pless P. Transesophageal pacing. *PACE* 1983;6:674–679.

85. Kerr CR, Chung DC, Cooper J. Improved transesophageal recording and stimulation utilizing a new quadripolar lead configuration. *PACE* 1986;9:644–651.

86. Gallagher JJ, Smith WM, Kerr CR, et al. Esophageal pacing: A diagnostic and therapeutic tool. *Circulation* 1982;65:336–341.

87. Dick M, Campbell RM, Jenkins JM. Thresholds for transesophageal atrial pacing. *Cath Cardiovasc Diag* 1984;10: 507–513.

88. Buchanan D, Clements F, Reves JG, et al. Atrial esophageal pacing in patients undergoing coronary artery bypass grafting: Effect of previous cardiac operations and body surface area. *Anesth Analg* 1988;69:595–598.

89. Backofen JE, Schauble JF, Rogers MC. Transesophageal pacing for bradycardia. *Anesth Analg* 1984;61:777–779.

90. Falk R, Werner M. Transesophageal atrial pacing using a pill electrode for the termination of atrial flutter. *Chest* 1987;92:110–114.

91. Lubell DL. Cardiac pacing from the esophagus. *Am J Cardiol* 1971;27:641–644.

92. Sadowski Z, Szwed H. The effectiveness of transesophageal ventricular pacing in resuscitation procedure of adults (abstract). *PACE* 1987;6:A–132.

93. Touborg P, Andersen HR, Pless P. Low-current bedside emergency atrial and ventricular cardiac pacing from the esophagus. *Lancet* 1982;1:166.

94. Benson DW, Dunnigan A, Benditt DG, Schneider SP. Transesophageal cardiac pacing: History, application, technique. *Clin Prog Pacing Electrophysiol* 1984;2:360–372.

95. Favale S, Di Biase M, Rizzo U, et al. Ventricular fibrillation induced by transesophageal atrial pacing in hypertrophic cardiomyopathy. *Eur Heart J* 1987;8:912–916.

96. Burack B, Furman S. Transesophageal cardiac pacing. *Am J Cardiol* 1969;23:469–472.

Techniques of Pacemaker Implantation

Jeffrey Brinker and Mark Midei

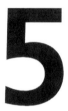

INTRODUCTION

A permanent pacing system consists of the pacemaker generator and the one or two leads that connect it to the endocardial or epicardial surface of the heart. Because of the initial mandate for epicardial lead placement, pacemaker implantation has traditionally been the task of the surgeon. Considerable evolution in technique and hardware has occurred over the past three decades,[1] however, which has greatly simplified the implantation procedure. The introduction of relatively simple and safe methods of central venous access has facilitated the almost universal adoption of transvenous leads, which are the most reliable means of pacing the heart. Associated with this has been a miniaturization of the power source and circuitry of the generator such that subcutaneous placement has become less demanding even in the very young or elderly. Now, compared to the need to formulate optimal programming prescriptions and interpret complex ECG–pacer–patient interactions, the implantation of a modern sophisticated pacemaker may be the least arduous aspect of pacing. Reflecting these changes has been the increasingly predominant role of the cardiologist, either alone or with a surgeon, in the implantation process. In this chapter, transvenous pacemaker implantation will be examined from a broad perspective emphasizing practical considerations that influence the safety and efficacy of this procedure.

PHYSICIAN QUALIFICATIONS

The practice of pacing overlaps a spectrum of the specialties and subspecialties of medicine and surgery. As suggested above, there has been increasing participation of nonsurgeons. Indeed, the subspecialty of electrophysiology has matured to such a degree that in many institutions much of the decision making concerning indications for pacemaker implantation, the procedure itself, and the follow-up has been assumed by this group. There remains, however, a large group of nonelectrophysiologist pacing enthusiasts who implant devices either alone or as part of a team (e.g., a surgeon obtains vascular access and makes a pocket while a physician places the lead, tests electrical parameters, and provides follow-up). Although some nonsurgeons are becoming more aggressive in learning to perform certain procedural variations such as inframammary or subpectoral dissections, most depend on their surgical colleagues for assistance in these more complicated situations.

Procedural success is determined by the skill and experience of the operator. Although the amount of "surgery" required for a transvenous implantation is modest, good surgical technique is essential. Experience is also necessary to ensure proper positioning of leads so that optimal stability and performance are obtained. A physician wishing to implant pacing systems independently should perform a sufficient number of procedures under the supervision of an accomplished operator to gain the skill and confidence necessary for independent work. The minimal number of cases to credential a physician depends on the physician's prior familiarity with intravascular catheterization, surgical technique, and knowledge of the principles of pacing. This experience should include single- and dual-chamber systems and use of both the subclavian and cephalic approaches for venous access. In addition to this initial exposure, there should be the expectation that a reasonable number of implantations will be performed over time to maintain a level of proficiency. Optimally, this number should be 30 procedures per year; a minimal number might be 10 to 15.[2] Recently,[3] guidelines for training in pacemaking have been published that, although directed at fellowship training, may serve as a more general model. Because fluoroscopic imaging is a necessary component of the implantation process, knowledge of the basics of radiation physics and safety is required to minimize risk to the patient and operator.[4]

If a team approach to implantation is taken, the role of each member must be clearly delineated. Although this may be obvious during the procedure, the responsibility for performance of periprocedural tasks such as writing orders, checking laboratory tests, adjusting the pacemaker, and arranging follow-up may be less clear.

Specialty assistance may be anticipated prior to a procedure in some cases, and appropriate consultation should be obtained. This might include enlisting the aid of a plastic surgeon for a procedure in a young woman or a pediatrician to help with a child. Implantation procedures are generally performed under conscious sedation, but, on occasion, there may be a need for support by anesthesiology. Operating physicians should be familiar with the principles of conscious sedation and the particular institutional guidelines under which they are employed, including acceptable drugs (dosages, reversibility), support personnel, monitoring equipment, and recovery procedures.

Quality assurance has become a necessary part of every hospital's activities. Procedures and physicians who perform them are most often examined. It is the responsibility of all physicians to be conscious of the quality of their work; those in administrative positions must ensure that proper databasing and performance evaluations are carried out. The objective of these practices is improved quality of care; this may be accomplished at many levels.[5]

LOGISTICAL REQUIREMENTS

The logistical requirements for pacemaker implantation are relatively modest.[6] The procedure may be carried out in an operating room, a catheterization laboratory, or a special procedure room with no compromise of success rate or difference in complications.[7] The room should be adequate in size and well lighted, and it should comply with all electrical safety requirements for intravascular catheterization. The radiographic equipment should function within accepted guidelines and appropriate shielding must be available and used.

In addition to the operator, staffing should include qualified individuals to monitor the ECG and help with the imaging equipment. A nurse (who may perform one of the aforementioned tasks) is required to prepare and administer medications. Often a representative of a pacemaker company is present to provide some assistance. These individuals may be a valuable source of information but should not substitute for a nurse or technologist during the implant procedure.

An adequate imaging system is an important requirement of the pacemaker laboratory. The image intensifier may be portable or fixed but must be capable of rotation so that oblique and lateral views of the areas of interest (which may extend from the neck to the groin) can be obtained. A mechanism for magnification is helpful for situations such as confirmation of extension of the helix of active fixation leads, lead removal procedures, and the identification of problems such as fractures of a retention wire.[8] Digital acquisition and storage capabilities have proven to be advantageous. Such technology can be used to "road-map" or superimpose real-time fluoroscopy on a stored image. This may facilitate venous access by storing an image of the subclavian vein (obtained by injecting contrast into an ipsilateral upper extremity vein) toward which the exploring needle is directed under fluoroscopic control (Figure 5.1). The use of pulsed digital fluoroscopy may reduce radiation exposure to patient and operator.

The patient's support should be flat, radiolucent, and configured in such a way that the operator may work on either side (and perhaps at either end). Movement of the imaging system about the support should be unhindered. A mechanism to assume Trendelenburg and reverse Trendelenburg positions is advantageous.

It is essential that the electrocardiogram be continuously monitored; a simultaneous multilead display that is easily visualized

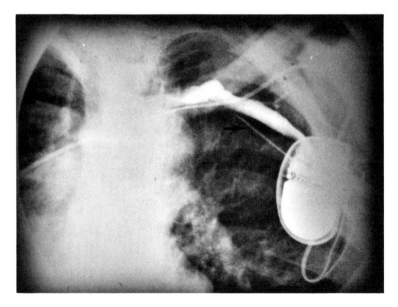

Figure 5.1 Venography may be helpful in documenting the patency of venous structures. In addition, road-mapping techniques facilitate needle (arrow) entry into the vein and avoidance of injury to preexisting leads.

is preferable. There should be an ability to obtain hard copy of the monitored rhythm strip as well as a complete 12-lead tracing if necessary. Leads placed on the chest or back should consist of radiolucent electrodes and wires. Special electrodes having the capability to monitor the ECG, deliver a direct current defibrillatory shock, or transcutaneously pace may be used. It is, of course, necessary that a defibrillator/cardioverter and temporary pacing system be available.

A mechanism for monitoring blood pressure throughout the procedure is necessary; this may be achieved by using an automated noninvasive device. Pulse oximetry may also be beneficial by providing information about the respiratory status of a heavily sedated patient or one in whom a complication (e.g., air embolism, pneumothorax) occurs. Pulse oximetry is necessary when heavy sedation is used.

The surgical instruments required for the procedure depend on the demands of the particular procedure and operator. A pacemaker tray may be derived from the hospital's surgical cutdown set supplemented in accordance to the specifics of the case. Add-ons include tear-away vascular introducer sets, appropriate cables to connect to a pacing system analyzer (PSA), suction, and electrocautery or battery-powered coagulators. The operator should be familiar with guidelines for electrocautery use to ensure safety, particularly when oxygen is being administered.

An adequate supply and variety of pacing hardware should be available, including not only pacemakers and leads but also sheaths, stylets, lead adapters, sterile lubricant and adhesive, disk electrodes for unipolarization, and the like. It is good practice to have at least two of every item on hand in case of accidental damage or loss of sterility.

The PSA (Figure 5.2) provides a mechanism to measure a variety of pacing parameters (capture and sensing threshold, lead impedance, electrograms, slew rate) that are essential in determining the adequacy of lead position and integrity. Direct digital readout and the capability to print a hard copy are desirable. These devices may also be used to evaluate the function of the pacing generator; because of inherent pacemaker diagnostic capabilities, however, this capability is now rarely used.

Equipment necessary for pericardiocentesis and emergency pacing must be at hand, and it is advantageous to have prompt access to a two-dimensional echocardiography machine. A crash cart containing resuscitative supplies (including those necessary to establish endotracheal intubation), an adequate supply of appropri-

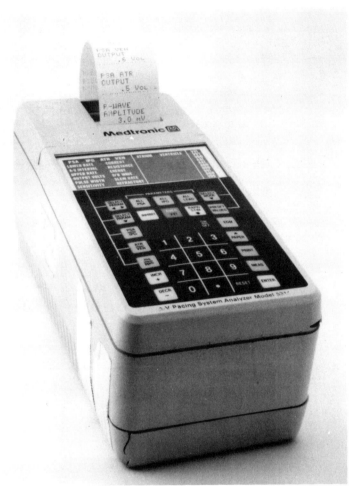

Figure 5.2 Medtronic Model 5311 Pacing System Analyzer (PSA). This device can measure capture and sensing thresholds and record intracardiac electrograms.

ate drugs, and experienced staff must be immediately available should complications occur.

ASSESSMENT OF THE PATIENT

The implantation process begins with an evaluation of the patient. This should include reviewing medical records, obtaining a pertinent history (including previous reactions to drugs and contrast

221

material), performance of a physical examination, and acquisition of basic laboratory tests. The indication for pacing should be clear and characterized in accordance with the American College of Cardiology/American Heart Association guidelines.[9] Documentation of the indication should be made in the patient's chart and should be supported by a relevant ECG tracing.

Consideration of the type of pacing system to be used should be part of the initial assessment so that a truly "informed" consent

---

Table 5.1 Consideration of Site and Approach for Implants

1. Recent or current pacer or central line
2. Infection or dermatitis
3. Anomalous venous drainage
4. Patient right- or left-handedness
5. Need for imminent thoracotomy (e.g., valve replacement)
6. Hemiparesis
7. Radiation therapy
8. Previous surgery (e.g., mastectomy)
9. Superior vena cava occlusion
10. Tricuspid valve replacement
11. History of clavicular fracture

Table 5.2 Consideration of Pacing Hardware

1. Active fixation lead
   A. Heart transplant
   B. Corrected transposition of great vessels
   C. Dilated right ventricle
   D. Tricuspid regurgitation
   E. Pulmonary hypertension
   F. Retained pacing lead in same chamber
   G. Outpatient procedure
   H. Post heart surgery (e.g., Mustard procedure)
2. Special leads
   A. Steroid-eluting (e.g., exit block, ? routine)
   B. Single-lead VDD system
   C. Sensor (e.g., temperature, oxygen saturation)
3. Small generator
   A. Child
   B. Anticipated difficulty with pocket
4. Lead adaptor/extender
   A. Interface preexisting lead with new generator
   B. Generator placement remote from venous access site

can be obtained. The decision on mode of pacing (e.g., atrial, ventricular, dual-chamber, single- or double-lead, rate-adaptive) is made on the basis of the underlying conduction disturbance, the presumed immediate and future need for pacing, and the hemodynamic status of the patient. Other factors that might influence the method of implantation, the operative site, or the type of hardware needed should be delineated prior to the procedure (Tables 5.1 and 5.2). Examples include need for an epicardial lead system in a patient with a previously documented venous anomaly, the use of active fixation ventricular leads in a patient with severe tricuspid regurgitation or corrected transposition of the great vessels, and the use of a steroid lead in a patient with a pacing history complicated by exit block.

COST-EFFECTIVENESS

Great emphasis is currently being placed on the cost-effectiveness of medical care, especially those aspects of care that are procedurally centered. Ideally, attention to cost-effectiveness is accompanied by increased quality of care. Clearly, length of hospital stay is of primary concern, but hospital administrators have increasingly focused on the throughput of patients, the cost of specific devices, and the level of patient satisfaction. Mechanisms of clinical practice improvement that may reduce cost yet increase the quality of care have been employed.[10] Practice guidelines, critical paths, and other methods of standardizing care will likely become more widespread. Physicians must continue to play a leading role in cost constraint without compromising optimal patient care.

INFORMED CONSENT

It is the implanting physician's responsibility to obtain informed consent from the patient (or the patient's family) prior to the procedure. An honest appraisal of the anticipated risks and benefits, acute and long-term, must be given along with an explanation of alternatives. There should be a discussion not only of why pacing is being offered but also of why a particular mode of pacing is being entertained. The need for lifelong follow-up should be emphasized, and mention should be made of the eventuality of generator (and possibly lead) replacement.

It is good practice for the physician to establish a rapport with the patient and the patient's family. One should ensure that all their questions are answered, and although fears concerning the procedure should be allayed, it is important that no guarantees regarding outcome be given. The participation of other physicians at the time of implantation or during follow-up should be described. The various members of the team should be in agreement about all aspects of the procedure so that the presentation to the patient is not confused.

PREIMPLANTATION ORDERS

Although outpatient pacemaker implantation can be performed, it is usual practice to admit the patient to the hospital. This may be done on the day of the procedure if the patient's medical condition does not in itself mandate prior hospitalization. Routine preimplant laboratory tests include posteroanterior and lateral chest x-rays, a 12-lead electrocardiogram, complete blood count, prothrombin and partial thromboplastin times, serum electrolytes, BUN, and creatinine.

Food is withheld for six to eight hours prior to the procedure. Hydration is maintained by the establishment of an intravenous line, preferably with a large-bore cannula in a vein of the upper extremity *ipsilateral* to the intended implant site. This will facilitate the injection of contrast should difficulty be encountered in achieving venous access. In general, the patient is allowed to continue whatever medication he or she has been taking, with the obvious exception of anticoagulants, which are stopped prior to the procedure (see below). The dosage of insulin or oral hypoglycemics may require temporary alteration.

Patients on oral anticoagulant therapy can be converted to intravenous heparin, which can be stopped four to six hours prior to implant if there is concern about the duration of time during which the patient is not effectively anticoagulated (e.g., mechanical heart valve procedure). Heparin may be restarted 8 to 12 hours after the procedure and warfarin may be reinitiated the day of the procedure or even the night before.

Antibiotic prophylaxis is controversial; however, there has been a suggestion that its use, either systemic or local, decreases the incidence of infection.[11-14] We routinely give a drug active against staphylococcus prior to the procedure and for 24 hours after the procedure. Procedures that are prolonged, complicated by potential breaches in sterility, or "redo" procedures are empirically given slightly longer courses of therapy (3–5 days).

The implant site (typically the area from above the nipple line to the angle of the jaw bilaterally) should be shaved and cleaned prior to the patient's arrival in the pacemaker laboratory. Mild sedation (e.g., 5–10 mg valium and 25–50 mg benadryl PO) is given augmented by intravenous sedatives/analgesics during the procedure (e.g., 0.5–1 mg midazolam, 25–50 µg fentanyl) as needed.

Care should be taken not to oversedate patients, especially the elderly. Drugs to reverse sedation should be readily available: flumazenil in 0.2 mg increments IV reverses midazolam; naloxone in 0.2 mg increments IV reverses fentanyl. On rare occasions for particular patients (children, emotionally disturbed persons, etc.), light general anesthesia may be needed. If such a situation is anticipated, appropriate arrangements with an anesthesiologist should be made in advance.

PATIENT PREPARATION

On entering the procedure room, the patient is placed on the support in such a way as to facilitate access to the specific operative site. Physiologic monitoring (ECG, automated blood pressure, and pulse oximetry) should be quickly established so that rhythm disturbances may be detected and treated. The operative site is prepared with an antiseptic solution, wiped dry, and a plastic adhesive sterile field is applied. Disposable towels and drapes are liberally applied to provide a large sterile work place and to minimize the risk of accidental contamination. A separate adhesive plastic pocket is affixed to the lateral aspect of the procedure site to collect draining fluid and sponges. A sterile plastic cap is placed over the image intensifier and leaded glass shield (if used) to avoid inadvertent contamination of the sterile field.

IMPLANT PROCEDURE
Site

Access to the right heart for permanent pacing has been achieved by introducing leads into any of a number of veins including the subclavian, cephalic, internal or external jugular, and iliofemoral.[15] Typically, the choice of venous entry site determines where the generator will be housed, although lead extenders can be used when necessary to allow a more remote positioning of the device. In most cases a cephalic or subclavian vein is used, and the pacemaker is placed subcutaneously in the adjacent subclavicular region.

On occasion, however, the generator may be implanted under the pectoral muscle or in an abdominal position. For women in whom there is a concern about cosmetic appearance, an inframammary incision may be performed and the pacemaker placed under the breast.[16] In such circumstances it may be wise to enlist the assistance of a plastic surgeon.

The site of implant is influenced by the factors listed in Table 5.1. Most often the left side is chosen because most patients are right handed and there is a less acute angle between the left subclavian and the innominate vein than exists on the right side. A disadvantage of utilizing the left side is the small (0.3–0.5 percent) incidence of persistent left superior vena cava with drainage into the coronary sinus, which complicates lead positioning. Suspicion of this anomaly may be raised by finding greater distention and a double A wave in the left jugular vein compared with that of the right vein, a left paramediastinal venous crescent on chest x-ray, and an enlarged coronary sinus on echocardiography.[17] Contrast echocardiography or catheterization will confirm the diagnosis. Although both single-chamber ventricular (Figure 5.3) and dual-chamber systems[18] have been placed through a persistent left superior vena cava via the coronary sinus, it is preferable to approach implantation from the right side when this anomaly exists.

Rarely, there is a coexistent absence of the right superior vena cava with all brachycephalic flow entering into the coronary sinus. Such a condition should be excluded before implantation is attempted from the right side in patients with a persistent left superior vena cava. Epicardial implants remain an option for patients with anomalous venous drainage.

Venous access: Figure 5.4 illustrates the two major easily identifiable landmarks (clavicle and deltopectoral groove) for implantation in a left infraclavicular site. Venous access into either the subclavian or cephalic vein is usually achieved through an incision that will also serve as the portal for subcutaneous generator placement. Local anesthetic is injected through a small-gauge needle along a line 4 to 6 cm in length and two fingerbreadths below and parallel to the clavicle. If the cephalic vein is used, the incision begins about 0.5 cm lateral to the deltopectoral groove and is extended medially; otherwise, the incision may be placed medial to the groove. This method provides adequate exposure for access to either the subclavian or cephalic vein. Some operators begin with a smaller incision specifically located to achieve venous access, after which

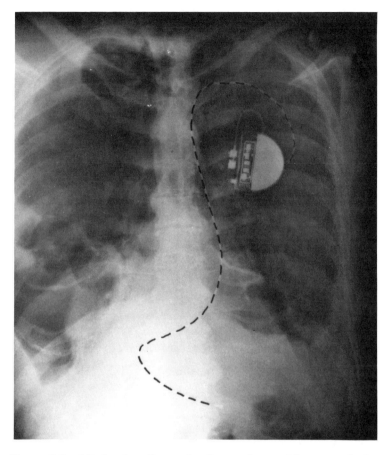

Figure 5.3 AP chest radiograph of a patient with a ventricular demand pacemaker placed through a congenitally persistent left superior vena cava.

the incision is extended or a new one is made for the pocket. This is obviously necessary when the internal or external jugular venous approach is chosen. In the latter situation, the leads are tunneled over or under the clavicle to the generator, which is placed in the usual pectoral position.

Pacing leads may be introduced through a venotomy in an exposed vein (cephalic, jugular, iliofemoral), or venous access may be achieved using the Seldinger technique. The latter approach provides easy access to a relatively large central vein, obviating the need for surgical dissection. In addition, the use of the dilator–

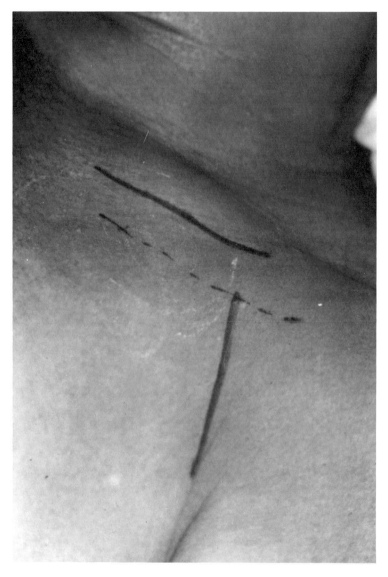

Figure 5.4 Surface landmarks in a patient about to undergo pace-maker implantation. The top solid line indicates the inferior margin of the left clavicle. The dashed line 2.0 cm beneath indicates site of incision, from which access to both the subclavian vein and the cephalic vein is possible. The more vertical solid line indicates the deltopectoral groove in which the cephalic veins are found.

sheath technique facilitates the introduction of multiple large leads and provides a means (via a retained guidewire) to reenter the venous system should that be necessary (e.g., if change from a passive to an active fixation lead is needed because a stable position is not found with the former). Nevertheless, the blind subclavian stick poses the risk of injury to nearby structures, including the artery, lung, thoracic duct, and nerves, and it is the most hazardous part of the implantation procedure.[2]

The subclavian method: The Seldinger approach to the subclavian vein has long been a popular method of gaining rapid access to the central venous circulation. The introduction of the tear-away sheath provided an effective means for the insertion of permanent pacemaker leads,[19-21] and this method is now the most frequently employed.[22] The efficacy and safety of subclavian entry is increased by taking measures to distend the vein (proper hydration, leg elevation) and place it in the proper position (by placing a wedge under the patient's shoulders and by adduction of the ipsilateral upper extremity).

An 18-gauge needle attached to a 10-ml syringe containing a few milliliters of local anesthetic is introduced through an incision that has been bluntly dissected to the underlying prepectoral fascia. The tip of the needle is advanced, bevel down, along this tissue plane at the level of the junction of the medial and middle thirds of the clavicle and directed toward a point just above the sternal notch. Small amounts of anesthetic may be injected along this course. On reaching the clavicle, the needle's angle of entry with respect to the thorax is increased until the tip slips under the bone. Negative pressure is exerted on the syringe as the needle is advanced so that blood is aspirated on entrance into the vein.

Once under the clavicle, the needle should not be redirected; doing so may lacerate underlying structures. If venous entry is not obtained, the needle should be withdrawn, cleared of any obstructing tissue, and reinserted in a slightly different direction. Inadvertent arterial entry is apparent with the appearance of pulsatile bright red blood. Prompt withdrawal of the needle and compression at its entry site under the clavicle is usually all that is necessary to close the entry point. Repeated unsuccessful attempts to enter the vein suggest a deviation in anatomy or occlusion of the vessel. In either situation, the risk of complication is increased with additional "blind" needle insertions; no more than three such attempts should be made, at which point one should consider a contrast injection to determine vessel patency and to provide a "road map" to its site.

Adequate opacification of the subclavian vein is achieved by the injection of a bolus of 20 to 40 cc of iodinated contrast through a large-bore cannula in an ipsilateral arm vein. This should be followed immediately by injection of saline to hasten transit of the contrast solution. The amount of fluid and rate of injection is gauged by fluoroscopic observation of the course of dye into the central veins. It is important that enough contrast be used and that adequate time be given for the contrast to fill the subclavian vein or collaterals. If the vessel is patent, there is often enough lingering contrast to allow an exploring needle to be directed at it.

It is helpful to record the injection on videotape or digitally so that the procedure may be reviewed. Some digital systems allow superimposition of real-time fluoroscopy on a stored contrast-filled image, which greatly facilitates the procedure (see Figure 5.1). This technique may be especially useful in upgrade procedures as a way to avoid needle damage to a preexisting lead. On occasion, a formal venogram may be obtained to document the status of the venous system prior to or after implantation (Figure 5.5).

On successful entry of the needle into a vessel, the character of the aspirated blood is examined. Dark nonpulsatile flow suggests a venous location; however, nonpulsatile flow does not exclude arterial entry, and pulsatile flow is sometimes noted from a vein (e.g., tricuspid regurgitation, right heart failure, cannon waves). Once vascular access is achieved, the syringe is detached (taking care to prevent air from entering the venous system) and a J-tipped guidewire is inserted through the needle and advanced under fluoroscopy to the inferior vena cava (IVC). If this is accomplished, inadvertent aortic entry is precluded; merely observing the guidewire coursing to the right of the sternum or even into a ventricular chamber does not exclude its presence in a tortuous ascending aorta or its passing retrograde into the left ventricle.

If resistance to advancement of the guidewire is encountered, the guidewire should be withdrawn through the needle with great care to prevent shearing off the distal wire by the needle tip. If any difficulty is encountered with withdrawal, either the wire and the needle should be withdrawn together or, if enough wire has been passed into the vein, the needle may be withdrawn and a small lumen plastic catheter advanced over the wire and into the vein. In the latter situation, contrast may then be injected through

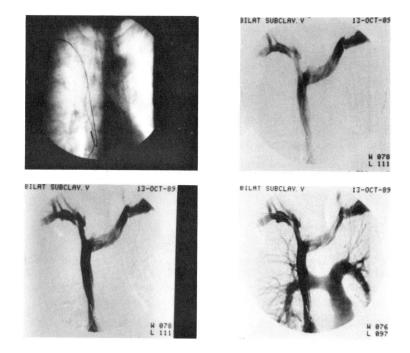

Figure 5.5 Digital imaging of simultaneous bilateral brachial venous injection of contrast provides excellent definition of subclavian venous anatomy and the superior vena cava. This patient was thought to have superior vena caval obstruction prohibiting the insertion of a replacement for fractured ventricular lead. Scout radiograph prior to contrast injection (top left). Sequential imaging (from top right, to bottom left and then bottom right) reveals patency of venous system. A new lead was then successfully placed via the subclavian venous approach.

the catheter to identify the problem and a more torqueable wire that may be directed appropriately can be introduced.

Once the wire is positioned in the IVC, a commercially available peel-away sheath–dilator combination (9–12 Fr) may be advanced over the wire into the superior vena cava, which will provide access for the introduction of pacing leads. The relatively stiff, straight dilator may be molded into a gentle curve by the operator prior to insertion. Advancement of the device under the clavicle may be facilitated by torquing it as if it were being screwed into place. Considerable resistance may be encountered if the subclavian vein has been entered medially through a fibrous or

231

calcified ligament. The use of a stiffer guidewire may be advantageous in such a situation, as might the passage of initially small, then progressively larger dilators. Entrance into such a location may be a marker for future lead entrapment, however, and one may consider seeking a more lateral entry site (see below). Excessive force should not be necessary once the sheath has entered the vein. Fluoroscopic confirmation of proper alignment of dilator and wire is necessary if resistance is encountered. On occasion, countertraction on the wire while advancing the dilator is helpful. The sheath should not be allowed to slide over the tapered tip of the dilator, nor should the dilator be unprotected by a guidewire during advancement.

Once properly positioned in the superior vena cava, the dilator is removed while the guidewire is retained within the sheath to allow for the introduction of a second sheath if necessary. A clamp may be applied to the end of the guidewire to prevent its accidental migration into the vein. Care should be taken to limit the possibility of the aspiration of air through the large-bore open sheath by pinching its orifice until the lead is inserted. The patient should not be heavily sedated and should be instructed to avoid inspiration during this process. Recently, tear-away sheaths with hemostatic valves have been introduced, which may be helpful in preventing air embolism. The pacing lead is introduced alongside the guidewire and advanced into the right atrium or IVC, at which time the sheath is withdrawn and peeled apart proximal to the venous entry site to prevent injury to the vessel. If a dual-chamber device is to be employed, the retained wire is used to introduce a second sheath. If only one lead is to be utilized, it is still wise to retain the guidewire so that venous reentry is facilitated should the lead prove inadequate. It has been suggested that the use of a larger single sheath may be beneficial by allowing the two leads to be introduced simultaneously.[20] The risk of air embolism would seem greater in this situation, however.

Recently, attention has been directed at the role that the lead insertion site may play in the development of lead failure. It has been suggested that medial access to the subclavian vein may result in entrapment of the lead between the subclavius muscle and the costoclavicular ligament.[23–25] Forces exerted on leads placed through this traditional subclavian technique may predispose to insulation failure. This has led to the development of techniques to access the axillary vein by direct needle stick.[26,27] Although these approaches are not yet generally employed, a more lateral access to the central venous circulation, which avoids the effects of the medial subclavicular musculotendinous complex, is relatively easily achieved by cephalic vein cutdown.

The cephalic vein approach: The cephalic vein resides in the space between the deltoid and pectoral muscles. This area is readily identified by palpation and is occupied by loose connective tissue and fat, which is easily separated to reveal the underlying vein that sometimes lies fairly deep in this groove. The consistent course of this vessel, its reasonable size, and the direct path it takes to the central venous system recommend it for lead placement. Prior to the introduction of the peel-away-sheath method to enter the subclavian vein, the cephalic approach was the most frequent route of venous access for endocardial pacing. On occasion, however, this vessel is small, consists of a plexus of tiny veins rather than a larger single channel, or takes a circuitous route to the subclavian vein. These conditions may make lead insertion difficult or impossible. In addition, the inability to insert two leads routinely into the cephalic vein has limited the opportunity to utilize this approach for dual-lead systems.

The greatest benefit of the cephalic approach is its margin of safety compared with that of the subclavian stick—there is almost no risk of pneumo- or hemothorax. One may take advantage of this method of accessing the central venous system by inserting a guidewire through a cephalic venotomy (which can be accomplished with a cephalic vein of almost any size). A dilator–introducer sheath combination may then be utilized as described above for the retained wire method in the subclavian approach.[28] Although the cephalic vein itself may be sacrificed by this procedure, it often dilates to accommodate the leads and remain intact. In either case, the guidewire provides virtually unlimited access to the subclavian vein.

Rarely, the cephalic vein takes an aberrant course or a pectoral vein is inadvertently accessed. In such cases the guidewire may easily enter the subclavian vein; however, it may not be possible to manipulate a sheath over the wire successfully, which necessitates abandoning the technique. In other cases the vein may spasm or be invaginated by passage of the dilator, which essentially traps the sheath. Application of a vasodilator (e.g., nitroglycerine) or actually cutting the constricting vein, exposed by pulling back on the dilator, may be necessary to fully insert the sheath. Despite these potential limitations of the cephalic technique, an experienced operator can successfully implant leads by this approach in most cases in which it is attempted.

THE PACEMAKER POCKET

The pacemaker is usually placed in a subcutaneous position near the site of venous entry. Generators have continued to decrease in size and can be placed quite easily in most patients, including those having a paucity of subcutaneous tissue. Most often, the device is placed in the infraclavicular area through the incision used to obtain venous access. Local anesthesia is applied to the subcutaneous tissue, which is then dissected down to the prepectoral fascia. A pocket directed inferomedially and large enough to accommodate both the generator and redundant lead is made in this tissue plane by blunt dissection using the fingers. Too small a pocket may result in tension exerted on the overlying tissue by the implanted hardware; too large a pocket invites future migration or "flipping over" of the generator. Augmentation of anesthesia with a rapidly acting parenteral agent is recommended during the brief period of time it takes for pocket creation because this may be the most uncomfortable part of the procedure for the patient. Attention to hemostasis is necessary, but significant bleeding rarely accompanies blunt dissection in the proper tissue plane. On completion of its formation, the pocket may be temporarily packed with radiopaque sponges soaked in antibacterial solution.

Pockets located at a distance from the site of lead insertion require that the leads (with or without extenders) be tunneled through subcutaneous tissue to its location. A simple method for tunneling leads from the infraclavicular site to a submammary pacemaker pocket utilizing a long needle, guidewire, and dilator–introducer sets has been described by Roelke et al.[29]

LEAD INSERTION

A variety of leads are available for endocardial placement. They differ in composition, shape, electrode configuration, and method of fixation. Special leads that contain steroid-eluting collars[30] or biosensors are also now available. Passive fixation leads have tines or fins that anchor them in the trabeculated right ventricle or atrial appendage; active fixation leads employ a helix that provides a mechanism for actually fixing the lead to the endocardium. The helix may be extrudable and retractable or may be fixed at the tip.

In the latter situation, the helix is covered with an absorbable agent to facilitate passage of the lead to its site of implantation, by which time absorption of the material exposes the helix and allows it to be fixed to the heart. Both active and passive types of leads have advantages[31–33] and disadvantages[34,35] (Table 5.3) and may be used for either atrial or ventricular placement (see Chapter 2). Steroid-eluting active fixation leads may offer some benefit in terms of lowered subacute and possibly chronic thresholds.[36] Despite the progress in lead design and their overall excellent performance, the failure over time of several models of these devices remains a cause for concern.[37]

Prior to introduction, leads should be inspected for imperfections and, if they are to be inserted through a sheath, to confirm that this can be done easily in the presence of a retained guidewire. Active fixation leads should be tested to ensure that the helix extrudes and retracts appropriately. Care should be taken to ensure that the screw does not pick up debris during this process. It is important to confirm that the connector pin of the lead is appropriate for the generator that has been selected (see Chapter 2, Figures 2.27 and 2.28). The suture sleeve should be positioned at the proximal portion of the lead and prevented from migrating distally during lead placement.

Stylets are used to supply a degree of stiffness and shapeability to the lead. The stylets may vary in stiffness and length and in some cases are specially configured to engage an active fixation mechanism. They must be matched for a specific purpose to the lead. Stylets should be kept clean and dry to facilitate insertion and

---

Table 5.3   Lead Characteristics

1. Active fixation lead
   A. Easy passage
   B. Low acute dislodgment rate
   C. Unrestricted positioning
   D. Easier removal of chronic implant
   E. Higher capture thresholds
2. Passive fixation lead
   A. Greater electrode variety
   B. Lower thresholds
   C. More difficult passage
   D. More difficult chronic removal
   E. Higher early dislodgment rate

withdrawal from the lead. Torque applied to a shaped stylet may help rotate the lead. Although not required to retract the lead, the stylet provides "body" and may be needed to advance the lead to optimize position.

Leads may be inserted directly into a venotomy or through a peel-away sheath. The venous system is usually traversed easily, and the lead placed in the IVC or right atrium pending introduction of a second lead or removal of the sheath. On occasion there may be difficulty in advancing the lead through the sheath. This is more common when there is a sharp angle to be negotiated and the sheath kinks. The temptation to force the lead through the sheath should be resisted to avoid damage to the lead. Withdrawing the sheath slightly, advancing the retained guidewire along with the lead, and sometimes withdrawing the stylet to soften the lead tip may prove helpful.

Although the retained-guidewire approach facilitates the insertion of two leads required for dual-chamber pacing, manipulation of one lead may affect the position of the other. There is also a potential for a lead or guidewire to be withdrawn accidentally if they are not attended to closely. It has been suggested that two independent sheaths be used and not withdrawn until both leads have been positioned, or that separate venous sites (e.g., cephalic and subclavian or two separate subclavian entry sites) be accessed for each lead. If a modicum of care is taken, however, two leads may be positioned by using the retained-guidewire technique, which is quicker and probably safer than the alternative approaches.

Although good fluoroscopic imaging is a key to successful lead implantation, in unusual situations, such as a pregnant patient, echocardiography has been used to position leads to limit radiation exposure.[38,39]

Ventricular lead positioning

In dual-chamber systems, the ventricular lead is usually positioned first because it may supply back-up pacing, its position is usually a bit less tenuous than that of the atrial lead, and it is usually considered the most important of the leads. On occasion the lead may seem to enter the right ventricle with little assistance from the operator, but more often some manipulation is necessary. Withdrawing the stylet a few inches allows one to catch the lead tip in the right atrium; further advancement will cause the formation of a J shape with the distal lead, which may then be rotated toward the tricuspid valve. Slight retraction results in prolapse into the right ventricle, at which time the lead can be either advanced into the pulmonary artery or directed down toward the apex by advancing the stylet while the lead is slowly pulled back. Entrance into the pulmonary artery confirms that the lead has traversed the right ventricle and is neither in the atrium nor in the coronary sinus. The lead may then be pulled back as the stylet is advanced (as described above).

Once the lead tip falls toward the apex, the patient is asked to inspire deeply and the lead is advanced into place. This procedure is often accompanied by ventricular ectopy, the absence of which suggests that the lead is not in the ventricle. An alternative method of gaining entry to the ventricle is to form the stylet into a dogleg or a J shape and use it to direct the lead across the tricuspid valve. Once in the right ventricle, the shaped stylet may be replaced with a straight one to facilitate positioning at the apex.

The proper fluoroscopic appearance of the ventricular endocardial lead is one in which the lead's tip is well to the left of the spine and is pointing anteriorly and caudal (Figures 5.6 and 5.7).

In the anteroposterior projection it may not be possible to distinguish whether a lead is in a posterior coronary vein, the left ventricle, or the right ventricular apex. Oblique views and the electrocardiographic pattern of ventricular activation during pacing may be helpful (Figures 5.8 and 5.9). In patients with left ventricular prominence and/or counterclockwise rotation of the heart, the lead tip may not appear to extend far enough to the left border of the cardiac silhouette. Imaging in the right anterior oblique position may be helpful in such circumstances; observing the position of the lead with respect to the tricuspid valve allows an estimation of how far the lead is in the ventricle.

Once in place, the tip should maintain a relatively stable position and not appear to be bouncing with cardiac contraction. A slight loop of lead is left in the atrium to avoid tension at the tip during deep inspiration. Too large a loop may predispose to ectopy, lead displacement, and possible chronic perforation at the tip. Lead position should be checked with the stylet withdrawn.

Although an apical position is preferred for reasons of stability, there are occasions when another location in the right ventricle is required (e.g., a retained ventricular lead, which might result in electrical potentials being generated between it and the new lead). Efforts to obtain a more physiologic activation sequence and, presumably, contraction from ventricular stimulation have led some to advocate positioning the lead in the right ventricular outflow tract

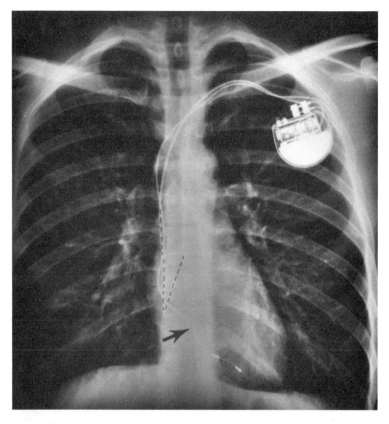

Figure 5.6 AP chest radiograph of a patient immediately after implantation of a dual-chamber pacemaker. The ventricular lead is positioned with the tip at the RV apex, well beyond the spine shadow, as shown here. A slight downward position of the tip is desirable. Some indentation of the ventricular lead at the level of the tricuspid valve is common (arrow). The atrial lead (enhanced) is positioned in the right atrial appendage. When it is positioned optimally, a deep inspiration opens the angle of the loop.

or at the ventricular septum. In these circumstances, the use of an active fixation lead is recommended. The benefits of seeking such a position compared with the stability of the traditional apical location require further study.

When a reasonable position is obtained, preliminary measurements of the electrical parameters are made. This is usually accomplished with the stylet withdrawn about halfway so as not to

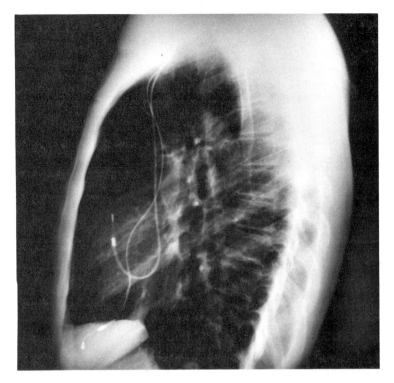

Figure 5.7   Lateral chest radiograph of the patient in Figure 5.6. RV apical position is confirmed by the extreme anterior location of the ventricular lead tip. The anterior position of the atrial lead is consistent with a location in the right atrial appendage.

interfere with the position of the lead tip and to facilitate movement of the lead body should that be necessary. When active fixation leads are used, such measurements may be taken before extensions of the helix and again after fixation. Active fixation leads vary in the ways they interface with the heart; the helix may be electrically active, the distal electrode may be active, or both the helix and a distal electrode may be active. Adequate pacing characteristics may not be found immediately after extension of the helix, possibly because the screw has not entered the myocardium, because the site is inadequate, or because local tissue injury has occurred. It is common for capture thresholds to decrease significantly 15 to 30 minutes after active fixation.[41]

If parameters are unacceptable, the helix may be retracted and a new site tested. At times one may be unable to retract the screw

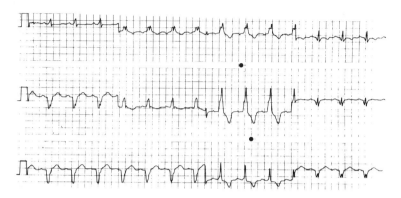

Figure 5.8 ECG-demonstrated pacing with right bundle branch block morphology. AP chest radiograph was consistent with RV apical position; however, the lateral radiograph demonstrated the lead in the left ventricle (see Figures 5.12 and 5.13).

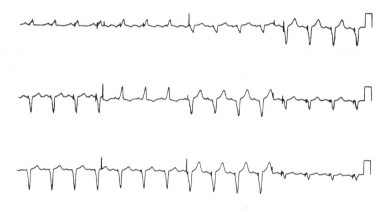

Figure 5.9 Left bundle branch block pattern with paced events was seen following repositioning of the lead into the right ventricle.

either because the mechanism has been damaged or because tissue has become impacted in the helix. It might still be possible to reposition the lead and fix it to the myocardium by rotating the entire lead (indeed, some active fixation leads have nonretractable screws); however, replacement of the lead with a new one remains an option.

Threshold parameters tested with a PSA define the electrical adequacy of lead position. This is accomplished using a set of connector cables, which can be configured for unipolar or bipolar leads. When testing unipolar leads, the anode is connected to tissue in the pacemaker pocket using a disk electrode or a clamp. Electrograms may be obtainable from the PSA or may be recorded using the chest (V) lead of a standard electrocardiograph machine. If satisfactory parameters (Table 5.4) are not obtained, alternative lead positions should be sought. Capture threshold may be influenced by a number of factors;[42] on occasion (e.g., diseased/infarcted myocardium, pharmacotherapy) optimal parameters may not be achieved, and acceptance of a position most closely approximating ideal is necessary. Because the short- and long-term success of the pacing system is related to initial lead position, effort should be expended to obtain the best possible initial location in terms of both stability and electrical performance. Rarely, a cardiac vein may prove the only site from which one may pace the ventricle reliably despite elevated thresholds.[43]

Atrial lead implantation

The right atrial appendage has become the preferred implant site for atrial leads because of its trabeculated nature. Studies have shown that reasonably good pacing parameters may be obtained and maintained from this location.[44] There has long been a perception, especially among physicians in the United States, that the atrium is a less reliable site for endocardial pacing. A number of studies have documented that dislodgement is not more common with atrial leads,[45] but reliance on an atrial appendage location may mandate the acceptance of less than ideal pacing characteristics that become unacceptable over time. Active fixation leads (especially those with steroid-eluting capabilities) would appear to be beneficial in this regard by allowing further exploration of the right atrium in the search for an optimal position.

A variety of leads (active, passive, J-shaped, straight) may be used for atrial pacing. A J-shaped stylet can be used to configure a

Table 5.4 Acceptable Electrical Parameters of Lead Placement

	Atrium	Ventricle
Capture threshold*	≤1.5 V	≤1.0 V
Sensed P/R wave	≥1.5 mV	≥4.0 mV
Slew rate	>0.3 V/sec	≥0.5 V/sec
Impedance	400–1000 ohms	400–1000 ohms

* At 0.5-msec pulse duration.

routine ventricular lead, which facilitates its entry into the append-age. When using active fixation leads, there are advantages and disadvantages to preformed devices. The non-J lead may be easier to place in areas other than the appendage; however, dislodgment may result in the lead's falling into the right ventricle and causing competitive pacing[46] or ectopy (Figures 5.10 and 5.11). The J-shaped active fixation lead may also be positioned almost anywhere in the atrium, but in some sites (e.g., low atrium) its shape may cause undue tension at the site of attachment to the endocardium.

A series of leads manufactured by Telectronics Pacing Systems, Inc. (Englewood, CO) utilized a distal flat J retention wire to achieve a J configuration. It has recently been shown that this

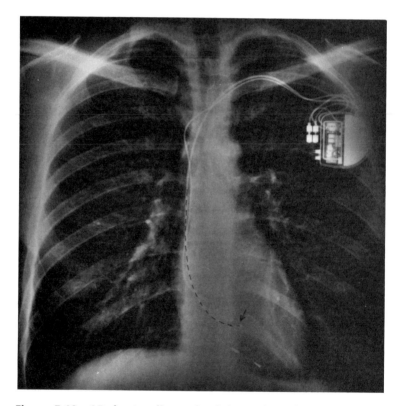

Figure 5.10 AP chest radiograph of the patient shown in Figures 5.6 and 5.7, three months postimplantation. Dislodgment of the straight atrial active fixation lead (arrow) previously placed in the right atrial appendage results in its falling into the right ventricle lumen. Pacing from this lead resulted in ventricular capture.

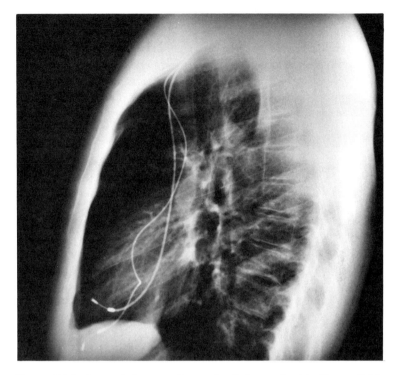

Figure 5.11   Lateral chest radiograph of the patient in Figure 5.10.

wire may fracture over time, presumably due to stress and strain. The fractured fragment may perforate the lead's insulation and lacerate the heart and other mediastinal structures or break off and embolize distally.[8] Although these leads have been taken off the market, management of the many patients who have had them implanted remains problematic.

The atrial lead is inserted into the venous system with a straight stylet to facilitate negotiation of the central veins. Positioning in the atrial appendage is attempted first. The lead is directed toward the tricuspid valve and allowed to take its J shape either by withdrawing the straight stylet (in preformed leads) or by inserting a J stylet. Slow retraction of the lead results in the tip's entering the appendage, where it will appear to catch and take on a characteristic to-and-fro motion with atrial activity. When well positioned, slight rotation of the lead should not dislodge the tip, and deep inspiration opens the curve to an L configuration but no further. In some patients the atrial appendage may be quite large and trabe-culae may be attenuated; in others, who have received cardiopul-monary bypass, the appendage may be oversewn. In either circumstance, placement of a preformed J lead may be difficult.

Acceptable electrical parameters for atrial pacing are listed in Table 5.4. As seen when positive fixation leads are used in the ventricle, there may be a significant improvement of the parameters during the first half hour; if borderline values are obtained initially, it may be worthwhile to remeasure them after a short wait.[47] If poor values are obtained initially, however, it is best to search for a new position. The better the electrical characteristics, the more probable that long-term pacing will be successful.

SINGLE-LEAD VDD PACING

The general principles of lead insertion are similar for the dual-chamber (VDD) systems that employ specially arrayed proximal atrial sensing electrodes as well as a tip electrode to sense and pace the ventricle on a single lead. It is important to have the atrial electrodes at an optimal position in the right atrium; one may have to choose among leads with varying distances between the tip and atrial electrodes. Care is necessary to ensure that atrial activity is intact and consistently sensed. Testing for atrial sensing during extremes of respiration and during cough is necessary. Although it may be necessary to accept low-amplitude P waves and program the device to be very sensitive, reasonable results are reported over a moderately long follow-up period.[48]

GENERATOR INSERTION

After both leads have been placed in an acceptable electrical posi-tion, their stability is confirmed with fluoroscopic observation during deep inspiration and cough. There should be just enough intravascular lead to prevent undue tension at the tip with inspira-tion. The suture sleeve is carefully advanced distally, with care not to pull on the lead. Frequent fluoroscopic checks are important during this process. The lead is tied down to the underlying muscle with two or three sutures of nonreabsorbable 2–0 or 3–0 material. Sutures should never be tied around the unprotected lead, and even with the suture sleeve, too tight a suture may compromise lead integrity. The sutures should be tight enough, however, to avoid lead migration. Electrical parameters and fluoroscopic position should be rechecked after suturing; if they are not optimal, the sutures may be removed and the lead repositioned.

Once the leads have been secured, the sponges that had been placed in the subcutaneous pocket are removed and the area is irrigated and checked for hemostasis. Fluoroscopy of the pocket area will reveal any radiopaque foreign body (e.g., sponge, needle) that has not been removed prior to generator insertion. The pacemaker should be preprogrammed to the desired initial settings while still in its sterile package, after which it is given to the operator for implantation. For dual-chamber devices it is important that the atrial and ventricular leads be identified easily and connected properly to the generator. Bifurcated leads are marked to ensure that the distal electrode is inserted into the cathodal portion of the connector block.

The proximal connector pin of the lead should be seen to pass the set screw(s) of the generator and remain there after tightening. Care should be taken that the screws are not overtorqued when tightened. A slight tug on the lead will confirm a tight connection. For in-line bipolar leads, both screws must be set correctly. Some pacemakers (i.e., unipolar, minute ventilation) may not function as programmed until placed within the pocket.

The generator is carefully placed in the pocket so that its markings face up. Redundant leads may be looped along the sides of the device or underneath it to avoid acute angulations. Some operators place the generator and leads in a polyethylene fabric pouch for implantation. Once in place, the pacemaker should function as programmed. Fluoroscopic examination of the entire system may be done prior to pocket closure.

The pocket is closed in layers using 4–0 polyglactin 910 subcutaneously. Care must be taken to avoid piercing a lead with the suture needle. The skin edges may be approximated with skin sutures, resorbable subcuticular sutures, or staples. An antibiotic ointment and dressing are then applied.

Prior to leaving the pacemaker laboratory, a final fluoroscopic check of the generator pocket and the course of the leads is made. The system is noninvasively interrogated to confirm adequacy of function and is programmed so that it temporarily overdrives the intrinsic heart rate. A 12-lead electrocardiogram is obtained (to demonstrate a paced rhythm), and overpenetrated anteroposterior and lateral (shot through the ipsilateral upper extremity) chest x-rays are performed to document lead position and the absence of a pneumothorax. A sling may help discourage excessive movement of the ipsilateral upper extremity during the first 12 to 24 hours.

POSTPROCEDURE MANAGEMENT

There has been some enthusiasm for outpatient implantation, but at present most patients are hospitalized at least overnight. Telemetry of the electrocardiogram is usually obtained for 12 to 24 hours. Longer hospitalization may be required because of ancillary medical problems. Analgesia may be necessary for a short period of time; however, it is rarely needed after the first day. The patient is advised to limit motion of the ipsilateral upper extremity for a time—specifically, to avoid raising it above the shoulder level or subjecting it to marked abduction for about two weeks.

Prior to the patient's discharge, the device is programmed in accordance with the patient's specific needs and a complete noninvasive assessment of the pacing system is performed. A rise in capture threshold over the first two to six weeks postimplantation is to be expected, and an adequate safety margin should be programmed into the generator to ensure successful pacing during this time. This is usually achieved with a voltage output of three to five times threshold at implant. Older patients have less rise in threshold,[49] and the use of steroid-eluting leads may be associated with a blunted subacute increase.[36] A copy of the programmed parameters should be given to the patient to keep in addition to the device registry card.

It is important that the physician register the generator and leads appropriately so that the patient may be tracked should recall of a device occur. Arrangements for follow-up care must be made by the implanting physician, and the patient should be counseled as to the importance of having the system checked at regular intervals. There is some controversy as to the need for antibiotic prophylaxis in patients with endocardial leads. Although there is a potential for endocarditis to occur, this has been reported infrequently.

Programming of the pacemaker is guided by two principles: 1) optimization of the patient's hemodynamic state and 2) maximal conservation of battery-energy expenditure. When these two factors are in opposition, the first should rule; however, opportunities to achieve the second should not be overlooked. This might include programming a longer AV interval to avoid fusion beats, a low resting minimal heart rate, and lower stimulation outputs (within an acceptable safety margin). Rate-adaptive parameters may be set prior to discharge or at a follow-up visit. This is commonly done empirically and tested by having the patient perform walking exercises.[50,51] The adequacy of pacing response may be judged by real-time telemetry or by using rate histograms stored in the pacer. Follow-up evaluation and possibly adjustment of programmed parameters, including rate adaptation, will be necessary.

COMPLICATIONS OF IMPLANTATION

Inherent with pacemaker therapy is the potential for the occurrence of an untoward event.[52] Skill, experience, and technique are all mitigating factors, but every operator should anticipate that eventually he or she will have to deal with a complication. Thus, the implanting physician must be concerned not only with measures to avoid complications but also with their recognition and treatment. Such untoward events associated with the introduction and physical presence of the generator and lead may be classified according to their etiology (Tables 5.5 and 5.6). With current technology, the complication rate encountered with dual-chamber pacing is similar to that associated with single-chamber systems.[53]

Venous access

By its very nature, the blind subclavian venous puncture has a potential for complication, the risk of which depends on both

---

Table 5.5   Acute Complications of Pacemaker Implantation

1. Venous access
    A. Secondary to Seldinger technique
        1. Pneumothorax
        2. Hemothorax
        3. Other (e.g., injury to thoracic duct, nerves, etc.)
    B. Secondary to sheath insertion
        1. Air or foreign body embolism
        2. Perforation of the heart or central vein
        3. Inadvertent entry into artery
2. Lead placement
    A. Brady-tachyarrhythmia
    B. Perforation of heart or vein
    C. Damage to heart valve
    D. Damage to lead
3. Generator
    A. Improper or inadequate connection of leads

Table 5.6   Delayed Complications of Pacemaker Therapy

A. Lead-related
1. Intravascular thrombosis ($+/-$ embolization)
2. Intravascular constriction (i.e., SVC obstruction)
3. Macro- or micro-lead dislodgment
4. Fibrosis at electrode–myocardial interface
5. Infection—endocarditis
6. Lead failure
   a. Insulation failure (inner/outer)
   b. Conductor fracture
7. Retention wire fracture
8. Chronic perforation
9. Pericarditis
B. Generator-related
1. Pain
2. Erosion
3. Infection—pocket
4. Migration
5. Premature failure
6. Damage from extrinsic energy (e.g., radiation, electrical shock, etc.)
C. Patient-related
1. Twiddler

operator and anatomy. Inadvertent damage by the exploring needle to structures that lie in proximity to the vein (e.g., lung, subclavian artery, thoracic duct, nerves) is the most frequent cause of significant complications encountered during the implantation process. Such complications may be evident immediately, or they may be recognized only after the procedure is completed.

Pneumothorax is often asymptomatic and discovered on the routine postprocedure chest x-ray. Rarely, it may be the cause of severe respiratory distress intraprocedurally. Pleuritic pain, cough (especially if productive of blood-tinged sputum), and difficulty in breathing suggest the diagnosis. The aspiration of air during attempted venous puncture may also raise concern about this possibility but is neither sensitive nor specific. The presence of apical cystic lung disease, variations in relationship between the clavicle and subclavian vein, and an uncooperative (poorly sedated) patient may increase the risk for this complication; repeated unsuccessful attempts at venous puncture certainly do. Symptoms arising during the procedure should prompt assessment of pulse, blood pressure, oximetry, and perhaps blood gas analysis. Fluoroscopic examination of both lung fields should also be performed.

Treatment of pneumothorax depends on its severity and associated symptoms. Respiratory distress during the procedure may necessitate the urgent/emergent insertion of a chest tube. The completion of the implantation will depend on the patient's status and the progress already made. Although there may be some controversy as to the need for evacuation of an asymptomatic pneumothorax seen on chest x-ray, if its extent is greater than 10 percent, a chest tube should be considered. If a small pneumothorax does not resolve or enlarges on serial x-rays, evacuation is indicated. Inspiration of 100% oxygen by face mask may help shrink a small pneumothorax.

Hemothorax, a less common complication of the subclavian approach, results from injury to the subclavian artery, vein, or other intrathoracic vessel. Penetration of the artery by the exploring needle is usually not productive of sequelae if the needle is withdrawn and slight pressure applied at the site of entry under the clavicle. Significant complication may occur, however, if the artery is lacerated by the cutting edge of the needle or if a large-bore dilator or sheath is inadvertently introduced. If a large sheath is mistakenly inserted into the artery, it should probably be left in place, pending emergency repair. Surgery should be considered although there may be a role for endovascular catheter-based intervention. The likelihood of a bleeding complication is increased if the coagulation system is impaired either intrinsically or by pharmacologic therapy. Angiographic evaluation and possible repair should be considered for severe or persistent bleeding from an uncertain source. A symptomatic hemothorax should be drained.

In addition to the above, injury to other structures (lymphatic system, nerves, etc.) has been reported to be a consequence of the Seldinger technique for venous access. Thus, although this methodology has facilitated endocardial lead placement, there is the potential for a variety of complications not encountered when the leads are directly inserted into an exposed vein.

Air embolism may occur when a central vein is accessed by a sheath regardless of the technique used to introduce it. The occurrence of this complication may be signaled by a hiss as air is sucked into the sheath by negative intrathoracic pressure. This may occur suddenly when a heavily sedated, snoring patient deeply inspires at a time when control over the sheath's orifice is not adequate. Air may be fluoroscopically tracked into the right ventricle and pulmonary outflow tract.[54] In most instances, the amount of air introduced is small and well tolerated, but respiratory distress, chest pain, hypotension, and arterial oxygen desaturation may occur if there is significant blockage to pulmonary flow. Treatment of symptomatic air embolism includes supplemental oxygen, attempted catheter aspiration, and inotropic cardiac support if necessary. These supportive measures will usually suffice until the air embolism breaks up and absorption occurs. Postural changes to prevent migration of air trapped in the right atrium or ventricle from reaching the pulmonary arteries may be considered although usually the latter occurs too rapidly for these maneuvers to be of much success. Preventive measures are listed in Table 5.7.

Lead placement

Arrhythmia: The introduction, manipulation, and positioning of the pacemaker leads in the heart may give rise to a number of complications. Arrhythmia may be a manifestation of the patient's underlying disease, or it may be procedurally related (Table 5.8). In a

---

Table 5.7   Avoidance of Air Embolism

1. Increase central venous pressure
   A. Hydrate well
   B. Elevate legs (Trendelenburg position)
   C. Have patient valsalva or "hum" when sheath is open
2. Awaken patient and caution against deep inspiration
3. Use smallest sheath compatible with task
4. Pinch or occlude neck of sheath when appropriate
5. Consider the use of sheaths with hemostatic valves

Table 5.8   Causes of Arrhythmia During Pacer Implantation

1. Bradyarrhythmia
   A. Patient's underlying electrophysiologic disorder
   B. Vagal reaction
   C. Lead "bruise" to the conduction system
   D. Inadvertent disruption of a pacing system
   E. Suppression of escape rhythm by anesthetic
2. Tachyarrhythmia
   A. Atrial/ventricle
      1. Underlying electrophysiology
      2. Irritation by lead/wire
      3. Ischemia, anesthesia, hypoxia

---

pacemaker-dependent patient, accidental interference with a preexisting pacing system—whether temporary or permanent—may cause asystole or symptomatic bradycardia. Other causes include a vagal reaction, excessive local anesthesia, and injury to the conduction system during lead manipulation (e.g., a bruise to the right bundle branch in a patient with left bundle branch block). Some have advocated the use of standby transcutaneous pacing devices for temporary support in such cases. Administration of isoproterenol or atropine may also be helpful until a lead can be successfully placed and pacing established.

Tachyarrhythmia may also occur; it is usually the result of stimulation of myocardium by a lead or guidewire. Supraventricular arrhythmias are most likely to occur in patients with atrial enlargement, heart failure, pulmonary disease, or other predisposing conditions such as sick sinus syndrome; they are usually transient. Atrial fibrillation occurring prior to or during atrial lead placement may be problematic in that atrial parameters cannot be tested unless the rhythm terminates either spontaneously or by cardioversion. Ventricular dysrhythmia is common as the lead is manipulated in this chamber; however, it is rarely sustained. Predisposing factors to more malignant arrhythmia include hypoxia, ischemia, pharmacologic therapy (e.g., sympathomimetics), and asynchronous pacing. Removal of the lead from an irritating position almost always terminates the ectopy. On occasion a retained guidewire or a temporary ventricular pacing lead is displaced and serves as an occult source of ventricular irritation that is not resolved by retraction of the permanent pacing lead.

Because the attention of the implanter may be focused on the fluoroscopic image during lead placement, another individual should be assigned to monitor the ECG during this time. Rarely, a permanent ventricular (or prolapsing atrial) pacing lead will be the cause of recurrent ventricular tachycardia.[55]

Perforation: The heart may be perforated internally (into another cardiac chamber) or externally (into the pericardial space) by the pacing lead. Right ventricular perforations are probably more common than reported because clinical sequelae may not occur. Poor sensing or capture thresholds may prompt withdrawal of the lead back into the ventricle with "self-sealing" of the perforation. On occasion, however, life-threatening tamponade may occur, and progressive hypotension during or after lead placement should be considered tamponade until proven otherwise by echo-

251

cardiography. Old age, steroid therapy, recent right ventricular infarction, and the use of stiff leads (stylets?) may be considered risk factors for perforation. Pericarditis and tamponade have also accompanied active fixation atrial lead implantation,[56] presumably due to perforation by the helix. Interference with normal coagulation predisposes to tamponade. Anticoagulants should be withheld for at least 8 to 12 hours and thrombolytics should be considered contraindicated in the immediate postimplant period. Pericardiocentesis with catheter drainage will rapidly reverse the pathophysiology of tamponade and may be the only therapy necessary.

Suspicion of perforation without tamponade may be aroused by an extreme distal location of the lead tip at the cardiac apex (especially if it seems to curve around the apex, tenting up the cardiac silhouette), or by the presence of a pericardial friction rub, chest pain, an ECG-pacing pattern of right bundle branch block, or an electrogram recorded from the lead tip.[57] Poor pacing and sensing thresholds may be seen. In such situations, two-dimensional echocardiography may be helpful in localizing the lead tip.[58] If perforation is confirmed, the lead should be withdrawn under hemodynamic monitoring at a facility capable of treating tamponade.

A transvenous pacing lead may enter the left heart through a communication between the atria, through the membranous septum separating the right atrium from the left ventricle, or through the muscular intraventricular septum.[59] The permanent pacing lead may also be inadvertently introduced into an artery and passed retrograde across the aortic valve into the left ventricle. The anteroposterior radiographic image of a lead positioned in the left ventricle may not be distinguishable from that of one placed in the right ventricular apical position (Figure 5.12). Oblique or lateral views, however, will demonstrate the posterior location of a left ventricular lead (Figure 5.13). In addition, pacing from the left ventricle will result in a right bundle branch block pattern (see Figure 5.8). Two-dimensional echocardiography can be used to trace the course of a lead.[60]

Early recognition of a lead in a systemic chamber should prompt its immediate repositioning because of the danger of thrombus formation and embolization.[61] A lead chronically implanted in such a location poses a more difficult problem because extraction may be technically more demanding and there may be greater risk of embolization during the removal process. Long-term

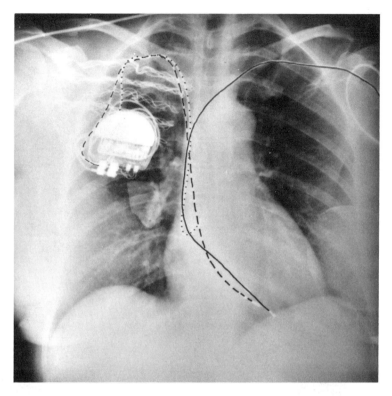

Figure 5.12 AP chest radiograph in a patient immediately after implantation of a dual-chamber pacemaker. Right bundle branch block pattern was noted with paced beats (see Figures 5.8 and 5.9). An abandoned ventricular lead (solid line) is seen to originate in the left infraclavicular area. The new ventricular lead (dashed line) appears to be positioned near the RV apex, and the atrial lead (dotted line) appears to be in a suitable position.

anticoagulation may be indicated in such patients,[61] or removal by open heart surgery may be considered.[62]

Other lead complications: Ordinarily, the presence of a pacing lead across the tricuspid orifice results in little or no valvular dysfunction.[63] On occasion, however, this structure may be interfered with[64] or acutely (or chronically) damaged. During insertion, the tines of a passive fixation lead may become entangled with the chordae tendineae, and rupture of the latter may result if vigorous lead withdrawal is attempted. The valve may be chronically injured

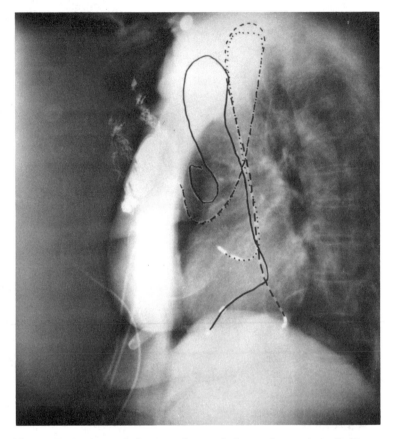

Figure 5.13 Lateral chest radiograph from the patient in Figure 5.12 shows a posterior diversion of the new ventricular lead at the atrial level. Echocardiography showed evidence of the lead within the left ventricle, and passage of the lead across a patent foramen ovale, across the mitral valve, and into the left ventricular apex was confirmed.

by the lead's lying across it; clot and adhesions may form between the two and serve as a nidus for infection.

The pacing lead itself may be damaged by the physical forces exerted upon it during the process of implantation, by entrapment by the muscular skeletal system, by retention ligatures, and by the stresses placed on it by the beating heart. Loss of integrity of the insulation (either inner or outer) is manifested by a low lead impedance that causes a high current drain; conductor fracture is associated with a high impedance. Lead fracture may be recognized radiographically (Figures 5.14 and 5.15). A defect in the insulation between the conductor wires of a bipolar lead may produce potentials resulting in transient inhibition of the pacemaker.[65] Such intermittent dysfunction may require the performance of provocative maneuvers for detection.

An all-too-frequent complication of lead placement is its subsequent displacement. This usually occurs early, before clot and fibrosis act to further anchor the device. Dislodgment rates are inversely related to the experience of the implanter, which suggests that inadequate initial positioning is a major risk factor. A unique cause of lead dislodgment is known as *Twiddler's syndrome*.[66,67] In these cases the (usually elderly) patient unwittingly turns the pace-

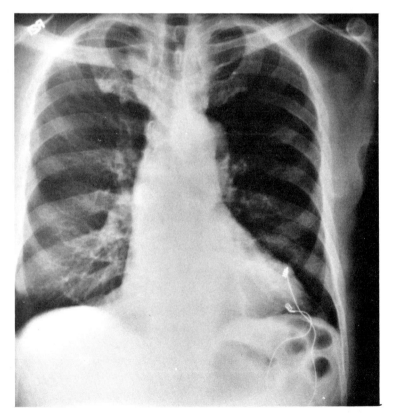

Figure 5.14 Chest radiograph of a patient with a normally functioning bipolar epicardial ventricular pacemaker.

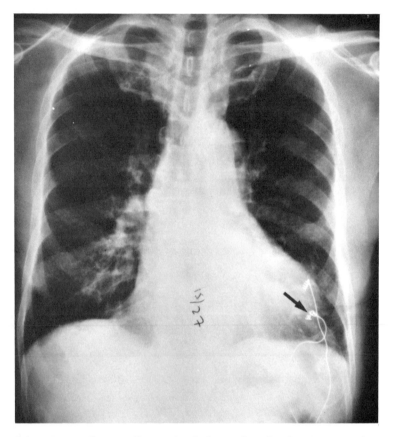

Figure 5.15 Chest radiograph of the patient in Figure 5.14 a few years later, when pauses in paced rhythm and syncope were noted. A fracture of the inferior lead (arrow) resulted in electrical chatter and pacemaker inhibition.

maker in such a way that the lead(s) are wound around it and, potentially, are withdrawn from the heart (Figure 5.16).

The incidence of lead dislodgment has been reduced with refinement of both active and passive fixation devices; it is now less than 2 or 3 percent. The risk of this complication is lessened by ensuring a stable position at implant, leaving a proper amount of intravascular lead so that tension is not exerted at the tip by respiration or arm motion, adequately anchoring the suture sleeve to underlying tissue, and by limiting abduction and elevation of the ipsilateral upper extremity for a time postimplantation.

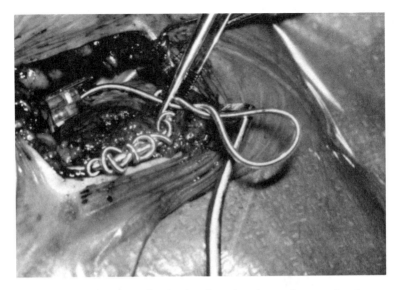

Figure 5.16 Photograph obtained at the time of operative intervention to reposition a lead dislodged due to Twiddler's syndrome. The lead can be seen to be tightly twisted upon itself; although this tangle can be straightened, the stresses imparted to both the conductor and the insulation make it unsafe to reuse this lead. A new lead should be inserted. (Courtesy of Dr. Paul Levine.)

Early recognition of lead dislodgment (often by deterioration in pacing parameters) should result in attempts at repositioning. This is usually accomplished with minimal effort because the lead has not fibrosed to endocardium or venous endothelium. Deterioration of the performance of one or more chronic leads may present a more difficult problem and it is often necessary to employ a new lead. If exit block is a problem, steroid–eluting leads may be beneficial.

Intravascular: The presence of intravascular leads may incite thrombosis. Isotope scans reveal a high incidence of asymptomatic venous thrombosis that appears to be related to the number of leads placed.[68] Clinically significant pulmonary embolization is surprisingly rare but may occur.[69] Symptomatic thrombosis of the brachiocephalic veins occurs on occasion and presents as a swollen, painful upper extremity two or more weeks after implant. Extension of the clot to involve contralateral structures[70] or the cerebral venous sinus[71] may occur. Venography will reveal the extent of thrombus and reveal collateral pathways.

Symptomatic thrombosis that is limited to the subclavian or axillary veins may be treated conservatively or with thrombolytics[72] (Figure 5.17). Thrombolytic therapy may be given in a large dose for a short time (e.g., 1 million units streptokinase during one hour) or during 12 to 24 hours (e.g., 200 to 500,000 units urokinase during one hour followed by 100,000 units per hour) with or without concomitant heparin. Thrombolytics need not be delivered directly into an ipsilateral arm vein. In our experience, thrombolytic therapy has been associated with rapid symptomatic and angiographic improvement. Prolonged therapy with either

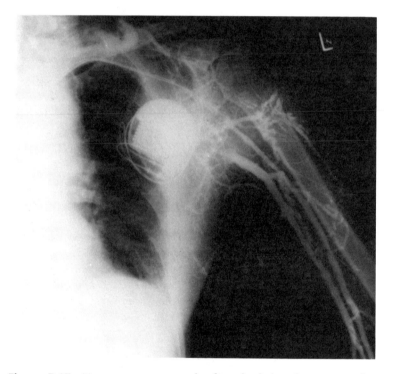

Figure 5.17 **Venogram one week after dual-chamber pacemaker implantation. The patient presented with swelling and pain in the left arm. Left axillary vein thrombosis is noted. The patient was treated with streptokinase, and a repeat venogram showed restoration of venous patency and disappearance of collaterals. (Reproduced with permission from** *Management of Cardiac Arrhythmias***, E.V. Platia (ed.), Philadelphia: J. B. Lippincott, 1987.)**

aspirin or oral anticoagulants may be considered. We have not observed a bleeding complication or clinical recurrence in patients treated in either fashion. Conservative therapy with heat and upper extremity elevation may also be satisfactory. This may allow for the development of adequate collateralization. A significant number of patients with endocardial leads develop silent thrombosis of the subclavian vein, which is revealed only when attempts are made to reenter the vessel (e.g., for upgrade to a dual-chamber unit). It is not necessary to treat asymptomatic occlusions.

Complete or partial occlusion of the superior vena cava has been reported as a complication of pacemaking.[73–75] This has been attributed to both thrombosis and fibrosis and may be treated with balloon dilatation[76] or surgical reconstruction.[77] A pedunculated clot on a pacing wire may occlude the tricuspid orifice and cause profound symptoms.[78] Treatment of lead-associated atrial thrombus with thrombolytic therapy has been reported.[79]

It is now generally accepted that a more subtle effect of pacing on the incidence of thromboembolism is ventricular pacing in patients with sinoatrial disease. Atrial fibrillation is thought to be more common in this situation, as is a propensity for thromboembolism.[80] This rationale has been used to support atrial or dual-chamber pacing in such patients.

Generator: Function of a pacing system depends on a proper connection between the leads and the generator. The terminal lead pin(s) are inserted into the connector block of the generator and are fixed into position by some mechanism, most commonly, set screws. If this is not done properly, the pin may either lose contact altogether (i.e., no electrical continuity, "open circuit") or intermittently contact the pacemaker terminal and produce spurious potentials that may be sensed by the pacemaker as intrinsic electrical activity, which will cause inhibition of pacer output. When dual-chamber systems are used, it is essential that the atrial and ventricular leads be connected correctly to their corresponding terminals (Figure 5.18).

Care should be exercised when using electrocautery; application in the vicinity of the generator may lead to inhibition of pacing or to abnormal tracking. Reprogramming of the device to a reversion mode[81] or the induction of a runaway pacemaker[82] may also result. Exposure to other sources of energy (e.g., direct-current defibrillation,[83] magnetic resonance imaging,[84] security systems,[85] high-dose radiation therapy,[86] cellular phones,[87] etc.) may also affect

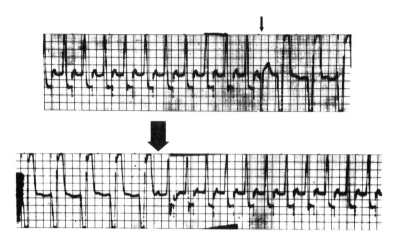

Figure 5.18 Continuous rhythm strip of a patient with a dual-chamber pacemaker in whom the leads were inadvertently reversed at the generator. R waves sensed on the atrial channel are tracked, resulting in atrial pacing with conduction through the AV node to the ventricle. A premature ventricular depolarization (small arrow) falling within the postventricular atrial refractory period is not sensed on the atrial channel, and dual-chamber pacing commences in reverse order. This occurs until a spontaneous P wave (large arrow) is sensed on the ventricular channel and inhibits both atrial and ventricular output long enough for normal conduction to occur. A normally conducted R wave is again sensed on the atrial channel and is "tracked," with reversion to initial rhythm.

pacemaker function. In some cases, pacemaker function can be restored by use of a special engineering programmer; in other situations, the device may be permanently damaged and require removal.

The generator is usually well tolerated in its subcutaneous pocket; however, on occasion its presence may be associated with pain. Most often this occurs because the pocket is small and tension is exerted on the overlying tissue. A low-grade infection not productive of significant effusion may also be etiologic. Pain attributed to neuralgia has been treated successfully with steroid injection. Swelling of the pacemaker pocket may be caused by infection, seroma, or hematoma. Unnecessary aspiration of the effusion should be discouraged because of the possibility of introducing infection.

Migration of the pacemaker under the breast or into the axilla may occur if the pocket is large, the surrounding tissue lax, and the device not secured. Movement of the generator may place tension on the leads or result in the assumption of a position (e.g., in the axilla) that is uncomfortable or predisposes to erosion. Internal erosion evidenced by the migration of a generator into the urinary bladder from an implantation site in the posterior rectus muscle has also been reported.[88]

Erosion of pacing hardware is caused by pressure necrosis of overlying tissue or infection. This is usually signaled by a preceding period of "preerosion," during which there is discomfort and discoloration of thinning tissue tensely stretched over a protrusion of the pacing apparatus (Figure 5.19). Risk factors for erosion include a paucity of subcutaneous tissue, the mass and configuration of the pacemaker, need for extra hardware (e.g., lead adaptor) in the pocket, the pocket's construction, and irritation caused by the patient or by articles of clothing. Identification of preerosion allows salvage of the pacing system by repositioning of the hardware under the pectoralis muscle or in an abdominal location.

If erosion occurs, the system is considered contaminated and current opinion favors removal of the generator and leads. There has been the suggestion that extensive debridement of the pocket

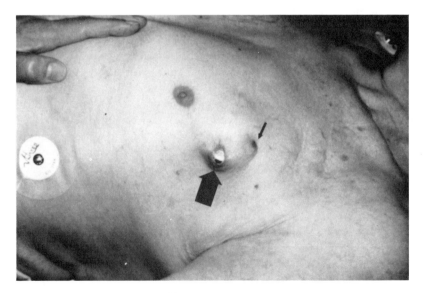

Figure 5.19 **Patient with a permanent pacemaker in whom areas of preerosion (small arrow) and erosion (large arrow) are present.**

and prolonged irrigation and antibiotic therapy may provide an alternate option to removal in cases of both erosion and frank infection.[89] This approach is not generally accepted. For localized erosions, some have suggested removing the generator, debriding the site, and cutting the leads but leaving them in situ. However, now that percutaneous lead removal has advanced to a relatively high degree, it would appear appropriate to try to remove leads rather than to leave them if sterility is questioned.

Bleeding into the pocket may occur when procedural hemostasis is inadequate, when there is a coexistent coagulopathy, or when anticoagulant or thrombolytic therapy is begun prematurely. On occasion this may compromise the pocket's integrity and may be a risk factor for infection.

Infection

A noneroded pacemaker implantation site may become infected. Diabetes mellitus and postoperative hematoma appear to be predisposing factors.[90] Acute infections (usually with *Staphylococcus aureus*) become manifest within the first few weeks of implantation and are often associated with the accumulation of pus. A more indolent infection caused by a less virulent agent such as *S. epidermidis* may present months or years after implantation.[91] A fungal infection may also occur.[92,93] One-third to one-half of infections complicate new implants; the rest are associated with reoperation for generator replacement or lead repositioning.[94] Staphylococci adhere to the plastic insulation of pacing hardware and form colonies that become covered with a secreted substance protecting the organism from host defense and antimicrobial drugs.[95] Antibiotic therapy alone is rarely sufficient to cure infection, and removal of the pacing system is usually indicated.[96] In such patients, a new system may be placed at the time of removal of the infected hardware or a two-step approach may be taken with temporary pacing bridging the time between explantation and the new implant.[97] Less frequently, a patient may develop sepsis without localizing signs, in which case endocarditis associated with a pacing lead should be excluded. Lead sepsis generally occurs later than pocket infection.[98] Two-dimensional echocardiography may be of help in these situations and transesophageal echocardiography may be superior to transthoracic echocardiography[99] in detecting vegetations. A recurrence of sepsis in a patient without a demonstrable etiology should prompt consideration of removal of the entire pacing system even if no vegetation is seen by echocardiography. Superficial infections of the suture line that do not extend to the pocket itself may be treated conservatively.

Lead removal

On occasion, consideration is given to the removal of implanted endocardial leads (Table 5.9). This may be accomplished percutaneously or via thoracotomy. Most pacing enthusiasts feel that if extraction is to be performed it should be done percutaneously. Some, however, argue the benefits of surgery.[100] There is some debate as to the breadth of indications for lead removal. Clearly, if the procedure could be performed without risk to the patient, all nonfunctional leads would probably be removed. There is, however, a risk to lead removal that correctly influences the aggressiveness with which one should pursue this approach.

Sepsis heads all hierarchical classifications of indications for lead removal; retained functionless hardware is usually least aggressively pursued. The latter poses little risk to the patient[101] but may complicate the placement of additional pacing leads either by adding to the venous obstruction (and the risk of thrombosis/embolization) or by generation of spurious electrical potentials between leads. Removal of superfluous leads would be ideal, but chronically implanted leads form adhesions to the heart and venous system and often cannot be easily extracted by standard traction techniques. Recent studies have suggested a risk of death of 0.6 percent and that of potentially life-threatening complication of 2.5 percent when vigorous percutaneous extraction is attempted.[102] Extraction of a chronically implanted lead should be undertaken only after careful consideration of the risk-benefit ratio.

Alternatively, one may abandon the lead by applying an insu-

Table 5.9   Indications for Lead Removal

1. Sepsis
2. Pocket infection/erosion
3. Ventricular/atrial ectopy (lead may be repositioned)
4. Retention wire fracture (may selectively remove wire)
5. Interference with tricuspid valve (may reposition)
6. Pain or preerosion caused by lead (may reposition)
7. Means of accessing central veins for new system
8. Perforation (may reposition)
9. Redundant nonfunctioning leads
10. Abandonment of entire pacing system

---

lating cap to the connector pin or by cutting excess lead at least 3 to 4 cm from the venous access site. The lead can be electrically isolated by pulling its insulation over the exposed end. If the latter method is chosen, care should be taken to leave enough lead accessible so that extraction may be possible if it becomes necessary. In either case, the lead is then sutured to underlying tissue to prevent retraction into the vascular system.

When a decision to extract a lead is made, a number of techniques may be applied. The traditional approach to lead removal without thoracotomy involves the application of traction on the proximal end, which is freed up to its venous entry by careful dissection. Tension on the lead should be sustained but not vigorous. Pain, ectopy, and fall in blood pressure suggest that too much traction is being exerted and that the ventricle may be invaginating. If success is not achieved intraoperatively, prolonged weighted traction has been suggested, but since the introduction of lead-extraction devices, this method is rarely used. Thicker silastic leads may be easier to remove than those insulated with polyurethane, although the latter is said to incite less thrombosis and, presumably, less fibrosis.[103] Breaks in the insulation of leads may occur with traction and the exposed conductor wire may offer an additional hazard when pulled.

A variety of new devices have been developed to assist in removal of pacing leads. Success rates of 85 percent for complete removal and 93 percent for complete or partial removal have been reported.[104,105] Atrial leads and active fixation leads appear more readily removed but risk may be increased in older patients, especially females. The technical difficulties encountered with these devices and potential for morbidity and mortality should not be underestimated. Such procedures should be performed only by physicians with experience and skill in intravascular catheterization techniques at institutions having access to immediate cardiovascular surgical support.

TECHNIQUE

Knowledge of the implanted system (e.g., type of lead, site of venous access, number of retention sutures), of the degree to which the patient is pacemaker-dependent, and of the necessity of complete removal is essential prior to the explanation attempt. The procedure is usually performed in the pacemaker laboratory at a time when cardiovascular surgical support is available if needed.

The patient is prepared as for an implantation. In addition, both groin areas are prepped and a small lumen catheter is placed in the left femoral artery to monitor blood pressure. A 6-Fr sheath is placed in the right femoral vein for venous access. Sterile drapes are liberally placed such that a sterile field is maintained from the neck to toes. If the patient is pacemaker-dependent, a temporary pacing wire is inserted through either a femoral or an internal jugular vein. A commercially available lead-extraction kit (e.g., Cook Pacemaker, Leechburg, PA) containing a variety of tools that may be needed for lead removal should be fully stocked and on hand. A pericardiocentesis tray should be readily available and there should be access to an echocardiography machine. The patient may be typed and crossmatched for blood.

The pocket is entered through the previous incision line. With a combination of sharp and blunt dissection, the generator and lead(s) are freed. The lead is traced to the venous entry point, the suture sleeve is identified, and all retention sutures are cut. An initial attempt at gentle traction is probably worthwhile; however, care must be taken not to damage the lead during this process if further effort with the interlocking lead-extraction device is contemplated. Active fixation leads appear to be easier to extract than passive leads, presumably because the tines provide a greater surface for adhesion. An attempt at unscrewing the former should be made prior to application of traction. If the retraction mechanism is not effective in unscrewing the helix, the entire lead should be rotated in a counterclockwise direction to unfix the lead tip from its attachment.

If the lead is not easily removable by the above approach, a standard lead stylet is inserted through the connector pin to demonstrate patency of the inner lumen. The stylet is withdrawn and the lead cut close to the terminal pin with wire cutters; care must be taken not to damage the distal lead, which may be held by a specially designed clamp. The central lumen of the lead is identified and carefully dilated with a coil-expander tool. The diameter of the lumen is then determined by the insertion of a series of gauge pins. A locking stylet (Figure 5.20) of a size corresponding to the largest gauge pin accepted by the lead is then advanced through the lumen to the lead tip. Slight clockwise torque may be applied to the stylet to facilitate its passage through the lead. On reaching the lead tip, one applies counterclockwise rotation to lock the stylet in place and provide a mechanism for traction to be delivered directly to the lead tip.

265

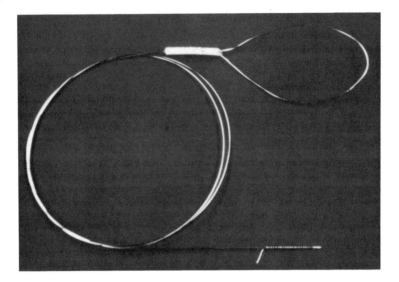

Figure 5.20 Locking guidewire stylet. (Reproduced courtesy of Cook Pacemaker Corporation.)

Accumulation of fibrous tissue attachments along the course of the lead may prevent removal by simple traction. Because leads are not isodiametric, withdrawal of the lead may result in the tip's being trapped in the intersuscepting fibrous sheath. In such cases, a variety of plastic and metal sheaths may be placed over the stylet and lead and slowly advanced into the venous system and heart to lyse the adhesions. Proper alignment of the sheaths and lead must be confirmed fluoroscopically to minimize perforation by the stiff sheaths. Correct positioning of the sheath provides a mechanism for countertraction to be applied to the lead to facilitate extraction. If the lead(s) are removed successfully, a new pacing system may be implanted at the same site (if circumstances permit) by using a guidewire inserted through the extraction sheath to facilitate venous entry.

On occasion, the lead cannot be removed completely by use of the superior approach, in which case a femoral technique is employed. With this method, a large (16-Fr) sheath serves as a "work station" through which a smaller sheath, a Dotter retrieval basket, and a tip-deflecting guidewire may be passed. Using this method, one cuts the lead proximally, which allows it to be pulled into the circulation where it can be captured by the basket and withdrawn into the sheath, which can then be advanced over the lead to apply countertraction. One may utilize a variety of catheters and snares to help capture the lead. A benefit of utilizing the femoral approach is that the proximal end of the lead can be relatively easily withdrawn through the endovascular fibrous sheath.

A unique problem has arisen recently in leads utilizing a J retention wire. As noted earlier in this chapter, fracture of this wire and its erosion through its insulating cover has the potential for patient injury (Figure 5.21). Management of these patients remains problematic with the options of lead removal, monitoring, or use of a procedure in which the protruding fractured wire fragment is snared, pulled free from the lead, and withdrawn into a sheath, which leaves the functioning lead in place.[106]

Percutaneous lead removal is of value in preventing thoracotomy for leads that must be removed. A variety of other methodologies have been employed for lead removal, including the use of a bioptome to grasp and remove the lead[107] and a lead-

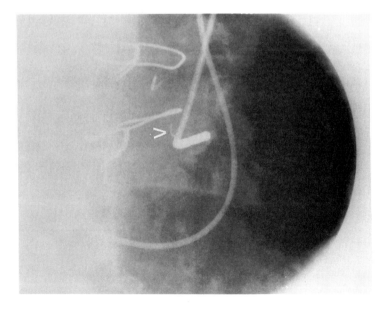

Figure 5.21 Cinefluoroscopy of Telectronics Pacing Systems model 330–801 Accufix atrial J lead in right anterior oblique projection showing protruding segment of retention wire fragment indicated by >.

transecting catheter[108] to cut it at the tip. Under development are additional techniques such as sheaths that employ laser energy to cut through adhesions and mechanical cutters. Currently, accumulated experience with the Cook extraction equipment is largest and makes that equipment the gold standard to which other techniques may be compared.

MEDICAL-LEGAL ASPECTS OF IMPLANTATION

As with many invasive procedures, the patient's expectations of pacemaker therapy may exceed the results obtained. As noted above, there is ample opportunity for even the most skilled and experienced operator to encounter a misadventure. The risk of litigation[109] is real and may be focused on any of several areas of physician responsibility (Table 5.10). Avoidance of litigation requires not only that the highest of standards be maintained but also that rapport be established with the patient and the patient's family. The best defense against successful litigation is full documentation in the patient's medical record of every aspect of the implantation (or extraction) process. This should include the indication for the procedure, the informed consent, a complete procedure note to include the pacing parameters achieved and any difficulties encountered, evidence of postprocedure evaluation, and arrangements for follow-up care. The removal of preexisting hardware and its disposition (e.g., returned to manufacturer for evaluation) must also be documented.

Pacemaker implantation implies much physician responsibility. As with any implantable device, there is a continued risk to the patient as long as he or she has the device. Somewhat unique to pacing and electrophysiologic systems is the knowledge that the power source has limited life and may need to be replaced. The North American Society of Pacing and Electrophysiology

---

Table 5.10   Responsibilities of an Implanting Physician

1. Establish and document accepted indications
2. Obtain a fully informed consent
3. Implant an indicated system
4. Avoid undo delay
5. Conform to accepted technique and standards
6. Obtain expert consultation when appropriate
7. Provide for follow-up care

(NASPE) and others have provided a service to physicians by creating guidelines to assist in patient management. Recently NASPE issued a policy statement on pacemaker follow-up,[110] which should be an important asset to those wishing to be involved with pacemaker services.

REFERENCES

1. Hanley PC, Vlietstra RE, Merideth J, et al. Two decades of cardiac pacing at the Mayo Clinic (1961–1981). *Mayo Clin Proc* 1984;59:268–274.
2. Parsonnet V, Bernstein AD, Lindsay B. Pacemaker-implantation complication rates: An analysis of some contributing factors. *J Am Coll Cardiol* 1989;13:917–921.
3. Hayes DL, Naccarelli GV, Furman S, Parsonnet V, and the NASPE Pacemaker Training Policy Conference Group. Report of the NASPE Policy Conference training requirements for permanent pacemaker selection, implantation, and follow-up. *PACE* 1994;17:6–12.
4. Brinker JA, Pepine CJ, Bonchek LI, et al. Use of radiographic devices by cardiologists. *J Am Coll Cardiol* 1995;25:1738–1739.
5. Schoenfeld MH. Quality assurance in cardiac electrophysiology and pacing: A brief synopsis. *PACE* 1994;17(Pt I):267–269.
6. Parsonnet V, Furman S, Smyth NPD, Bilitch M. Optimal resources for implantable cardiac pacemakers. Intersociety commission for heart disease resources (JCHD). *Circulation* 1983;68:227A–244A.
7. Hess DS, Gertz EW, Morady F, et al. Permanent pacemaker implantation in the cardiac catheterization laboratory: The subclavian approach. *Cath Cardiovasc Diag* 1982;8:453–458.
8. Lloyd MA, Hayes DL, Holmes DR. Atrial "J" pacing lead retention wire fracture: Radiographic assessment, incidence of fracture, and clinical management. *PACE* 1995;18(Pt I):958–964.
9. Dreifus LS, Fisch C, Griffin JC, et al. Guidelines for implantation of cardiac pacemakers and antiarrhythmic devices. A report of the American College of Cardiology/American Heart Association Task Force on Pacemaker Implantation. *Circulation* 1991;84:455–467.
10. National Quality of Care Forum. Bridging the gap between

theory and practice: Exploring clinical practice guidelines. *J Qual Improve* 1993;19:384–400.

11. Muers MF, Arnold AG, Sleight P. Prophylactic antibiotics for cardiac pacemaker implantation: A prospective trial. *Br Heart J* 1981;46:539–544.

12. Ramsdale DR, Charles RG, Rowlands DB. Antibiotic prophylaxis for pacemaker implantation: A prospective randomized trial. *PACE* 1984;7:844–849.

13. Bluhm G, Jacobson B, Ransjo U. Antibiotic prophylaxis in pacemaker surgery: A prospective trial with local or systemic administration of antibiotics at generator replacements. *PACE* 1985;8:661–670.

14. Mounsey JP, Griffith MJ, Tynan M, et al. Antibiotic prophylaxis in permanent pacemaker implantation: A prospective randomized trial. *Br Heart J* 1994;72(4):339–343.

15. Ellestad MH, French JH. Iliac vein approach to permanent pacemaker implantation. *PACE* 1989;12:1030–1103.

16. Bellot PH, Bucko D. Inframammary pulse generator placement for maximizing cosmetic effect. *PACE* 1983;6:1241–1244.

17. Spearman P, Leier DV. Persistent left superior vena cava: Unusual wave contour of left jugular vein as a presenting feature. *Am Heart J* 1990;120:999–1022.

18. Zardo F, Nicolosi GL, Burelli C, Zanuttini D. Dual chamber transvenous pacemaker implantation via anomalous left superior vena cava. *Am Heart J* 1986;112:621–622.

19. Littleford PO, Spector SD. Device for the rapid insertion of a permanent endocardial pacing electrode through the subclavian vein: Preliminary report. *Ann Thorac Surg* 1979;7:265–271.

20. Bognolo DA, Vijaynagar R, Eckstein PF, Janss B. Two leads in one introducer technique for AV sequential implantations. *PACE* 1982;5:358–539.

21. Belott PH. Retaining guidewire, introducer technique for unlimited access to the central circulation: A review. *Clin Prog Pacing Electrophysiol* 1983;1:363–373.

22. Parsonnet V, Bernstein AD, Galasso D. Cardiac pacing practices in the United States in 1985. *Am J Cardiol* 1988;62:71–77.

23. Jacobs DM, Fink AS, Miller RP, et al. Anatomical and morphological evaluation of pacemaker lead compression. *PACE* 1993;16(Pt I):434–444.

24. Magney JE, Flynn DM, Parsons JA, et al. Anatomical mechanisms explaining damage to pacemaker leads, defibrillator leads, and failure of central venous catheters adjacent to the sternoclavicular joint. *PACE* 1993;16:445.
25. Magney JE, Parsons JA, Flynn DM, Hunter DW. Pacemaker and defibrillator lead entrapment: Case studies. *PACE* 1995;18:1509–1517.
26. Byrd CL. Safe introducer technique for pacemaker lead implantation. *PACE* 1992;15:262–267.
27. Moran SG, Peoples JB. The deltopectoral triangle as a landmark for percutaneous infraclavicular cannulation of the subclavian vein. *Angiology* 1993;44:683–686.
28. Ong LS, Barold SS, Lederman M, et al. Cephalic vein guidewire technique for implantation of permanent pacemakers. *Am Heart J* 1987;4:753–756.
29. Roelke M, Jackson G, Harthorne JW. Submammary pacemaker implantation: A unique tunneling technique. *PACE* 1994;17(Pt I):1793–1796.
30. King DH, Gillette PC, Shannon C, Cuddy TE. Steroid-eluting endocardial pacing lead for treatment of exit block. *Am Heart J* 1983;106:1428–1440.
31. Ward DE, Clarke B, Schofield PM, et al. Long-term transvenous ventricular pacing in adults with congenital abnormalities of the heart and great arteries. *Br Heart J* 1983;50:325–329.
32. Snow N. Elimination of lead dislodgement by use of tined transvenous electrodes. *PACE* 1982;5:571–574.
33. Madigan NP, Mueller KJ, Curtis JJ, Walls JT. Stability of permanent transvenous dual-chamber pacing electrodes during cardiopulmonary resuscitation. *PACE* 1983;6:1234–1240.
34. Chew PH, Brinker JA. Oversensing from electrode "chatter" in a bipolar pacing lead: A case report. *PACE* 1990;13:808–811.
35. Ong LS, Barold SS, Craver WL, et al. Partial avulsion of the tricuspid valve by tined pacing electrode. *Am Heart J* 1988;102:798–799.
36. Brinker JA, Crossley G, Reynolds D, et al. Chronic performance of a new bipolar steroid eluting active fixation lead: A multi-center randomized trial (abstract). *PACE* 1994;17(Pt II):853.
37. Brinker JA. Endocardial pacing leads: The good, the bad, and the ugly. *PACE* 1995;18:953–954.

38. Jordaens LJ, Vandenbogaerde JF, VandeBruquene P, DeBuyzere M. Transesophageal echocardiography for insertion of a physiological pacemaker in early pregnancy. *PACE* 1990;13:955–957.

39. Guldal M, Kervancioglu C, Oral D, et al. Permanent pacemaker implantation in a pregnant woman with guidance of ECG and two-dimensional echocardiography. *PACE* 1987; 10:543–545.

40. Kosowsky BD, Scherlag BJ, Damato AN. Re-evaluation of the atrial contribution to ventricular function: Study using His bundle pacing. *Am J Cardiol* 1968;21:518–524.

41. deBuitleir M, Kou WH, Schmalz S, Morady F. Acute changes in pacing threshold and R- or P-wave amplitude during permanent pacemaker implantation. *Am J Cardiol* 1990;65:999–1003.

42. Dohrmann ML, Goldschlager NF. Myocardial stimulation threshold in patients with cardiac pacemakers: Effect of physiologic variables, pharmacologic agents, and lead electrodes. *Cardiol Clinics* 1985;3:527–537.

43. Bai Y, Strathmore N, Mond H, et al. Permanent ventricular pacing via the great cardiac vein. *PACE* 1994;17:678–683.

44. Timmis G, Westveer D, Gadowski G, et al. The effect of electrode position on atrial sensing for physiologically responsive cardiac pacemakers. *Am Heart J* 1984;108:909–916.

45. Parsonnet V, Crawford CC, Bernstein AD. The 1981 United States survey of cardiac pacing practices. *J Am Coll Cardiol* 1984;3:1321–1332.

46. Barber K, Amikam S, Furman S. Atrial lead malposition in a dual chamber (DDD, M) pacemaker. *Chest* 1983;84:766–767.

47. Shandling AH, Castellanet MJ, Thomas LA, et al. Variation in P wave amplitude immediately after pacemaker implantation: Possible mechanism and implications for early reprogramming. *PACE* 1989;12:1797–1805.

48. Antonioli GE. Single lead atrialsynchronous ventricular pacing: A dream come true. *PACE* 1994;17:1531–1547.

49. Brandt J, Schuller H. Inverse relation between patient age and chronic stimulation threshold in permanent endocardial ventricular pacing. *Am Heart J* 1985;109:816–820.

50. Langenfeld H, Schneider B, Grimm W, et al. The six-minute walk—An adequate exercise test for pacemaker patients? *PACE* 1990;13(Pt II):1761–1765.

51. Hayes DL, Von Feldt L, Higano ST. Standardized informal

exercise testing for programming rate-adaptive pacemakers. *PACE* 1991;14:1772–1776.

52. Phibbs B, Marriott HJL. Complications of permanent transvenous pacing. *N Engl J Med* 1985;312:1428–1432.
53. Mueller X, Hossein S, Kappenberger L. Complications after single versus dual chamber pacemaker implantation. *PACE* 1990;13:711–714.
54. Rotem CE, Greig JH, Walters MB. Air embolism to the pulmonary artery during insertion of transvenous endocardial pacemaker. *J Thorac Cardiovasc Surg* 1967;53:562–565.
55. Pinakatt T, Leska Y, Rozanski JJ, et al. A permanently implanted endocardial electrode complicating ventricular tachycardia with a second VT. *PACE* 1983;6:26–32.
56. Glikson M, Von Feldt LK, Suman VJ, et al. Clinical surveillance of an active fixation, bipolar, polyurethane insulated pacing lead. Part I: The atrial lead. *PACE* 1994;17:1399–1404.
57. Barold SS, Center S. Electrocardiographic diagnosis of perforation of the heart by pacing catheter electrode. *Am J Cardiol* 1969;24:274–278.
58. Gondi B, Nanda NC. Real-time two-dimensional echocardiographic features of pacemaker perforation. *Circulation* 1981;64:97–106.
59. Chang AC, Atiga WL, McAreavey D, Fananapazir L. Relief of left ventricular outflow tract obstruction following inadvertent left ventricular apical pacing in a patient with hypertrophic cardiomyopathy. *PACE* 1995;18:1450–1454.
60. Reeves WC, Nanda NC, Barold SS. Echocardiographic evaluation of intracardiac pacing catheters: M-mode and two-dimensional studies. *Circulation* 1978;58:1049–1056.
61. Sharifi M, Sorkin R, Lakier JB. Left heart pacing and cardioembolic stroke. *PACE* 1994;17:1691–1696.
62. Liebold A, Aebert H, Muscholl M, Birnbaum DE. Cerebral embolism due to left ventricular pacemaker lead: Removal with cardiopulmonary bypass. *PACE* 1994;17(Pt I):2353–2355.
63. Morgan DE, Norman R, West RO, Burggraf G. Echocardiographic assessment of tricuspid regurgitation during ventricular demand pacing. *Am J Cardiol* 1986;58:1025–1029.
64. Gibson TC, Davidson RC, DeSilvey DL. Presumptive tricuspid valve malfunction induced by a pacemaker lead: A case

report and review of the literature. *PACE* 1980;3:88–90.

65. Brinker JA, Zimmern S, Gentzler R, et al. Coaxial bipolar leads–potential for internal insulation problem (abstract). *PACE* 1991;14:639.

66. Bayliss CE, Beanlands DS, Bair RJ. The pacemaker-Twiddler's syndrome: A new complication of implantable transvenous pacemakers. *Can Med Assoc J* 1968;99:371–373.

67. Kumar A, McKay CR, Rahimtoola SH. Pacemaker Twiddler's syndrome: An important cause of diaphragmatic pacing. *Am J Cardiol* 1985;56:797–799.

68. Pauletti M, DiRicco G, Solfanelli S, et al. Venous obstruction in permanent pacemaker patients: An isotopic study. *PACE* 1981;4:36–41.

69. Pasquariello JL, Hariman RJ, Yudelman IM, et al. Recurrent pulmonary embolization following implantation of transvenous pacemaker. *PACE* 1984;7:790–793.

70. Fitzgerald SP, Leckie WJH. Thrombosis complicating transvenous pacemaker lead presenting as contralateral internal jugular vein occlusion. *Am Heart J* 1985;109:593–595.

71. Girard DE, Reuler JB, Mayer BS, et al. Cerebral venous sinus thrombosis due to indwelling transvenous pacemaker catheter. *Arch Neurol* 1980;37:113–114.

72. Bradof J, Sands MJ, Lakin PC. Symptomatic venous thrombosis of the upper extremity complicating permanent transvenous pacing: Reversal with streptokinase infusion. *Am Heart J* 1982;104:1112–1113.

73. Blair RP, Seibel J, Goodreau J, et al. Surgical relief of thrombotic superior vena cava obstruction caused by endocardial pacing catheter. *Ann Thorac Surg* 1982;33:511–515.

74. Youngson GG, McKenzie TN, Nichol PM. Superior vena cava syndrome: Case report. *Am Heart J* 1980;99:503–505.

75. Yakirevich V, Algem D, Papo J, Vidne BA. Fibrotic stenosis of the superior vena cava with widespread thrombotic occlusion of its major tributaries: An unusual complication of transvenous cardiac pacing. *J Thorac Cardiovasc Surg* 1983; 85:632–638.

76. Montgomery JH, S'Souza VJ, Dyer RB, et al. Nonsurgical treatment of the superior vena cava syndrome. *Am J Cardiol* 1985;56:829–830.

77. Odell JA, Keeton GR, Millar RNS, Beningfield SJ. Pace-

maker induced superior vena cava obstruction: Management by spiral vein graft. *PACE* 1995;18(Pt I):739–742.

78. Bogart DB, Collins RH, Montgomery MA, et al. Shock later after implantation of a permanent transvenous cardiac pacemaker. *Am J Cardiol* 1985;55:1241.

79. Cooper CJ, Dweik R, Gabbay S. Treatment of pacemaker-associated right atrial thrombus with 2-hour rtPA infusion. *Am Heart J* 1993;126:228–229.

80. Camm AJ, Katritis D. Ventricular pacing for sick sinus syndrome: A risky business. *PACE* 1990;13:695–699.

81. Belott PH, Sands S, Warren J. Resetting of DDD pacemakers due to EMI. *PACE* 1984;7:169–172.

82. Heller L. Surgical electrocautery and the runaway pacemaker syndrome. *PACE* 1990;13:1084–1085.

83. Altamura G, Bianconi L, Lo Bianco F, et al. Transthoracic DC shock may represent a serious hazard in pacemaker dependent patients. *PACE* 1995;18(Pt II):194–198.

84. Lauck G, Von Smekal A, Wolke S, et al. Effects of nuclear magnetic resonance imaging on cardiac pacemakers. *PACE* 1995;18:1549–1555.

85. Lucas EH, Johnson D, McElroy BP. The effects of electronic article surveillance systems on permanent cardiac pacemakers: An in vitro study. *PACE* 1994;17(Pt II):2021–2026.

86. Souliman SK, Christie J. Pacemaker failure induced by radiotherapy. *PACE* 1994;17(Pt I):270–273.

87. Barbaro V, Bartolini P, Donato A, et al. Do European GSM mobile cellular phones pose a potential risk to pacemaker patients? *PACE* 1995;18:1218–1224.

88. Baumgartner G, Nesser HJ, Jurkovic K. Unusual cause of dyspnea: Migration of a pacemaker generator into the urinary bladder. *PACE* 1990;13:703–704.

89. Hurst LM, Evans HB, Winale B, Klein GJ. The salvage of infected cardiac pacemaker pockets using a closed irrigation system. *PACE* 1986;9:785–792.

90. Kaul Y, Mohan JC, Gopinath N, Bhatia ML. Permanent pacemaker infections: Their characterization and management—A 15-year experience. *Indian Heart J* 1983;35:345–349.

91. Wohl B, Peters RW, Carliner N, et al. Late unheralded pacemaker pocket infection due to staphylococcus epidermidis: A new clinical entity. *PACE* 1982;5:190–195.

92. Mooran JR, Steenbergen C, Durack DT. Aspergillus infec-

tion of a permanent ventricular pacing lead. *PACE* 1984; 7:361–366.

93. Cole WJ, Slater J, Kronzon I, et al. Candida albicans-infected transvenous pacemaker wire: Detection by two-dimensional echocardiography. *Am Heart J* 1986;111:417–418.

94. Choo MH, Holmes DR, Gersh BJ, et al. Permanent pacemaker infections: Characterization and management. *Am J Cardiol* 1981;48:559–564.

95. Peters G, Saborowski F, Locci R, Pulverer G. Investigations on staphylococcal infection of transvenous endocardial pacemaker electrodes. *Am Heart J* 1984;108:359–365.

96. Morgan G, Ginks W, Siddons H, Leatham A. Septicemia in patients with an endocardial pacemaker. *Am J Cardiol* 1979;44:221–230.

97. Lewis AB, Hayes DL, Holmes DR, et al. Update on infections involving permanent pacemakers. *J Thorac Cardiovasc Surg* 1985;89:758–763.

98. Kennelly BM, Piller LW. Management of infected transvenous permanent pacemakers. *Br Heart J* 1974;36:1133–1140.

99. Vilacosta I, Sarria C, San Roman JA, et al. Usefulness of transesophageal echocardiography for diagnosis of infected transvenous permanent pacemakers. *Circulation* 1994;89: 2684–2687.

100. Abad C, Manzano JJ, Quintana J, et al. Removal of infected dual-chambered transvenous pacemaker and implantation of a new epicardial dual chambered device with cardiopulmonary bypass: Experience with seven cases. *PACE* 1995;18:1272–1275.

101. Zerbe F, Ponizynski A, Dyszkiewicz W, et al. Functionless retained pacing leads in the cardiovascular system: A complication of pacemaker treatment. *Br Heart J* 1985;54:76–79.

102. Smith HJ, Fearnot NE, Byrd CL, and the U.S. Lead Extraction Database Investigators. Five-year experience with intravascular lead extraction. *PACE* 1994;17(Pt II):2016–2020.

103. Palatianos GM, Dewanjee MK, Panoutsopoulos G, et al. Comparative thrombogenicity of pacemaker leads. *PACE* 1994;17:141–145.

104. Fearnot NE, Smith HJ, Goode LB, et al. Intravascular lead extraction using locking stylets, sheaths, and other techniques. *PACE* 1990;13:1864–1870.

105. Sellers TD, Smith HJ, Fearnot NE, and the U.S. Lead Extraction Database Investigators. Intravascular lead extractions: Technique tips and U.S. database results (abstract). *PACE* 1993;16 (Pt II):1538.

106. Lloyd MA, Hayes DL, Stanson AW, Holmes DR. Snare removal of a Telectronics Accufix atrial J retention wire. *Mayo Clin Proc* 1995;70:376–379.

107. Roberts DH, Bellamy DM, Ramdale DR. Removal of a fractured temporary pacemaker electrode using endomyocardial biopsy forceps. *PACE* 1989;12:1835–1836.

108. Witte J, Munster W. Percutaneous pacemaker lead–transsecting catheter. *PACE* 1988;11:298–301.

109. Dreifus LS, Cohen D. Implanted pacemakers: Medicolegal implications. *Am J Cardiol* 1975;36:266–268.

110. Bernstein AD, Irwin ME, Parsonnet V, et al. Report of the NASPE policy conference on antibradycardia pacemaker follow-up: Effectiveness, needs, and resources. *PACE* 1994;17(Pt I):1714–1729.

Pacemaker Timing Cycles

David L. Hayes and Paul A. Levine

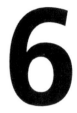

INTRODUCTION

Understanding various pacing modes and paced electrocardiograms requires a thorough understanding of pacemaker timing cycles. Pacemaker timing cycles include all potential variations of a single complete pacing cycle. This could mean the time from paced ventricular beat to paced ventricular beat; from paced ventricular beat to an intrinsic ventricular beat, whether it be a conducted R wave or a premature ventricular contraction (PVC); from paced atrial beat to paced atrial beat; from intrinsic atrial beat to paced atrial beat; from intrinsic ventricular beat to paced ventricular beat; and so forth. Various aspects of each of these cycles would include events sensed, events paced, and periods when the sensing circuit or circuits are refractory. Each portion of the pacemaker timing cycle should be considered in milliseconds (msec) and not in paced beats per minute (ppm). Although it may be easier to think of the patient's pacing rate in paced beats per minute, portions of the timing cycle are too brief to be considered in any unit but milliseconds.

If one knows the relation between the various elements of the paced electrocardiogram, understanding pacemaker rhythms becomes less complicated. Although a native rhythm may be affected by multiple unknown factors, each timing circuit of a pacemaker can function in only one of two states. A given timer can proceed until it completes its cycle; completion results in either the release of a pacing stimulus or the initiation of another timing cycle. Alternatively, a given timer can be reset, at which point it starts the timing period all over again.

PACING SYSTEM CODE

To make this chapter more readable and to facilitate clarity, a series of abbreviations is used to designate native and paced events and portions of the timing cycle. These abbreviations are listed in Table 6.1. P indicates a native atrial depolarization, A an atrial paced event, R a native ventricular depolarization, and V a paced ventricular output. I represents an interval. From this, PR refers to a native complex that completely inhibits the pacemaker on both the atrial and the ventricular channels. AV refers to pacing sequentially in both the atrium and the ventricle. If an atrial paced complex is followed by native ventricular depolarization that inhibits the ventricular output of the pacemaker, the designation is AR. If a native atrial complex is followed by a paced ventricular depolarization, P-synchronous pacing, the designation is PV. Because there are more portions of the pacemaker timing cycle to consider in dual-chamber pacing than in single-chamber pacing, more time will be

Table 6.1 Abbreviations for Native and Paced Events and Portions of the Timing Cycle

P	Native atrial depolarization
A	Atrial paced event
R	Native ventricular depolarization
V	Ventricular paced event
I	Interval
AV	Sequential pacing in the atrium and ventricle
AVI	Programmed atrioventricular pacing interval
AR	Atrial paced event followed by intrinsic ventricular depolarization
ARP	Atrial refractory period
PV	Native atrial depolarization followed by a paced ventricular event, P-synchronous pacing
AEI	Interval from a ventricular sensed or paced event to an atrial paced event, the VA interval
LRL	Lower rate limit
URL	Upper rate limit
MTR	Maximum tracking rate
MSR	Maximum sensor rate
PVARP	Postventricular atrial refractory period
RRAVD	Rate-responsive atrioventricular delay
VA	Ventriculoatrial interval: interval from a sensed or paced ventricular event to an atrial paced event
VRP	Ventricular refractory period

devoted to understanding dual-chamber timing cycles, specifically those of DDD pacing systems.

A three-letter code describing the basic function of the various pacing systems was first proposed in 1974 by a combined task force from the American Heart Association and the American College of Cardiology. Since that time, responsibility for periodically updating the code has been assumed by a committee consisting of members of the North American Society of Pacing and Electrophysiology (NASPE) and the British Pacing and Electrophysiology Group (BPEG). The code is designated the NBG code for pacing nomenclature.[1] The code has five positions, but the fifth position is rarely used. It is a generic code and, as such, does not describe specific or unique functional characteristics of each device. (Even though the first three positions are restricted to bradycardia support pacing, the code can describe all devices used for rhythm management. However, a more specific code is now used for implantable cardioverter-defibrillators.)[2] The NBG code will be used extensively in this chapter.

The first position reflects the chamber or chambers in which stimulation occurs. A refers to the atrium; V indicates the ventricle; and D means dual chamber, or both atrium and ventricle.

The second position refers to the chamber or chambers in which sensing occurs. The letters are the same as those for the first position. Manufacturers also use S in both the first and the second positions to indicate that the device is capable of pacing only a single cardiac chamber. Once the device is implanted and connected to a lead in either the atrium or the ventricle, S should be changed to either A or V in the clinical record to reflect the chamber in which pacing and sensing are occurring.

The third position refers to the mode of sensing, or how the pacemaker responds to a sensed event. An I indicates that a sensed event inhibits the output pulse and causes the pacemaker to recycle for one or more timing cycles. T means that an output pulse is triggered in response to a sensed event. D, in a manner similar to that in the first two positions, means that there are dual modes of response. This designation is restricted to dual-chamber systems. An event sensed in the atrium inhibits the atrial output but triggers a ventricular output. Unlike in the single-chamber triggered mode, in which an output pulse is triggered immediately on sensing, there is a delay between the sensed atrial event and the triggered ventricular output to mimic the normal PR interval. If a native ventricular signal or R wave is sensed, it will inhibit the ventricular output and possibly even the atrial output, depending on where sensing occurs.

The fourth position of the code reflects both programmability and rate modulation. O indicates that none of the settings of the pacing system can be noninvasively altered. P is simple programmability; one or two variables can be changed, but this code does not specify which ones. M is multiparameter programmability, which means that three or more parameters can be changed. C reflects the ability of the pacemaker to communicate with the programmer; namely, it has telemetry. By convention, it also means that the pacemaker has multiparameter programmability. An R in the fourth position indicates that the pacemaker incorporates a sensor to control the rate independently of intrinsic electrical activity of the heart. Virtually all pacemakers with a sensor also have extensive telemetric and programmable capabilities. There is not sufficient space within the code to indicate which sensor is being utilized. From a practical standpoint, R is the only indicator commonly used in the fourth position.

The fifth position is restricted to antitachycardia functions and is rarely used.

PACING MODES

Ventricular asynchronous pacing, atrial asynchronous pacing, and AV sequential asynchronous pacing

Ventricular asynchronous (VOO) pacing is the simplest of all pacing modes because there is no sensing and no mode of response. The timing cycle is shown in Figure 6.1. Irrespective of any other events, the ventricular pacing artifacts occur at the programmed rate. The timing cycle cannot be reset by any intrinsic event. In the absence of sensing, there is no defined refractory period.

Atrial asynchronous (AOO) pacing behaves exactly like VOO, but the pacing artifacts occur in the atrial chamber.

Dual-chamber, or AV sequential asynchronous (DOO), pacing has an equally simple timing cycle. The interval from atrial artifact to ventricular artifact (atrioventricular interval, AVI) and the interval from the ventricular artifact to the subsequent atrial pacing artifact (VA or atrial escape interval, AEI) are fixed. The intervals never change, because the pacing mode is insensitive to any atrial or ventricular activity, and the timers are never reset (Figure 6.2).

281

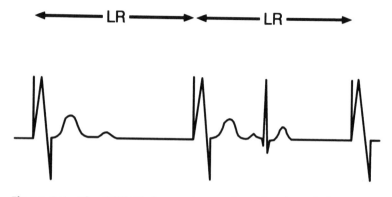

Figure 6.1 The VOO timing cycle consists of only a defined rate. The pacemaker delivers a ventricular pacing artifact at the defined rate regardless of intrinsic events. In this example, an intrinsic QRS complex occurs after the second paced complex, but because there is no sensing in the VOO mode, the interval between the second and the third paced complex remains stable.

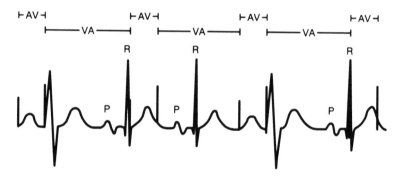

Figure 6.2 The DOO timing cycle consists of only defined AVI and VV intervals. The VA interval is a function of the AV and VV intervals. An atrial pacing artifact is delivered and the ventricular artifact follows at the programmed AVI. The next atrial pacing artifact is delivered at the completion of the VA interval. There is no variation in the intervals because no activity is sensed; that is, nothing interrupts or resets the programmed cycles.

Ventricular inhibited pacing

By definition, ventricular inhibited (VVI) pacing incorporates sensing on the ventricular channel, and pacemaker output is inhibited by a sensed ventricular event (Figure 6.3). VVI pacemakers are refractory for a period after a paced or sensed ventricular event, the ventricular refractory period (VRP). Any ventricular event occurring within the VRP is not sensed and does not reset the ventricular timer (Figure 6.4).

Atrial inhibited pacing

Atrial inhibited (AAI) pacing, the atrial counterpart of VVI pacing, incorporates the same timing cycles, with the obvious differences that pacing and sensing occur from the atrium and pacemaker

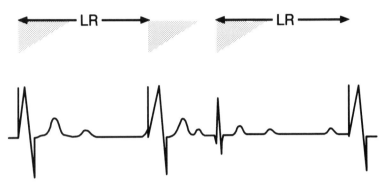

Figure 6.3 The VVI timing cycle consists of a defined lower rate limit (LRL) and a ventricular refractory period (VRP, represented by triangle). When the LRL timer is complete, a pacing artifact is delivered in the absence of a sensed intrinsic ventricular event. If an intrinsic QRS occurs, the LRL timer is started from that point. A VRP begins with any sensed or paced ventricular activity.

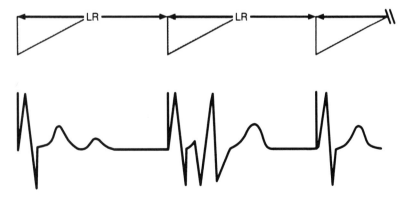

Figure 6.4 If, in the VVI mode, a ventricular event occurs during the VRP (represented by triangle), it is not sensed and therefore does not reset the LRL timer.

output is inhibited by a sensed atrial event (Figure 6.5). An atrial paced or sensed event initiates a refractory period during which nothing is sensed by the pacemaker. Confusion can arise when multiple ventricular events occur while there is atrial pacing. For example, in addition to the intrinsic QRS that occurs in response to the paced atrial beat, if a premature ventricular beat follows, it does not inhibit an atrial pacing artifact from being delivered (Figure 6.6). When the AA timing cycle ends, the atrial pacing artifact is delivered regardless of ventricular events, because an AAI pacemaker should not sense anything in the ventricle. The single exception to this rule is far-field sensing; that is, the ventricular signal is large enough to be inappropriately sensed by the atrial lead (Figure 6.7). In this situation, the atrial timing cycle is reset. Sometimes this anomaly can be corrected by making the atrial channel less sensitive or by lengthening the refractory period.

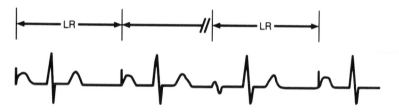

Figure 6.5 The AAI timing cycle consists of a defined lower rate limit (LRL) and an atrial refractory period (ARP). When the LRL timer is complete, a pacing artifact is delivered in the atrium in the absence of a sensed atrial event. If an intrinsic P wave occurs, the LRL timer is started from that point. An ARP begins with any sensed or paced atrial activity.

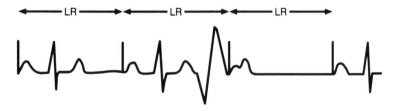

Figure 6.6 In the AAI mode, only atrial activity is sensed. In this example, it may appear unusual for paced atrial activity to occur so soon after intrinsic ventricular activity. Because sensing occurs only in the atrium, ventricular activity would not be expected to reset the pacemaker's timing cycle.

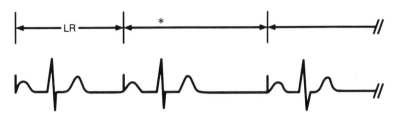

Figure 6.7 In this example of AAI pacing, the AA interval is 1000 msec (60 ppm). The interval between the second and the third paced atrial events is >1000 msec. The interval from the second QRS complex to the subsequent atrial pacing artifact is 1000 msec. This occurs because the second QRS complex (*) has been sensed on the atrial lead (far-field sensing) and has inappropriately reset the timing cycle.

Single-chamber triggered-mode pacing

Initially developed as a way to defeat the problem associated with oversensing in the inhibited demand mode, the triggered mode has its own unique advantages as well as disadvantages. In single-chamber triggered-mode pacing, the pacemaker releases an output pulse every time a native event is sensed. This feature increases the current drain on the battery, accelerating its rate of depletion. This mode of pacing also deforms the native signal, compromising interpretation of the electrocardiogram. However, it can serve as an excellent marker for the site of sensing within a complex. It can also prevent inappropriate inhibition from oversensing when the patient does not have a stable native escape rhythm. In addition, it can be used for noninvasive electrophysiologic studies, with the already implanted pacemaker tracking chest wall stimuli created by a programmable stimulator. The one special requirement if one is to use the triggered mode for noninvasive electrophysiologic studies is to shorten the refractory period intentionally, allowing the implanted pacemaker to track the external chest wall stimuli to rapid rates and close coupling intervals. Normally, the refractory mode is at or near 400 msec to minimize the chance of sensing its own T wave and triggering another output pulse into the vulnerable zone of myocardial repolarization.

Rate-modulated pacing

Before various rate-modulated pacing modes are discussed, two terms—*sensor* and *sensed*—need clarification. Both are used in cardiac pacing and are commonly confused because they sound alike;

actually, they reflect markedly different events. *Pacemaker sensing* refers to the pacemaker's recognition of a native depolarization in either the atrium or the ventricle. The behavior of the pacemaker with respect to a sensed event is described by the third position of the NBG code. The "sensor function of the pacemaker" refers to a modulation of rate in response to an input signal other than the presence or absence of a native depolarization. Sometimes, a portion of the QRS-ST complex, such as the area of the evoked potential of the stimulus to the T-wave interval, serves as the sensor. Other sensors include vibration or acceleration associated with physical activity, central venous temperature, central venous oxygen saturation, QT interval, and impedance signals measuring minute ventilation.

Single-chamber rate-modulated pacing: Single-chamber pacemakers capable of rate-modulated (SSIR) pacing can be implanted in the ventricle (VVIR) or atrium (AAIR). The timing cycles for SSIR pacemakers are not significantly different from those of their non–rate-modulated counterparts. The timing cycle includes the basic VV or AA interval and a refractory period from the paced or sensed event. The difference lies in the variability of the VV or AA interval (Figure 6.8). Depending on the sensor incorporated and the level of exertion of the patient, the basic interval will shorten from the programmed lower rate limit (LRL). Shortening requires that an upper rate limit (URL) be programmed to define the absolute shortest cycle length allowable. Most approved SSIR pacemakers incorporate a fixed refractory period; that is, regardless of whether the pacemaker is operating at the LRL or URL, the refractory period remains the same. Thus, at the higher rates under sensor drive, the pacemaker may effectively become SOOR, since the alert period during which sensing can occur is so abbreviated. Native beats falling during the refractory period are not sensed. Hence, in SSIR pacing systems, if the refractory period is programmable, it should be programmed to a short interval to maximize the sensing period at both the low and the high sensor-controlled rates. Rate-variable or rate-adaptive refractory period as a programmable option—that is, as the cycle length shortens, the refractory period shortens appropriately, analogous to the QT interval of the native ventricular depolarization—is likely to become more commonly available in subsequent generations of SSIR pacemakers.

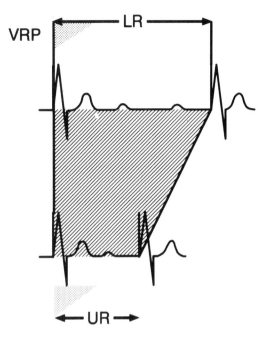

Figure 6.8 The VVIR timing cycle consists of a lower rate limit (LRL), an upper rate limit (UR), and a ventricular refractory period (VRP, represented by triangle). As indicated by sensor activity, the VV cycle length shortens accordingly. (The striped area represents the range of sensor-driven VV cycle lengths.) In most VVIR pacemakers, the VRP remains fixed despite the changing VV cycle length. In selected VVIR pacemakers, the VRP shortens as the cycle length shortens.

Single-chamber rate-modulated asynchronous and dual-chamber rate-modulated asynchronous pacing: The asynchronous pacing modes, that is, AOO, VOO, and DOO, as explained above, have fixed intervals that are insensitive to all intrinsic events, and the timers are never reset. If rate modulation is incorporated in an asynchronous pacing mode, the basic cycle length is altered by sensor activity. In the single-chamber rate-modulated asynchronous (AOOR and VOOR) pacing modes, any alteration in cycle length is due to sensor activity and not to the sensing of intrinsic cardiac depolarizations. In the dual-chamber rate-modulated asynchronous (DOOR) pacing mode, the pacing rate changes in response to the sensor input signal but not to the native P or R wave. In some pacemakers, the AVI may be programmed to shorten progressively as the rate increases, whereas in other units, it remains fixed at the initial programmed setting.

AV sequential, ventricular inhibited pacing: AV sequential, ventricular inhibited (DVI) pacing is rarely used as the preimplantation pacing mode of choice. However, this pacing mode is a programmable option in most available dual-chamber pacemakers. In addition, a small number of patients still have dedicated DVI pacemakers. For these reasons, it is important to understand the timing cycles for DVI pacing.[3,4]

By definition, DVI provides pacing in both the atrium and the ventricle (D) but sensing only in the ventricle (V). The pacemaker is inhibited and reset by sensed ventricular activity but ignores all intrinsic atrial complexes. The DVI units in the first generation were large and bulky and had two relatively large bipolar leads. The bipolar output pulses were small, and with the highly localized sensing field associated with the bipolar design, the ventricular sense amplifier remained alert when the atrial stimulus was released and throughout the AVI. Thus, a native R wave during the AVI was sensed, so that the ventricular output was inhibited and the AEI was reset (Figure 6.9a). For both atrial and ventricular stimuli to be inhibited, the sensed R wave would have to occur during the AEI. Improvements in circuit design enabled the manufacturers to reduce the size of the pulse generator. They also made the next generation unipolar to facilitate venous access for the two leads. The large unipolar atrial stimulus could be sensed on the ventricular channel. This would be sensed by the pacemaker as a ventricular event and inhibit ventricular output. This is known as crosstalk, which is potentially catastrophic if concomitant AV block is present. To prevent crosstalk, the second generation of DVI pacemakers initiated the ventricular refractory period on completion of the AEI timer. Thus, once there was an atrial output pulse, the ventricular sense amplifier was refractory and the pacemaker was obligated to release a ventricular output pulse, regardless of whether it was physiologically necessary. This event was termed *committed AV sequential pacing* (Figure 6.10). It caused significant confusion, because a normally functioning system might demonstrate functional undersensing and functional noncapture in both atrium and ventricle simultaneously.

The present generation of devices still requires a period of ventricular refractoriness, "ventricular blanking period," to minimize the chance of crosstalk, but this is now a very brief interval,

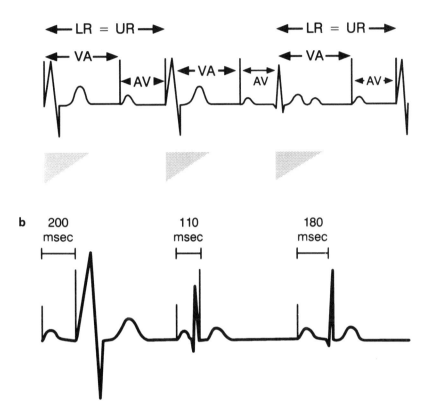

Figure 6.9 (a) In the noncommitted version of DVI, the components of the timing cycle are the same as those for DVIC (see Figure 6.10). However, if ventricular activity is sensed after the atrial pacing artifact, ventricular output will be inhibited; that is, a ventricular pacing artifact is not committed to the previous atrial pacing artifact. (b) In the modified or partially committed version of DVI, ventricular events sensed within the nonphysiologic AVI do not inhibit ventricular output, and a ventricular pacing stimulus occurs at the end of the interval. Ventricular events occurring within the physiologic AV interval inhibit pacemaker function. In this example, the first paced atrial and ventricular events represent normal DVI pacing. The second paced atrial and intrinsic ventricular complex demonstrates a spontaneous ventricular event occurring within the nonphysiologic AV interval and resulting in a ventricular pacing stimulus. In the third event shown, after an atrial paced event, a spontaneous ventricular event falls within the physiologic AV interval, resulting in inhibition of ventricular pacing function.

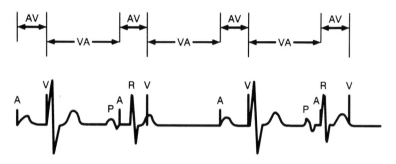

Figure 6.10 The timing cycle in DVIC consists of a lower rate limit (LRL), an AVI, and a VRP. The VRP is initiated with any sensed or paced ventricular activity. (By definition, there is no atrial sensing and, therefore, no defined atrial refractory period.) The VA interval is equal to the VV or LRL interval minus the AVI. In a committed system, a ventricular pacing artifact follows an atrial pacing artifact at the AVI regardless of whether intrinsic ventricular activity has occurred. In this example, the LRL is 1000 msec, or 60 ppm, and the AVI is 200 msec. At the end of the VA interval, 800 msec after a ventricular event, if no ventricular activity has been sensed, the atrial pacing artifact is delivered. A ventricular pacing artifact occurs 200 msec later irrespective of any intrinsic events.

between 12 and 125 msec; in many pacemakers its duration is programmable. If the atrial stimulus were to coincide with a native R wave, for example, a PVC, and the intrinsic deflection of the native complex fell outside the blanking period, the R wave would be sensed and ventricular output inhibited. In this situation, the pacemaker would behave like the earlier noncommitted systems. If, however, the intrinsic deflection coincided with the blanking period, the R wave would not be seen and the pacemaker would release a ventricular output pulse at the end of the AVI in a manner analogous to that of the committed systems. This operation has been termed *modified* or *partially committed* to reflect the fact that the devices may demonstrate both noncommitted and committed functions as part of their normal behavior[5] (Figure 6.9b).

The timing cycle (VV) consists of the AV and VA intervals. The basic cycle length (VV), or LRL, is programmable, as is the AVI. The difference, VV − AV, is the VA interval, or AEI. During the initial portion of the VA interval, the sensing channel is refractory. (The refractory period is almost always a programmable interval.) After the refractory period, the ventricular sensing channel is again operational, or "alert." If ventricular activity is not sensed by the expiration of the VA interval, atrial pacing occurs, followed by the AVI. If intrinsic ventricular activity occurs before the VA interval is completed, the timing cycle is reset. (Additional discussion of crosstalk, the ventricular blanking period, and ventricular safety pacing can be found in the subsequent section specifically discussing the AVI.)

AV sequential, non–P-synchronous pacing with dual-chamber sensing: AV sequential pacing with dual-chamber sensing, non–P-synchronous (DDI) pacing can be thought of as an upgrade of DVI noncommitted pacing or a downgrade of DDD pacing, that is, DDD pacing without atrial tracking.[6] The difference between DVI and DDI is that DDI incorporates atrial sensing as well as ventricular sensing. This prevents competitive atrial pacing that can occur with DVI pacing. The DDI mode of response is inhibition only; that is, no tracking of P waves can occur. Therefore, the paced ventricular rate cannot be greater than the programmed LRL. The timing cycle consists of the LRL, AVI, postventricular atrial refractory period (PVARP), and VRP. The PVARP is the period after a sensed or paced ventricular event during which the atrial sensing circuit is refractory. Any atrial event occurring during the PVARP will not be sensed by the atrial sensing circuit. If a P wave occurs after the PVARP and is sensed, no atrial pacing artifact is delivered at the end of the VA interval. The subsequent ventricular pacing artifact cannot occur until the VV interval has been completed; that is, the LRL cannot be violated (Figure 6.11).

It bears repeating that because P-wave tracking does not occur with the DDI mode, the paced rate is never greater than the programmed LRL. A slight exception to this statement occurs when an intrinsic ventricular complex takes place after the paced atrial beat (AR) and inhibits paced ventricular output before completion of the programmed AVI; that is, AR < AV. In this situation, the cycle length from A to A is shorter than the programmed LRL by the difference between the AR and the AVI (see Figure 6.17, top).

AV sequential, non–P-synchronous, rate-modulated pacing with dual-chamber sensing: The timing cycles for non–P-synchronous, rate-modulated AV sequential (DDIR) pacing are the same as those described above for DDI pacing except that paced rates can exceed the programmed LRL through sensor-driven

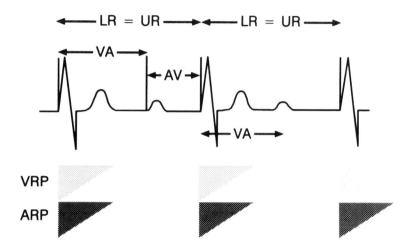

Figure 6.11 The timing cycle in DDI consists of an LRL, an AVI, a VRP, and an ARP. The VRP is initiated by any sensed or paced ventricular activity, and the ARP is initiated by any sensed or paced atrial activity. DDI can be thought of as DDD pacing without the capability of P-wave tracking or DVI without the potential for atrial competition by virtue of atrial sensing. The LRL cannot be violated even if the sinus rate is occurring at a faster rate. For example, the LRL is 1000 msec, or 60 ppm, and the AVI is 200 msec. If a P wave occurs 500 msec after a paced ventricular complex, the AVI is initiated; but at the end of the AVI, 700 msec from the previous paced ventricular activity, a ventricular pacing artifact cannot be delivered, because it would violate the LRL.

activity. Depending on the sensor incorporated and the level of exertion of the patient, the basic cycle length will shorten from the programmed LRL. This requires that a URL be programmed to define the absolute shortest cycle length allowable.

Even though there is no P-wave tracking in a DDIR system, it is possible for an intrinsic P wave to inhibit the atrial pacing artifact and give the appearance of P-wave tracking if an appropriately timed intrinsic atrial depolarization falls within the atrial sensing window (see "Dual-Chamber Rate-Modulated Pacemakers: Effect on Timing Cycles," below).

Atrial synchronous (P-tracking) pacing: Atrial synchronous (P-tracking) (VDD) pacemakers pace only in the ventricle (V), sense in both atrium and ventricle (D), and respond both by inhibition of ventricular output by intrinsic ventricular activity (I) and by ventricular tracking of P waves (T). (When the mode of response includes both I and T, the NBG code designation is D.) This mode of pacing is a programmable option in many dual-chamber pacemakers.[7] The VDD mode has also become increasingly available as a single-lead pacing system. In this system, a single lead is capable of pacing in the ventricle in response to sensing atrial activity by way of a remote electrode situated on the intra-atrial portion of the ventricular pacing lead.

The timing cycle is composed of LRL, AVI, PVARP, VRP, and URL. A sensed atrial event initiates the AVI. If an intrinsic ventricular event occurs before the termination of the AVI, ventricular output is inhibited and the LRL timing cycle is reset. If a paced ventricular beat occurs at the end of the AVI, this beat resets the LRL. If no atrial event occurs, the pacemaker escapes with a paced ventricular event at the LRL; that is, the pacemaker displays VVI activity in the absence of a sensed atrial event (Figure 6.12).

Dual-chamber pacing and sensing with inhibition and tracking:
Although it involves more timers, standard dual-chamber pacing and sensing with inhibition and tracking (DDD) is reasonably easy to comprehend if one understands the timing cycles already dis-

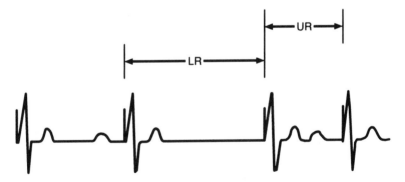

Figure 6.12 The timing cycle of VDD consists of an LRL, an AVI, a VRP, a PVARP, and a URL. A sensed P wave initiates the AVI (during the AVI, the atrial sensing channel is refractory). At the end of the AVI, a ventricular pacing artifact is delivered if no intrinsic ventricular activity has been sensed, that is, P-wave tracking. Ventricular activity, paced or sensed, initiates the PVARP and the VA interval (the LRL interval minus the AVI). If no P-wave activity occurs, the pacemaker escapes with a ventricular pacing artifact at the LRL.

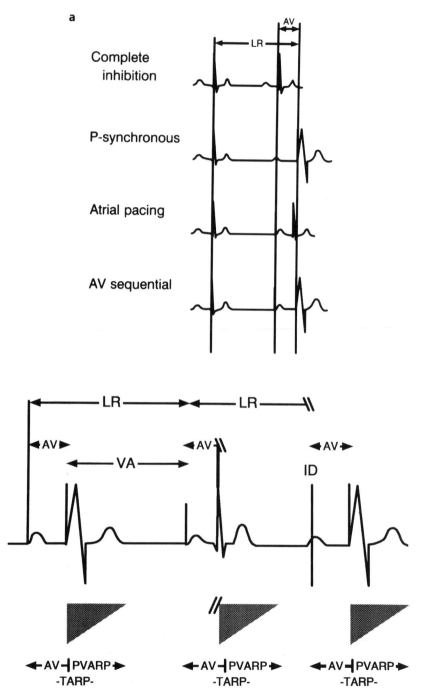

cussed.[7–12] The basic timing circuit associated with LRL pacing is divided into two sections. The first is the interval from a ventricular sensed or paced event to an atrial paced event. This is the AEI, or VA interval. The second interval begins with an atrial sensed or paced event and extends to a ventricular event. This interval may be defined by a paced AVI, PR interval, AR interval, or PV interval. An atrial sensed event that occurs before completion of the AEI promptly terminates this interval and initiates an AVI, and the result is P-wave synchronous ventricular pacing.[8] If the intrinsic sinus rate is less than the programmed LRL, AV sequential pacing at the programmed rate or functional single-chamber atrial (AR) pacing occurs (Figure 6.13a).

PORTIONS OF PACEMAKER TIMING CYCLES
Refractory periods

Every pacemaker capable of sensing must include a refractory period in its basic timing cycle. Refractory periods prevent the sensing of early inappropriate signals, such as the evoked potential and repolarization (T wave). Refractory period terminology is confusing to many students of pacemaker timing cycles, but it need not be.

◄───────────────────────────

Figure 6.13 (a) The timing cycle in DDD consists of an LRL, an AVI, a VRP, a PVARP, and a URL. There are four variations of the DDD timing cycle. If intrinsic atrial and ventricular activity occur before the LRL times out, both channels are inhibited and no pacing occurs (first panel). If a P wave is sensed before the VA interval is completed (the LRL minus the AVI), output from the atrial channel is inhibited. The AVI is initiated, and if no ventricular activity is sensed before the AVI terminates, a ventricular pacing artifact is delivered, that is, P-synchronous pacing (second panel). If no atrial activity is sensed before the VA interval is completed, an atrial pacing artifact is delivered, which initiates the AVI. If intrinsic ventricular activity occurs before the termination of the AVI, the ventricular output from the pacemaker is inhibited, that is, atrial pacing (third panel). If no intrinsic ventricular activity occurs before the termination of the AVI, a ventricular pacing artifact is delivered, that is, AV sequential pacing (fourth panel). (b) Potential pacing combinations that can occur in the DDD pacing mode. The intrinsic P wave is sensed during the early portion of the P wave. The AVI is initiated at the point of the intrinsic deflection (ID) of atrial activity, as seen on the atrial electrogram. (Modified from Medtronic, Minneapolis, MN.)

295

In a DDD system, a sensed or paced atrial event initiates an atrial refractory period (ARP) and also initiates the AVI (Figure 6.13b). During this portion of the timing cycle, the atrial channel is refractory to any sensed event; nor will atrial pacing occur during this period. A sensed or paced ventricular event initiates a VRP. (A VRP is always part of the timing cycle of any pacing system with ventricular pacing and sensing.) The VRP prevents sensing of the evoked potential and the resultant T wave on the ventricular channel of the pacemaker. A sensed or paced ventricular event also initiates a PVARP.[13,14] The PVARP prevents atrial sensing of a retrograde P wave (see "Endless-Loop Tachycardia," below) and also prevents sensing of far-field ventricular events. The combination of the PVARP and the AVI forms the total atrial refractory period (TARP). The TARP, in turn, is the limiting factor for the maximum sensed atrial rate that the pacemaker can reach. For example, if the AVI is 150 msec and the PVARP is 250 msec, the TARP is 400 msec, or 150 ppm. In this case, a paced ventricular event initiates the 250-msec PVARP, and only after this interval has ended can an atrial event be sensed. If an atrial event is sensed immediately after the termination of the PVARP, the sensed atrial event initiates the AVI of 150 msec. On termination of the AVI, in the absence of an intrinsic R wave, a paced ventricular event will occur, resulting in a VV cycle length of 400 msec, or 150 ppm. Programming a long PVARP limits the upper rate by limiting the maximum sensed atrial rate[15,16] (Figure 6.14). If the native atrial rate were 151 beats per minute (bpm), every other P wave would coincide with the PVARP, not be sensed, and hence not be tracked, so that the effective paced rate would be approximately 75 ppm, or half the atrial rate.

Atrioventricular interval

The AVI, often poorly understood, should be considered as a single interval with two subportions[17] (Figure 6.15a). The blanking period accounts for the earliest portion of the AVI. The blanking period can be defined as the time during and after a pacemaker stimulus when the opposite channel of a dual-chamber pacemaker is insensitive. The purpose of this is to avoid sensing the electronic event of one channel in the opposite channel.[18–20]

If the atrial pacing artifact were sensed by the ventricular sensing circuit, ventricular output inhibition would result. This is termed *crosstalk*. To prevent this, the leading edge of the atrial pacing artifact is masked, or blanked, by rendering the ventricular

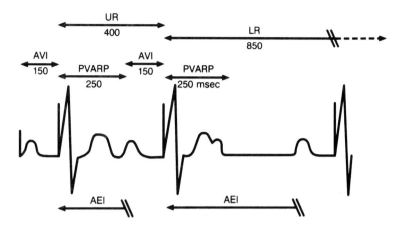

Figure 6.14 In the DDD pacing mode, the upper rate (UR) is limited by the AVI and the PVARP. In this example, the AVI is 150 msec and the PVARP is 250 msec for a TARP of 400 msec (this is equal to 150 ppm). As shown, after the first paced ventricular complex, a P wave occurs just after the completion of the PVARP. This P wave is sensed, initiates the AVI, and is followed by another paced ventricular complex. The subsequent P wave occurs within the PVARP and is therefore not sensed. The DDD response is to wait for the next intrinsic P wave to occur, as in this example, or for the AEI to be completed, whereupon AV sequential pacing occurs.

sensing circuit refractory during the very early portion of the AVI (Figure 6.15b). In current DDD pacemakers, the blanking period may be programmable, ranging from 12 to 125 msec. The blanking period is traditionally of short duration because it is important for the ventricular sensing circuit to be returned to the "alert" state relatively early during the AVI so that intrinsic ventricular activity can inhibit pacemaker output if it occurs before the AVI ends. The potential exists for signals other than those of intrinsic ventricular activity to be sensed and inhibit ventricular output. The greatest concern is crosstalk.[19,21] Even though the leading edge of the atrial pacing artifact is effectively ignored because of the blanking period, the trailing edge of the atrial pacing artifact occurring after the blanking period can at times be sensed on the ventricular channel. In a pacemaker-dependent patient, inhibition of ventricular output by crosstalk would result in asystole. A safety mechanism is present to prevent such an outcome.

If activity is sensed on the ventricular sensing circuit in a given portion of the AVI immediately after the blanking period (this—

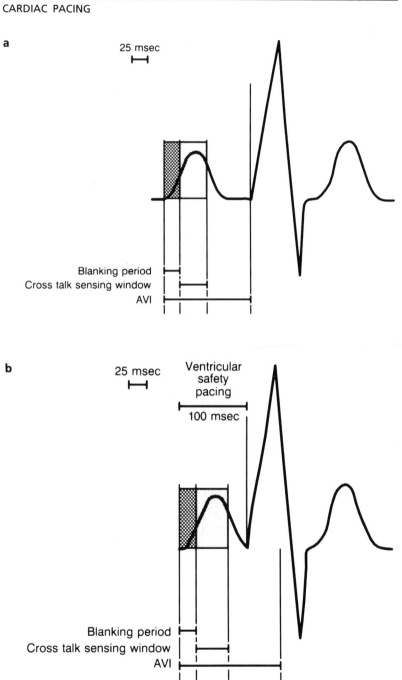

a

25 msec

Blanking period
Cross talk sensing window
AVI

b

25 msec

Ventricular
safety
pacing

100 msec

Blanking period
Cross talk sensing window
AVI

c

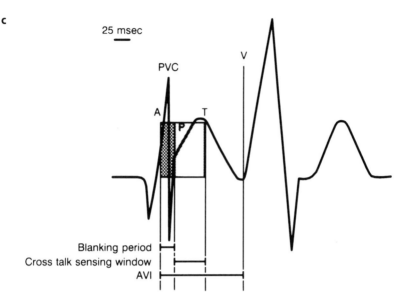

25 msec

PVC

V

A   T

P

Blanking period
Cross talk sensing window
AVI

Figure 6.15   (a) The AVI should be considered as a single interval with two subportions. The entire AVI corresponds to the programmed value, that is, the interval following a paced or sensed atrial beat allowed before a ventricular pacing artifact is delivered. The initial portion of the AVI is the blanking period. This interval is followed by the crosstalk sensing window. (b) If the ventricular sensing circuit senses activity during the crosstalk sensing window, a ventricular pacing artifact is delivered early, usually at 100 to 110 msec after the atrial event. This has been referred to as "ventricular safety pacing," "110-msec phenomenon," and "nonphysiologic AV delay." (c) The initial portion of the AVI in most dual-chamber pacemakers is designated as the blanking period. During this portion of the AVI, sensing is suspended. The primary purpose of this interval is to prevent ventricular sensing of the leading edge of the atrial pacing artifact. Any event that occurs during the blanking period, even if it is an intrinsic ventricular event, as shown in this figure, is not sensed. In this example, the ventricular premature beat that is not sensed is followed by a ventricular pacing artifact delivered at the programmed AVI and occurring in the terminal portion of the T wave.

the second—portion of the AVI has been called the "ventricular triggering period' or the "crosstalk sensing window"), it is assumed that crosstalk cannot be differentiated from intrinsic ventricular activity. To prevent catastrophic ventricular asystole, a ventricular pacing artifact is delivered early, that is, at an AVI of 100 to 120 msec, although in some units this interval is programmable for

50 to 150 msec[22] (Figure 6.15c). If the signal sensed is indeed crosstalk, a paced ventricular complex at the abbreviated interval prevents ventricular asystole. If, on the other hand, intrinsic ventricular activity occurs during the early portion of the AVI, the safety mechanism results in delivery of a ventricular pacing artifact within or immediately after the intrinsic beat. This delivery is safe because the ventricle is refractory, no depolarization results from the pacing artifact, and the pacing artifact is delivered too early to coincide with ventricular repolarization or a vulnerable period. This event has been referred to as "ventricular safety pacing," "nonphysiologic AV delay," or the "110-msec phenomenon."

After the blanking period and the nonphysiologic AV delay, the ventricular sensing circuit remains alert and will be reset by any activity sensed.

Differential AVI: If there is a consistent difference between AVIs initiated by a sensed event and those initiated by a paced event, the likely explanation is a differential AVI. As noted in the introduction to this section, this is an attempt to provide an interatrial conduction time of equal duration whether atrial contraction is paced or sensed. The PV interval initiated with atrial sensing commences at the time of atrial depolarization. Conversely, the AVI initiated with atrial pacing commences with the pacing artifact, not with atrial depolarization. The AVI following a sensed atrial event should therefore be shorter than that following a paced atrial event (Figure 6.16). The AVI differential is programmable in some pacemakers and preset in others.

One manufacturer uses the term *AV delay hysteresis* to describe the differential AVI.[23] This DDD pacemaker automatically calculates the AVI differential between paced and sensed atrial events. When an atrial paced event occurs, the AR interval is measured. When an atrial sensed event follows an atrial paced event, a new PR interval is measured. The AV delay hysteresis is set equal to the maximum value (AR or PR) minus the PR interval (Figure 6.17).

Rate-variable or rate-adaptive AVI: Many DDDR pacemakers have the capability of shortening the AVI during AV sequential sensor-driven pacing (Figure 6.18). Rate-adaptive or rate-variable AVI is intended to optimize cardiac output by mimicking the normal physiologic decrease in the PR interval that occurs in the normal

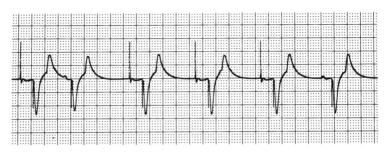

Figure 6.16 Electrocardiographic tracing demonstrating differential AVI. The AVI is 50 msec longer than the PV interval. (From *Relay Models 293-03 and 294-03. Intermedics Cardiac Pulse Generator Physician's Manual*. Angleton, TX: Intermedics, 1992. By permission of Intermedics.)

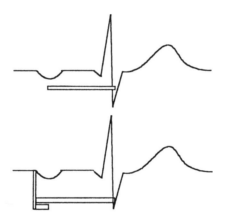

AV Delay Hysteresis = A-R Interval - P-R Interval

Figure 6.17 Schematic diagram of one manufacturer's differential AVI, designated "AV delay hysteresis." (Modified from *Chorus II Model 6234, 6244 Dual Chamber Pulse Generator Physician's Manual*. Minnetonka, MN: ELA Medical, 1994.)

heart as the atrial rate increases.[24–26] The rate-related shortening of the AVI may also improve atrial sensing by shortening the TARP and thereby extending the time for the atrial sensing window.

Rate-adaptive AVI may be designed in several ways. The method becoming more common is to allow linear shortening of the AVI from a programmed baseline AVI to a programmed minimum AVI. A second method allows a limited number of

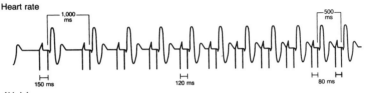

Figure 6.18 As heart rate increases, AV delay dynamically adapts to the change in cycle length. (From Hayes DL, Ketelson A, Levine PA, et al. Understanding timing systems of current DDDR pacemakers. *Eur JCPE* 1993;3[1]:70–86. By permission of Mayo Foundation.)

stepwise shortenings of the AVI. These steps may or may not be programmable. The least commonly used method is single-step or one-step shortening of the AVI at a given rate.

AVI hysteresis: This term has been used to represent several different variations of the AVI. Some use it synonymously with differential AVI (see "Differential AVI," above). Others have used this term to describe alterations in the paced AVI relative to the patient's intrinsic AV conduction. For example, a longer paced AVI is permitted to allow maintenance of intrinsic AV conduction. However, once the intrinsic PR or AR interval triggers the programmed AV hysteresis interval, consistent AV pacing at the programmed AVI occurs.

One manufacturer uses the designation "DDD/AMC™ pacing mode" for variations in AVI relative to the patient's intrinsic AV nodal conduction status.[23] When normal AV conduction is intact, the pacemaker functions in the AAI mode and monitors AV conduction (Figure 6.19a). Each PR or AR interval is monitored. When an atrial event is detected, a ventricular surveillance window (VSW) is activated that is equal to an average of the last eight PR or AR intervals (or both) plus 31 msec. If a spontaneous ventricular event occurs before the end of the VSW, the pacemaker calculates a new VSW and remains in the AAI mode. If a ventricular event is not sensed before the end of the VSW, the pacemaker switches to the DDD mode (Figure 6.19b). The ventricle is paced at the end of the VSW, and an AVI is initiated with the next atrial event. After the return of spontaneous atrial or ventricular activity or after 100 paced ventricular events, the AVI is lengthened by 31 msec to promote intrinsic AV conduction. If 16 consecutive cycles of spontaneous ventricular activity are detected after the 31-msec extension, the pacemaker returns to the AAI mode. If five consecutive paced ventricular events occur, the 31-msec extension is subtracted from the AVI, the pacemaker remains in the DDD mode, and the process is reinitiated.

BASE RATE BEHAVIOR

The way a pacemaker behaves in response to a sensed ventricular signal varies among manufacturers and among devices from the same manufacturer. Dual-chamber pacemakers may have a ventricular-based timing system, an atrial-based timing system, or a hybrid of these two systems.[4,27] Designation of a pacemaker's tim-

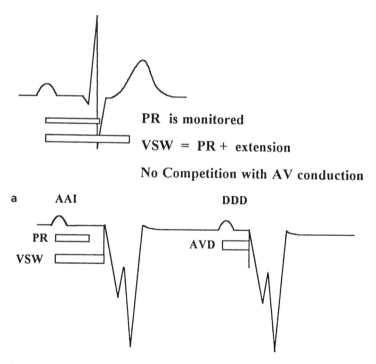

PR is monitored

VSW = PR + extension

No Competition with AV conduction

a   AAI   DDD

PR

VSW   AVD

b   When AV block occurs the pacemaker
           automatically switches from AAI to DDD.

Figure 6.19(a and b) DDD/AMC mode by ELA, Inc. (Minnetonka, MN). See text for explanation. (Modified from *Chorus II Model 6234, 6244 Dual Chamber Pulse Generator Physician's Manual*. Minnetonka, MN: ELA Medical, 1994.)

ing system as atrial- or ventricular-based has gained increased importance with the advent of rate-adaptive pacing. A description of pure atrial- and ventricular-based timing systems appears below. The difference between atrial- and ventricular-based dual-chamber pacemakers was of little clinical significance in non–rate-adaptive pacemakers, although the difference created some minor confusion in interpretation of paced electrocardiograms. By contrast, the difference in timing systems is of greater importance when DDDR behavior is examined.

Ventricular-based timing

In a ventricular-based timing system, the AEI is "fixed." A ventricular sensed event occurring during the AEI resets this timer, causing it to start all over again (Figure 6.20, top). A ventricular sensed event occurring during the AVI both terminates the AVI and initiates an AEI (Figure 6.21, top). If there is intact conduction through the AV node after an atrial pacing stimulus such that the AR interval (atrial stimulus to sensed R wave) is shorter than the programmed AVI, the resulting paced rate will accelerate by a small amount. This is demonstrated in Figure 6.21 (top).

This phenomenon is best understood by example. Assume that a pacemaker is programmed to an LRL of 60 bpm (a pacing interval of 1000 msec). With a programmed AVI of 200 msec, the AEI is 800 msec (AEI = LRL − AVI). If AV nodal function permits conduction in 150 msec (ARI = 150 msec), the conducted or sensed R wave inhibits the ventricular output. This, in turn, resets the AEI, which remains stable at 800 msec. The resulting interval between consecutive atrial pacing stimuli is 950 msec (AEI + ARI). This is equivalent to a rate of 63 bpm, which is slightly faster than the programmed LRL. When a native R wave occurs, for example, a ventricular premature beat during the AEI, the AEI is also reset. The pacemaker then recycles, resulting in a rate defined by the sum of the AEI and AVI. This escape interval is therefore equal to the LRL (Figure 6.20, top). In both cases, the sensed ventricular event, an R wave, regardless of where it occurs, resets the AEI.

Atrial-based timing

In an atrial-based timing system, the AA interval is fixed. This is in contrast to a ventricular-based system, in which the AEI is fixed. As long as there is stable LRL pacing, there will be no discernible difference between the two timing systems.

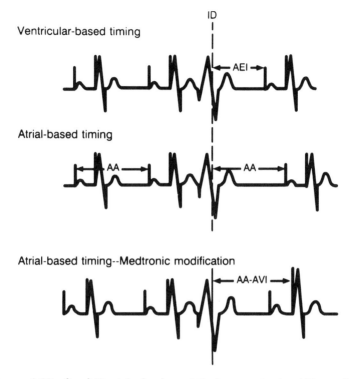

Figure 6.20 **(top)** Ventricular-based timing resets the AEI, so that the recycled pacing interval is equal to the programmed base rate. **(middle)** Atrial-based timing resets the AA interval and then adds the AVI. Thus, the interval from the sensed R wave to the next paced ventricular beat exceeds the base rate interval, a form of obligatory hysteresis. **(bottom)** Medtronic modification of the AA timing subtracts the AVI from the AA interval. The resulting rhythm is identical to that seen with ventricular-based timing. (From Levine PA, Hayes DL, Wilkoff BL, Ohman AE. *Electrocardiography of Rate-Modulated Pacemaker Rhythms.* Sylmar, CA: Siemens-Pacesetter, 1990. By permission of Siemens-Pacesetter.)

In a system with pure atrial-based timing, a sensed R wave occurring during the AVI inhibits the ventricular output but does not alter the basic AA timing. Hence, the rate stays at the programmed LRL (Figure 6.21, bottom) during effective single-chamber atrial pacing. When a ventricular premature beat is sensed during the AEI, the timers are also reset, but now it is the AA interval rather than the AEI that is reset. The pacemaker counts out an AA interval and then adds the programmed AVI, attempting to

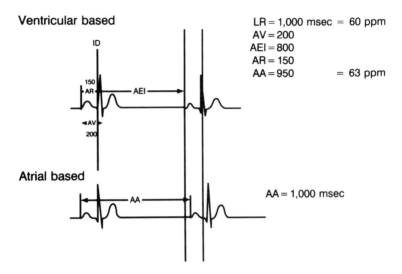

Figure 6.21 (top) With ventricular-based timing in patients with intact AV nodal conduction after atrial (AR) pacing, the sensed R wave resets the AEI. The base pacing interval consists of the sum of the AR and the AEI; thus, it is shorter than the programmed minimum rate interval. (bottom) With atrial-based timing in patients with intact AV nodal conduction after AR pacing, the sensed R wave inhibits the ventricular output but does not reset the basic timing of the pacemaker. There is atrial pacing at the programmed base rate. (From Levine PA, Hayes DL, Wilkoff BL, Ohman AE. *Electrocadiography of Rate-Modulated Pacemaker Rhythms.* Sylmar, CA: Siemens-Pacesetter, 1990. By permission of Siemens-Pacesetter.)

mimic the compensatory pause commonly seen in normal sinus rhythm with ventricular ectopy—a form of obligatory hysteresis (Figure 6.20, middle).

Other manufacturers have chosen to modify an atrial timing system. One DDDR pulse generator primarily uses modified atrial, or AA, timing, in which, in most instances, an atrial sensed or paced event resets the timing cycle of the device (much like the sinus node itself).[28] However, in certain situations (for example, after a PVC), an exception is made and ventricular (VA) timing is used. Another manufacturer uses an atrial timing system that ignores the sensed R wave during stable AR pacing, which eliminates the rate acceleration that would be seen with ventricular-based timing designs.[29] This is modified when a native R wave or sensed premature ventricular event occurs after the VRP is completed. The AA interval is reset but only after the AVI is first subtracted (Figure 6.22).

Comparison of atrial- and ventricular-based systems

When the heart rate is considered, usually the ventricular rate is paramount, because it, not the atrial rate, causes the effective (hemodynamic) pulse. During periods of 2:1 AV block at the lower rate, a ventricular-based timing system alternates between the programmed rate (AV pacing state) and a slightly faster rate (AR pacing state), as shown in Figure 6.23 (top).

In an atrial-based system, the alternation of the longer AVI with the shorter AR interval results in ventricular rates that are both faster and slower than the programmed base rate. This is shown in Figure 6.23 (bottom).

Although ventricular-based timing may result in an increase in the paced rate during AR pacing (see "Effects of Ventricular- and Atrial-Based Timing Systems on DDDR Timing Cycles," below), the LRL is never violated. This is not the case in atrial-based

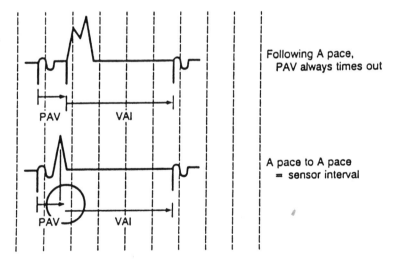

Figure 6.22   Atrial escape timing after an atrial (A) pace. The AVI after atrial pacing (PAV) always times out, regardless of ventricular inhibition. The escape interval from one atrial pace to the next is equal to the sensor interval. VAI, interval from ventricular sensed or paced event to atrial paced event. (From Hayes DL, Ketelson A, Levine PA, et al. Understanding timing systems of current DDDR pacemakers. *Eur JCPE* 1993;3[1]:70–86. By permission of Mayo Foundation.)

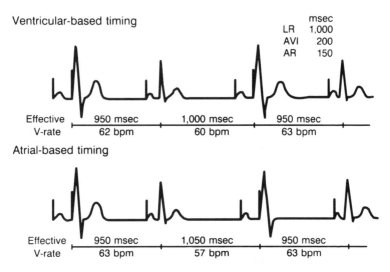

Figure 6.23 Diagrammatic representations of 2:1 AV block during base rate pacing. (top) With a ventricular-based timing system, the interval between consecutive AV and AR paced complexes is slightly shorter; hence, the rate is slightly faster than the programmed base rate. The interval between consecutive AR and AV paced complexes results in ventricular pacing at the base rate for that pacing cycle. (bottom) In an atrial-based timing system, the effective ventricular paced rate alternates between rates that are faster and slower than the programmed rate. The cycle between an AR and AV complex results in a ventricular rate that is slower than the programmed rate, a form of hysteresis. Meanwhile, the cycle between an AV and an AR complex causes the ventricular rate to be faster than the programmed rate. Atrial pacing is stable at the programmed rate, but it is the ventricular contraction that induces cardiac output. (From Levine PA, Hayes DL, Wilkoff BL, Ohman AE. *Electrocardiography of Rate-Modulated Pacemaker Rhythms.* Sylmar, CA: Siemens-Pacesetter, 1990. By permission of Siemens-Pacesetter.)

timing. When an AV complex follows an AR complex, the effective paced ventricular rate for that cycle falls below the programmed LRL. A 2:1 AV block in an atrial-based timing system induces alternating cycles that are either faster or slower than the programmed base rate but never are the same (Figure 6.23, bottom).

When one is asked to interpret an electrocardiogram of a patient with a dual-chamber pacemaker, it is helpful to know if the pace-maker has atrial- or ventricular-based timing. With a ventricular-based timing system, a pair of calipers set to the VA interval can be used to measure backward from an atrial paced stimulus to the point of ventricular sensing, because a ventricular event, paced or sensed, always initiates the VA interval.

A similar technique can be used in an atrial-based timing system, but only when a sensed ventricular complex occurs after the VRP ends. The calipers must be set to the AA interval before measuring backward from the atrial paced event that follows a ventricular sensed event. If one were to misidentify an atrial-based timing system as a ventricular-based system, an otherwise normal rhythm might be misinterpreted as T-wave oversensing or some other form of oversensing (Figure 6.20, middle).

Upper rate behavior

In the DDD mode of operation, whether atrial- or ventricular-based, acceleration of the sinus rate results in the sensed P wave terminating the AEI and initiating an AVI. This is P-wave synchronous ventricular pacing. (If the PR interval is shorter than the PV interval—the time from an intrinsic P wave to a paced ventricular depolarization—the pacemaker is completely inhibited.) P-wave synchronous pacing occurs in a 1:1 relationship between the programmed LRL and the programmed URL. This is the same as saying that when the interval between consecutive native atrial events is longer than the TARP, each P wave occurs in the atrial alert period and is therefore sensed. The atrial output is inhibited while simultaneously triggering a ventricular output after the AVI. However, when the interval between consecutive native atrial events is shorter than the TARP, some P waves are not sensed because, by definition, they fall into the TARP. The pacemaker goes into an abrupt fixed-block (2:1, 3:1, etc.) response, sensing only every other or every nth P wave, depending on the native atrial rate (Figure 6.24). Programming a long PVARP results in the fixed-block response occurring at a relatively low tracking rate. The abrupt change in pacing rate when the fixed block occurs can result in significant symptoms and frequently did in early generation DDD pacemakers.

To modulate the upper rate behavior better, there is an additional timing circuit, known as the maximum tracking rate (MTR) interval.[9,15] (The MTR interval has also been referred to as "upper rate limit" and "ventricular tracking limit.") This timing period defines the maximum paced ventricular rate or the shortest interval initiated by a sensed P wave at which a paced ventricular

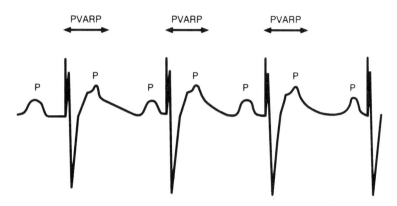

Figure 6.24 If the sinus rate becomes so rapid that every other P wave occurs within the PVARP, effective 2:1 AV block occurs; that is, every other P wave is followed by a ventricular pacing artifact.

beat can follow a preceding paced or sensed ventricular event. The pacemaker has an upper rate behavior that mimics AV nodal Wenckebach behavior. The appearance is that of group beating, progressive lengthening of the PV interval, and intermittent pauses on the electrocardiogram when the native atrial rate exceeds the programmed MTR interval (Figure 6.25). In these pacing systems, two timers must each complete their cycles for a ventricular stimulus to be released. These are the AVI and the MTR interval. A sensed P wave initiates an AVI. If, on completion of the AVI, the MTR interval has been completed, a pacemaker stimulus is released at the programmed AVI. If the MTR interval has not yet been completed, the release of the ventricular output pulse is delayed until the MTR interval ends. This delay has the functional effect of lengthening the PV interval. It also places the ensuing ventricular paced beat closer to the next P wave. Both the PVARP and the MTR interval are initiated by a paced or sensed ventricular event. During Wenckebach upper rate behavior, a P wave eventually coincides with the PVARP, is not sensed, and is therefore ignored by the pacemaker. This results in a relative pause. The MTR interval is then able to complete its timing period such that, depending on the atrial rate and programmed base rate, either the P wave that follows the unsensed P wave is tracked (restarting the cycle at the programmed AVI) or the pause is terminated by AV sequential pacing.

Thus, upper rate behavior can demonstrate Wenckebach-like

behavior or go into abrupt fixed block (e.g., 2:1). It will demonstrate 2:1 block behavior when the P wave falls into the TARP. If the MTR interval is longer than the TARP (TARP = AVI + PVARP), Wenckebach-like behavior will occur. This can be summarized by the following equation:

$$\text{Wenckebach interval} = \text{MTR interval} - \text{TARP}$$

Therefore, if a positive number results, Wenckebach-like behavior will occur, and if a negative number results, fixed 2:1 AV block will occur. For example, if a patient's pacemaker is programmed to an AVI of 250 msec, a PVARP of 225 msec, and an MTR of 400 msec, by the above equation the Wenckebach interval would be 400 − (250 + 225), or a negative number. Therefore, when the atrial rate reaches 401 msec, a 2:1 AV upper rate response will be seen. On the other hand, if this patient's AVI is reprogrammed to 125 msec, by the equation the Wenckebach interval would be 400 − (125 + 225), or a positive number (+50 msec). In the latter instance, when the atrial rate is 351 msec, Wenckebach-like conduction will be seen for a 50-msec interval. Once the atrial rate increases still further to 401 msec, 2:1 AV block will be noted.

Rate Smoothing™, a variation of upper rate behavior, was introduced by Cardiac Pacemakers, Inc. (St. Paul, MN) as a

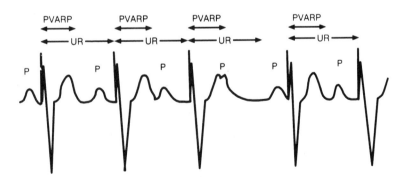

Figure 6.25 In the DDD pacing mode, the programmed upper rate limit (UR) cannot be violated regardless of the sinus rate. When a P wave is sensed after the PVARP, the AVI is initiated. If, however, delivering a ventricular pacing artifact at the end of the AVI would violate the UR, the ventricular pacing artifact cannot be delivered. The pacemaker would wait until completion of the UR and then deliver the ventricular pacing artifact. This action would result in a prolonged AVI.

method of preventing marked changes in cycle length not only at the URL of a DDD pacemaker but also any time that the sinus rate is accelerating or decelerating.[30] (With Rate Smoothing, the pacemaker is programmed to a percentage change that will be allowed between VV cycles, that is, 3, 6, 9, or 12 percent. For example, if the VV cycle length is stable at 900 msec during P-synchronous pacing, Rate Smoothing is "on" at 6 percent and the sinus rate suddenly accelerates; the subsequent VV cycle cannot accelerate by more than 54 msec, which is 6 percent of 900 msec.) The ventricular rate is therefore relatively smooth, but sometimes at the expense of uncoupling AV synchrony (Figure 6.26).

Because Wenckebach upper rate behavior results in the loss of a stable AV relationship and some patients may be symptomatic with both this and the resultant pauses that occur when a P wave coincides with the PVARP and is not tracked, another upper rate behavior—fallback—is available in some devices. When the atrial rate exceeds the programmed MTR, the pacemaker continues to

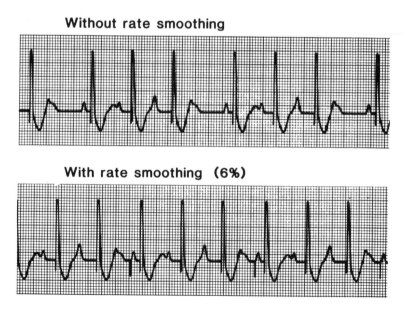

Figure 6.26 Electrocardiogram demonstrating DDD pacing with true Rate Smoothing capabilities (6 percent of the preceding RR interval). With true Rate Smoothing, the Wenckebach interval is allowed to lengthen only 36 msec over the preceding RR interval, at a maximum tracking rate of 100 ppm. (Reprinted with permission from Cardiac Pacemakers, Inc., St. Paul, MN.)

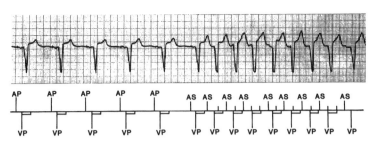

Figure 6.27 Resting electrocardiographic tracing demonstrating AV sequential pacing at lower rate (55 ppm) followed by paroxysmal atrial flutter with ventricular tracking at MTR (110 ppm). Diagram shows atrial paced events (AP), atrial sensed events (AS), and ventricular paced events (VP), with the PVARP noted by the rectangle. Short, unlabeled ticks represent atrial activity that occurs in the PVARP and is not sensed. (Diagram is based on Marker Channel™, Medtronic, Inc., Minneapolis, MN.) (From Levine PA, Hayes DL, Wilkoff BL, Ohman AE. *Electrocardiography of Rate-Modulated Pacemaker Rhythms*. Sylmar, CA: Siemens-Pacesetter, 1990. By permission of Siemens-Pacesetter.)

sense atrial activity but uncouples the native atrial rhythm from the ventricular paced complexes. The ventricular paced rate then slowly but progressively decreases to either an intermediate rate or the programmed base rate. This avoids the abrupt pauses that occur with both the Wenckebach and the fixed-block behaviors. When the atrial rate slows below either the MTR or the fallback rate, depending on the design of the system, the desired AV relationship is restored.

Mode switching

Mode switching refers to the ability of the pacemaker to automatically change from one mode to another in response to an inappropriately rapid atrial rhythm. Automatic mode switching, AMS™, was introduced by Telectronics, Inc. (Englewood, CO).[31] With AMS, when the pacemaker is functioning in the DDDR mode, the algorithm automatically reprograms the pacemaker to the VVIR mode if specific criteria for a pathologic atrial rhythm are met. Mode switching is particularly useful for patients with paroxysmal supraventricular rhythm disturbances. In the DDD or DDDR pacing mode, if a supraventricular rhythm disturbance occurs and the pathologic atrial rhythm is sensed by the pacemaker, rapid ventricular pacing may occur (Figure 6.27). Any pacing mode that

313

eliminates tracking of the pathologic rhythm, for example, DDI, DDIR, DVI, or DVIR, also eliminates the ability to track normal sinus rhythm, which is usually the predominant rhythm. Mode switching avoids this limitation (Figure 6.28).

Mode switching is now available in some DDD pacemakers with switching to VVI[32] and in a DDDR device that switches from DDDR to DDIR instead of VVIR, from DDD to DDIR, and from VDD to VVIR.[33]

The original AMS was successful, but in some instances the mode-switching criteria were too easily fulfilled, resulting in frequent mode switching. Refinement of subsequent algorithms has made this a very successful feature (Figure 6.29). Lau et al.[34] recently proved the effectiveness of this algorithm in preventing rapid irregular response to chest wall stimulation simulating atrial tachycardia.

AMS functions by measuring intervals between atrial events.[35] In some pacemakers, the rate at which mode switching occurs is now a programmable feature. The pacemaker utilizes a counter that considers a short interval to be one that is shorter than the programmed mode-switching rate and a long interval one that is longer than the programmed rate. When the counter accrues a

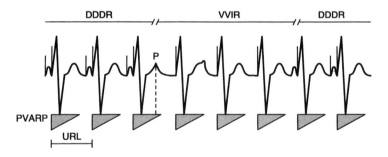

Figure 6.28 Electrocardiographic appearance of mode switching. The first three cardiac cycles are due to sensor-driven AV sequential pacing, that is, DDDR pacing. After the third paced ventricular complex, a P wave occurs during the PVARP (triangles) and initiates mode switching to the VVIR mode because the atrial rate has exceeded the URL. The pacing mode reverts to DDDR when the atrial rate falls below the programmed URL; that is, P waves fall outside the PVARP. (From Hayes DL. Timing cycles of permanent pacemakers. *Cardiol Clin* 1992;10:593–608. By permission of WB Saunders Company.)

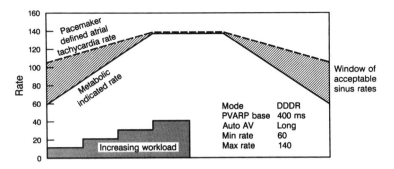

Figure 6.29 Diagram of the method by which the META DDDR pacemaker monitors the atrial rate to determine whether it is physiologic or nonphysiologic. The shaded area identifies tracked sinus rates. Sinus rates below the metabolic indicated rate (solid line) elicit atrial pacing, sinus rates within the shaded area elicit atrial tracking, and sinus rates above the atrial tachycardia rate (dashed line) result in automatic switching of the mode to VVIR. Auto AV, automatic alteration of the atrioventricular interval; PVARP, postventricular atrial refractory period. (From Hayes DL, Ketelson A, Levine PA, et al. Understanding timing systems of current DDDR pacemakers. *Eur JCPE* 1993;3[1]:70–86. By permission of Mayo Foundation.)

specified number of short intervals, the pacemaker reprograms to the VVIR mode and remains in this mode until a specified number of long intervals have occurred and altered the counter, at which point mode switching reverts.

Another device switches modes when the mean atrial rate exceeds approximately 180 bpm. Once the mode switch has occurred, the ventricular rate is gradually changed to the sensor-indicated rate. When the mean atrial rate drops below approximately 180 bpm or five consecutive atrial paced events occur, the pacemaker switches back to the programmed atrial tracking mode.[33]

Atrial tachycardia response, ATR™, is another programmable option that provides automatic mode switching from DDDR to VVIR when detected atrial activity exceeds the URL[36] (Figure 6.30). Like AMS, this feature has the objective of limiting the time that the paced ventricular rate is at the URL in response to pathologic atrial arrhythmias.

The operation of atrial tachycardia response is controlled by two programmable variables: duration and fallback time. Atrial

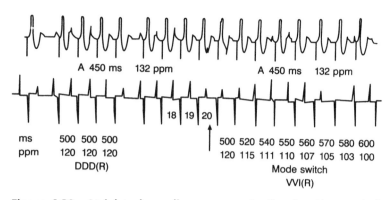

Figure 6.30 Atrial tachycardia response. In the duration period, the number of cycles (e.g., 20, arrow) is counted from the onset of the tachyarrhythmia. When duration is met, the device switches the mode to VVIR and the rate begins to decrease. A, atrial. (From Hayes DL, Ketelson A, Levine PA, et al. Understanding timing systems of current DDDR pacemakers. *Eur JCPE* 1993;3[1]:70–86. By permission of Mayo Foundation.)

tachycardia duration allows the physician to determine the number of cycles that occur above the URL before the ventricular rate begins decreasing to the LRL. Atrial tachycardia fallback time determines how quickly the rate will decrease from the URL to the LRL. During fallback, the pulse generator operates in the VVIR mode.

At the onset of an atrial tachycardia above the URL, the pacemaker begins to count AA intervals less than the URL interval. When the counter reaches eight consecutive intervals, atrial tachycardia duration begins. During the detection and duration period, the pulse generator continues to exhibit normal URL behavior—typically a Wenckebach block. As duration elapses, the pacemaker continues to count AA intervals; the counter must remain above eight for the duration tally to continue. When duration is satisfied, the pulse generator automatically switches to the VVIR mode, and fallback begins. The ventricular paced rate gradually decreases until the higher of the sensor-driven rate and the LRL is reached. Once mode switching occurs, the pacemaker searches for eight consecutive intervals of cycle lengths greater than the URL interval. After the eighth interval, the mode automatically switches back to DDDR.

Conventional ventricular tracking limit, CVTL™, is another method available to avoid inappropriate tracking of atrial rhythm disturbances.[28] When the pacemaker is programmed "on," the maximum pacing rate in the DDDR or VDDR pacing mode is limited to 35 ppm above the programmed pacing rate (but never less than 80 bpm) if sensor-driven signals indicating exercise are absent. During exercise, this interim limit is overridden and the programmed maximum pacing rate is in effect (Figure 6.31).

Dual-chamber rate-modulated pacemakers: effect on timing cycles

Dual-chamber rate-modulated (DDDR) pacemakers are capable of all the variations described for DDD pacemakers (Figure 6.13). In addition to using P-synchronous pacing as a method for increasing

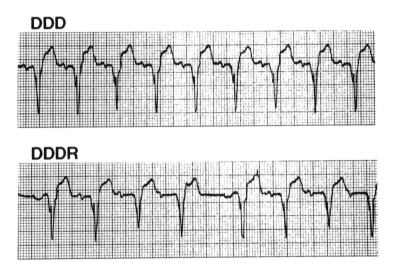

DDD

DDDR

Figure 6.31 Electrocardiographic tracings from a patient with an Intermedics Relay DDDR pacemaker with conditional ventricular tracking limit. In both tracings, the patient is at rest despite the rapid sinus rate. In the upper panel, P-wave tracking occurs with a sinus rate of 100. In the lower panel, the pacemaker is programmed DDDR, with a lower rate of 70 bpm. Because the patient is resting, the sensor indicates that a slower ventricular rate is appropriate. Because the atrial sensed events are more than 35 bpm faster than the lower rate limit, the pacemaker operates in pseudo-Wenckebach behavior. (An artifact is present during the fifth T wave.) (From Hayes DL. DDDR timing cycles: Upper rate behavior. In SS Barold, J Mugica (eds.). *New Perspectives in Cardiac Pacing*. Mount Kisco, NY: Futura, 1993, pp 233–257. By permission of the publisher.)

the heart rate, the sensor incorporated in the pacemaker may increase the heart rate. The rhythm may therefore be sinus-driven (alternatively called "atrial-driven" or "P-synchronous") or sensor-driven (Figure 6.32).

A significant difference in the timing cycle between DDD and DDDR pacing is the ability to pace the atrium during the PVARP in the DDDR mode (Figure 6.33). This does not occur in the DDD mode because paced atrial activity does not occur until the LRL has been completed, which, by definition, must be at some

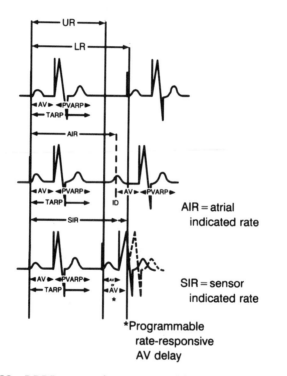

AIR = atrial indicated rate

SIR = sensor indicated rate

*Programmable rate-responsive AV delay

Figure 6.32 DDDR pacemakers are capable of all pacing variations previously described for DDD pacemakers (see Figure 6.13). When the device is functioning above the programmed LRL, it may increase the heart rate on the basis of the AIR or SIR. In current DDDR pacemakers, the PVARP remains fixed regardless of cycle length. A programmable feature in one DDDR pacemaker allows the length of the AVI to vary with the SIR; that is, as the SIR increases, the AVI shortens (Meta™ DDDR). Because a rate-responsive AV delay is incorporated, the TARP may shorten by virtue of the changing AVI even though the PVARP does not change at faster rates.

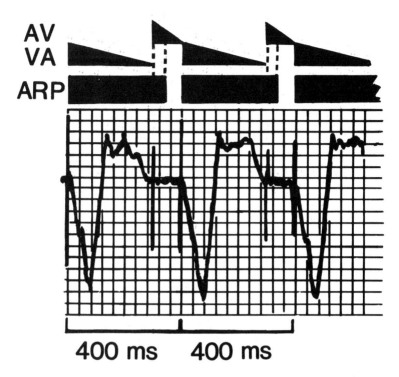

Figure 6.33 In this electrocardiographic example from a DDDR pacemaker, the maximum sensor rate is 150 ppm (400 msec), the atrial refractory period (ARP) is 350 msec, and the AVI is 100 msec. As illustrated in the block diagrams above the electrocardiogram, the two sensor-driven atrial pacing artifacts both occur during the terminal portion of the PVARP. Even though no atrial sensing can occur during the PVARP, as can be seen in this example by the intrinsic P wave that occurs immediately after the first paced ventricular depolarization, a sensor-driven atrial pacing artifact will not be prevented by the PVARP. Whether a sensor-driven atrial pacing artifact is delivered depends on the sensor-indicated rate at that time and not on the PVARP. (From Hayes DL, Higano ST. DDDR pacing: Follow-up and complications. In SS Barold, J Mugica (eds.). *New Perspectives in Cardiac Pacing*. Mount Kisco, NY: Futura, 1991, pp 473–491. By permission of the publisher.)

point after the PVARP. In the DDDR mode, however, even though the atrial sensing channel is refractory during the PVARP, sensor-driven atrial output can still occur[37] (Figure 6.33).

DDDR pacing systems further increase the complexity of the upper rate behavior because the pacemaker can be driven by intrinsic atrial activity to cause PV pacing or by a sensor whose input signal is not identifiable on the electrocardiogram, or by both, to result in AV or AR pacing.[4,27] The eventual upper rate also depends on the type of sensor incorporated in the pacemaker and how the sensor is programmed.[38] Between the programmed LRL and the programmed URL, there may be stable P-wave synchronous pacing, P-wave synchronous pacing alternating with AV sequential pacing, or stable AV sequential pacing at rates exceeding the base rate[39] (see Figure 6.36). AV sequential pacing rates may increase as high as the programmed maximum sensor rate (MSR).

Although the MSR and MTR are closely related, they are not identical. The tracking rate refers to the rate when the pacemaker is sensing and tracking intrinsic atrial activity. The MTR is the maximum ventricular paced rate that is allowed in response to sensed atrial rhythms. This may result in fixed-block, Wenckebach, fallback, or rate-smoothing responses, depending on the design of the system. The sensor-controlled rate is the rate of the pacemaker that is determined by the sensor-input signal. The MSR is the maximum rate that the pacemaker is allowed to achieve under sensor control.

Whether at the MTR or during rate acceleration below the MTR, the rhythm that results may be in part sensor driven and in part sinus driven (P-wave tracking) and not purely one or the other (see Figure 6.32). Which of these mechanisms predominates depends on the integrity of the sinus node and the sensor and how the pacemaker is programmed. DDDR pacing can result in a type of rate smoothing. If the sensor is optimally programmed, then as the atrial rate exceeds the MTR, the RR interval will display minimal variation between sinus-driven and sensor-driven pacing.[39] As shown in Figure 6.34, the variation in RR interval is markedly lessened with the sensor "on" (DDDR) rather than "passive" (DDD). In the DDDR mode, the RR interval is allowed to lengthen only as much as the difference between the MTR and the activity sensor rate interval. For example, if a device is programmed to a P-wave tracking limit of 120 ppm and the patient's atrial rate exceeds this, the pacemaker will operate in a Wenckebach-type block. If the sensor-indicated rate at this time is 100 ppm, the paced rate will decrease from 120 ppm (500 msec) to an AV sequential paced rate of 100 ppm (600 msec) for the Wenckebach cycle and then return to P-wave tracking at a rate of 120 ppm. This situation

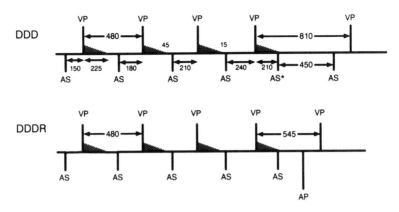

Figure 6.34 This diagram illustrates the difference in DDD and DDDR behavior when the intrinsic atrial rate increases. In the upper panel, DDD pacing is illustrated. The sensed atrial events (AS) occur increasingly closer to the PVARP, which is programmed to 225 msec (shown by the triangles) until the fifth AS event (*) occurs at 210 msec after the preceding ventricular paced event (VP) and within the PVARP and is not sensed. This is followed by another AS and VP after the programmed AVI of 150 msec. The resultant cycle length is 810 msec, significantly longer than the preceding cycles of 480 msec. In the lower panel, DDDR pacing is illustrated. The intervals are programmed to the same values as in the upper panel. When the fifth AS event occurs within the PVARP, it is, by definition, not sensed. However, the escape event is a sensor-driven atrial pacing artifact followed by a VP after the AVI. The sensor-indicated cycle length is 545 msec. Therefore, only a 65-msec difference exists between the programmed upper rate limit and the sensor-indicated rate—a minor difference in cycle lengths. (Modified from Markowitz HT. Dual chamber rate responsive pacing [DDDR] provides physiologic upper rate behavior. *PhysioPace* 1990;4[1]:1–4.)

usually shortens the DDD Wenckebach interval, but this interval depends on the atrial rate and the programmed values for the MTR and the TARP.

Maximal sensor-driven rate smoothing requires optimal programming of the sensor variable. If the rate-responsive circuitry is programmed to mimic the native atrial rate, the paced ventricular rate will not demonstrate the 2:1 or Wenckebach-type behavior. Conversely, if the rate-responsive circuitry is programmed to very low levels of sensor-driven pacing, little or no rate smoothing will take place. This rate response is illustrated diagrammatically in

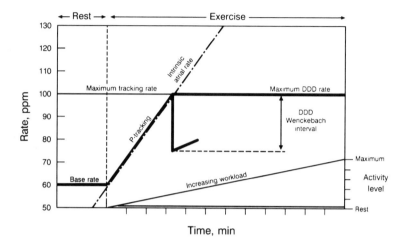

Figure 6.35   Diagram of the rate response of a DDD pacemaker with Wenckebach-type block at the upper rate limit (100 ppm). The dashed-dotted line represents the intrinsic atrial rate, and the heavy black line represents the ventricular paced rate, assuming complete heart block. Note the varying RR intervals during Wenckebach-type block as the atrial rate exceeds the maximum tracking rate. (From Higano ST, Hayes DL, Eisinger G. Sensor-driven rate smoothing in a DDDR pacemaker. *PACE* 1989;12:922–929. By permission of Futura Publishing Company.)

Figures 6.35 and 6.36. Figure 6.34 shows the sensor "passive" (DDD) response to exercise-induced increases in atrial rate, assuming complete heart block, an MTR of 100 ppm, and a Wenckebach-type response at the MTR. The ventricular and atrial rate responses to exercise are shown. As the MTR is exceeded, there is a transition from 1:1 P-synchronous function to Wenckebach upper rate behavior. Figure 6.36 shows the response that occurs with the sensor "on" (DDDR) and a maximum sensor rate of 120 ppm. The ventricular rate response to exercise, along with the atrial and sensor rates, is shown. Below the maximum P-wave tracking rate, the ventricle is paced in a P-synchronous fashion, similar to sensor "passive" (DDD) function. However, with the sensor "on" (DDDR), there is a transition from P-synchronous to AV sequential pacing through a period of Wenckebach-type block as the atrial rate exceeds the MTR. The Wenckebach interval is shortened by sensor-driven pacing. Note that the sensor rate response curve can be relocated almost anywhere on the graph by sensor parameter programming. Maximum sensor-driven rate smoothing requires optimal programming of these variables. Thus, sensor-modulated rate smoothing occurs only when the activity sensor is driving the pacemaker, when the intrinsic atrial rate exceeds the programmed MTR.

Another aspect of DDDR timing cycles is the atrial sensing window (ASW). The portion of the RR cycle that is not part of the PVARP or the AVI is the period during which the atrial sensing channel is alert, the ASW. If the PVARP or AVI (or both) is extended, there may effectively be no ASW and even a DDD pacemaker will function as a DVI system. Conversely, if a DDDR

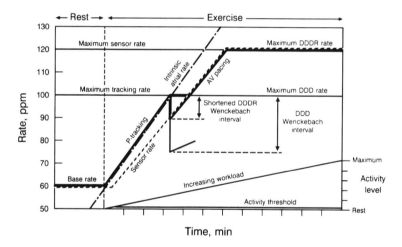

Figure 6.36 Diagram illustrating the rate response of the DDDR pacemaker and its behavior at both the maximum tracking and the maximum sensor rates. The dashed-dotted line represents the intrinsic atrial rate, and the diagonal dashed line represents the sensor rate during progressively increasing workloads. The heavy black line shows the ventricular paced rate, assuming complete heart block, as it progresses from the P-tracking mode to AV sequential pacing through a period of Wenckebach-type block. Note that the DDD Wenckebach interval is shortened by sensor-driven pacing, that is, "sensor-driven rate smoothing." Maximal shortening of the Wenckebach period is accomplished by optimal programming of the sensor rate-response variables (threshold and slope programming for an activity-driven sensor). (From Higano ST, Hayes DL, Eisinger G. Sensor-driven rate smoothing in a DDDR pacemaker. *PACE* 1989;12:922–929. By permission of Futura Publishing Company.)

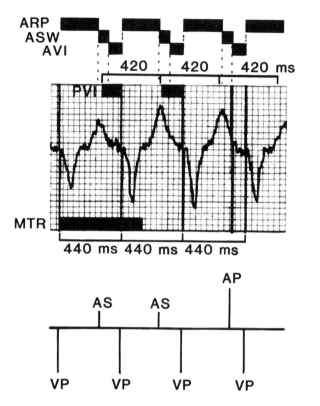

Figure 6.37 Diagram showing how an appropriately timed P wave can inhibit the sensor-driven A spike and result in apparent P-wave tracking above the maximum tracking rate (MTR). In this example, the MTR is 100 ppm, or 600 msec. The second and third complexes are preceded by intrinsic P waves that occurred during the atrial sensing window. This resulted in A-spike inhibition, or P-wave tracking above the MTR. The fourth complex was initiated by atrial pacing, because the preceding native P wave occurred outside the atrial sensing window in the atrial refractory period (ARP = 275 msec). Note the short P-stimulus interval produced by the subsequent atrial spike. Also shown are the atrial sensing window (ASW = 65 msec), AV interval (AVI = 100 msec), and variable PV interval (PVI). The intrinsic atrial rate is 143 bpm (420 msec). The sensor rate is 136 ppm (440 msec). A diagram in Marker Channel (Medtronic, Inc., Minneapolis, MN) fashion demonstrates the electrocardiographic findings. AP, atrial paced events; AS, atrial sensed event; VP, ventricular paced event. (From Higano ST, Hayes DL. P wave tracking above the maximum tracking rate in a DDDR pacemaker. *PACE* 1989;12 [Pt I]:1044–1048. By permission of Futura Publishing Company.)

pacemaker has exceeded the programmed MTR and is pacing at faster rates based on sensor activation, an appropriately timed intrinsic P wave can still inhibit the sensor-driven atrial pacing artifact and give the appearance of P-wave tracking at rates greater than the MTR[40] (Figure 6.37). Although the MTR is programmed to a single value in DDDR pacing, it behaves as if it were variable and equal to the sensor-driven rate when the sensor-driven rate exceeds the programmed MTR if a P wave occurs during the ASW to inhibit output of an atrial pacing artifact.

Effects of ventricular- and atrial-based timing systems on DDDR timing cycles

In a ventricular-based timing system, the effective atrial paced rate could theoretically be significantly higher than the programmed MSR if AR conduction were present[4] (Figure 6.38, top). Assume that the maximum sensor-controlled rate is 150 ppm (a cycle length of 400 msec). With a programmed AVI of 200 msec, the AEI would also be 200 msec. If AV conduction were intact such that the AR interval was 150 msec, the actual pacing interval would be ARI + AEI, or 150 + 200 msec, or 350 msec. A cycle length of 350 msec is equal to 171 ppm, which is significantly higher than the programmed MSR of 150 ppm. Although this potentially achievable faster rate may not be a problem or may even be advantageous for some patients, it could create problems for other patients (Figure 6.38, middle).

Rate acceleration can also be minimized in a DDDR ventricular-based timing system by incorporating a rate-responsive AV delay (RRAVD).[27,41] As the sinus or sensor-driven rate progressively increases, RRAVD causes the PV and AVIs to shorten progressively (Figure 6.38, bottom). Shortening the AVI with RRAVD results in a shorter TARP (shorter AVI + PVARP). This increases the intrinsic atrial rate that can be sensed, reducing the likelihood of both a fixed-block upper rate response and functional atrial undersensing. It also minimizes the chance of an inappropriately long PV interval at the higher rate, which may occur with a fixed AV delay when the fixed AV delay is programmed appropriately for lower rate behavior. In this case, the AV delay may be too long at higher rates. In a DDDR system, when the AVI shortens, the ventricular rate drive is held to that governed by the sensor, so that the time subtracted from the AVI is added to the AEI. Thus, at a rate of 150 ppm and pacing interval of 400 msec, if the RRAVD causes the AVI to shorten by 75 msec from an initially

Ventricular-based timing--fixed AV delay

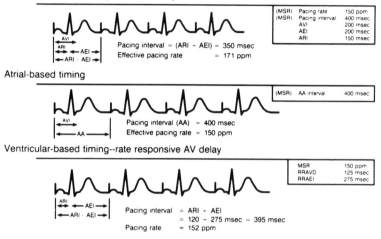

Figure 6.38 Effect of different timing systems on maximum sensor rate with intact stable AV nodal conduction (AR pacing). (top) In a ventricular-based timing system, there is a significant theoretical increase in the paced atrial rate exceeding that programmed by the physician. In the example shown, even though the maximum sensor rate programmed is 150 ppm, or 400 msec, the effective pacing rate achieved is 171 ppm, because the effective pacing rate is the sum of the ARI and the AEI; that is, 150 + 200 = 350 msec (171 ppm). (middle) In an atrial-based system, the R wave sensed during the AVI alters the basic timing during stable AR pacing. This results in atrial pacing at the sensor-indicated rate. (bottom) The addition of rate-responsive AV delay to a ventricular-based timing system minimizes the increase in the paced atrial rate above the programmed sensor-indicated rate. (From Levine PA, Hayes DL, Wilkoff BL, Ohman AE. *Electrocardiography of Rate-Modulated Pacemaker Rhythms.* Sylmar, CA: Siemens-Pacesetter, 1990. By permission of Siemens-Pacesetter.)

programmed AVI of 200 msec, the AVI shortens to 125 msec. Since the overall ventricular timing is held constant, the 75 msec subtracted from the AVI is added to the AEI, increasing it to 275 msec.

The RRAVD provides a more physiologic AVI at the faster rate while minimizing the degree of rate increase over the programmed MSR if AR conduction is intact. Assuming that the rate is 150 ppm and the initial AVI is 200 msec, the RRAVD is 125 msec, resulting in AV sequential pacing at the sensor programmed rate when the AR interval is 140 msec. If intact AV conduction is present at 120 msec, the overall shortening of the pacing interval is only 5 msec more than that seen at 150 bpm, a rate of 152 bpm (Figure 6.38, bottom).

Another manufacturer has modified the ventricular-based timing by automatically extending the VA interval as needed to control the AA pacing rate according to the programmed MSR (Figure 6.39). This extension results in adaptive-rate pacing, regardless of AV conduction status, that is equal to, but does not exceed, the desired MSR.

ENDLESS-LOOP TACHYCARDIA

Endless-loop tachycardia is not a portion of the timing cycle, but understanding the timing cycle of dual-chamber pacing is crucial to understanding endless-loop tachycardia and vice versa. Endless-loop tachycardia had also been referred to as "pacemaker-mediated tachycardia," "pacemaker-mediated reentry tachycardia," and "pacemaker circus movement tachycardia."[9] Endless-loop tachycardia has been defined as a reentry arrhythmia in which the dual-chamber pacemaker acts as the antegrade limb of the tachycardia and the natural pathway acts as the retrograde limb.[42,43]

If AV synchrony is uncoupled—that is, if the P wave is

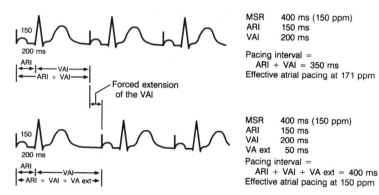

Figure 6.39   Pacing at maximum sensor rate (MSR): Timing algorithm provides effective pacing at MSR with intrinsic conduction to the ventricle. ARI, interval from atrial stimulus to sensed R wave; VA, ventriculoatrial; VAI, ventriculoatrial interval. (From Hayes DL, Ketelson A, Levine PA, et al. Understanding timing systems of current DDDR pacemakers. *Eur JCPE* 1993;3[1]:70–86. By permission of Mayo Foundation.)

displaced from its normal relation to the QRS complex—the subsequent ventricular event may result in retrograde atrial excitation if retrograde or VA conduction is intact.[42,43] If the retrograde P wave is sensed, the AVI of the pacemaker will be initiated. On termination of the AVI and MTR interval, a ventricular pacing artifact is delivered, which could once again be conducted in a retrograde fashion. Once established, this reentrant mechanism continues until interrupted or until the retrograde limb of the circuit is exhausted. The paced VV interval cannot violate the programmed maximum or URL of the pacemaker, and the endless-loop tachycardia often occurs at the URL. Many mechanisms have been adopted to prevent or minimize endless-loop tachycardia.[44]

SUMMARY

A clear understanding of the components of the pacemaker timing cycles is crucial to understanding and interpreting paced electrocardiograms. The information in this chapter provides basic rules for timing cycles for pacing modes currently in use (VVI, AAI, VVIR, AAIR, DDI, DDD, DDDR, DDIR) and for pacing modes less frequently used or of historic interest but critical in understanding how timing cycles have developed (VOO, AOO, DOO, DVIC, DVI, VDD).

Each pacemaker manufacturer may take license and alter or add some nuance to the timing cycle of a particular pacemaker. Although understanding basic timing cycles allows interpretation of most paced electrocardiograms, manufacturers' alterations require that one be intimately familiar with the design of each pacemaker to be interpreted.

REFERENCES

1. Bernstein AD, Camm AJ, Fletcher RD, et al. The NASPE/BPEG generic pacemaker code for antibradyarrhythmia and adaptive-rate pacing and antitachyarrhythmia devices. *Pacing Clin Electrophysiol* 1987;10:794–799.
2. Bernstein AD, Camm AJ, Fisher JD, et al. The NASPE*/BPEG** defibrillator code. *Pacing Clin Electrophysiol* 1993;16:1776–1780.
3. Barold SS, Falkoff MD, Ong LS, Heinle RA. Interpretation of electrocardiograms produced by a new unipolar

multiprogrammable "committed" AV sequential demand (DVI) pulse generator. *Pacing Clin Electrophysiol* 1981;4:692–708.

4. Levine PA, Sholder JA. *Interpretation of Rate-Modulated, Dual-Chamber Rhythms: The Effect of Ventricular Based and Atrial Based Timing Systems on DDD and DDDR Rhythms.* Sylmar, CA: Siemens-Pacesetter, 1990, pp 1–20.

5. Calfee RV. Dual-chamber committed mode pacing. *Pacing Clin Electrophysiol* 1983;6:387–391.

6. Floro J, Castellanet M, Florio J, Messenger J. DDI: A new mode for cardiac pacing. *Clin Prog Pacing Electrophysiol* 1984;2(3):255–260.

7. Levine PA, Lindenberg BS, Mace RC. Analysis of AV universal (DDD) pacemaker rhythms. *Clin Prog Pacing Electrophysiol* 1984;2(1):54–70.

8. Levine PA. Normal and abnormal rhythms associated with dual-chamber pacemakers. *Cardiol Clin* 1985;3:595–616.

9. Furman S. Comprehension of pacemaker timing cycles. In S Furman, DL Hayes, DR Holmes Jr (eds.), *A Practice of Cardiac Pacing* (2nd ed.). Mount Kisco, NY: Futura, 1989, pp 115–166.

10. Furman S, Hayes DL. Implantation of atrioventricular synchronous and atrioventricular universal pacemakers. *J Thorac Cardiovasc Surg* 1983;85:839–850.

11. Hauser RG. The electrocardiography of AV universal DDD pacemakers. *Pacing Clin Electrophysiol* 1983;6:399–409.

12. Barold SS, Falkoff MD, Ong LS, Heinle RA. Timing cycles of DDD pacemakers. In SS Barold, J Mugica (eds.), *New Perspectives in Cardiac Pacing.* Mount Kisco, NY: Futura, 1988, pp 69–119.

13. Levine PA. Postventricular atrial refractory periods and pacemaker mediated tachycardias. *Clin Prog Pacing Electrophysiol* 1983;1(4):394–401.

14. Barold SS. Management of patients with dual chamber pulse generators: Central role of the pacemaker atrial refractory period. *Learning Center Highlights* 1990;5(4):8–16.

15. Furman S. Dual chamber pacemakers: Upper rate behavior. *Pacing Clin Electrophysiol* 1985;8:197–214.

16. Barold SS, Falkoff MD, Ong LS, Heinle RA. Upper rate response of DDD pacemakers. In SS Barold, J Mugica (eds.), *New Perspectives in Cardiac Pacing.* Mount Kisco, NY: Futura, 1988, pp 121–172.

17. Hayes DL, Osborn MJ. Pacing: Antibradycardia devices. In ER Giuliani, V Fuster, BJ Gersh, et al. (eds.), *Cardiology: Fundamentals and Practice* (2nd ed.). St. Louis: Mosby–Year Book, 1991, pp 1014–1079.

18. Hayes DL. Programmability. In S Furman, DL Hayes, DR Holmes Jr (eds.), *A Practice of Cardiac Pacing* (2nd ed.). Mount Kisco, NY: Futura, 1989, pp 563–596.

19. Batey RL, Calabria DA, Shewmaker S, Sweesy M. Crosstalk and blanking periods in a dual chamber (DDD) pacemaker: A case report. *Clin Prog Electrophysiol Pacing* 1985;3(4):314–318.

20. Barold SS, Ong LS, Falkoff MD, Heinle RA. Crosstalk of self-inhibition in dual-chambered pacemakers. In SS Barold (ed.). *Modern Cardiac Pacing.* Mount Kisco, NY: Futura, 1985, pp 616–623.

21. Brandt J, Fahraeus T, Schuller H. Far-field QRS complex sensing via the atrial pacemaker lead. II. Prevalence, clinical significance and possibility of intraoperative prediction in DDD pacing. *Pacing Clin Electrophysiol* 1988;11:1540–1544.

22. Barold SS, Belott PH. Behavior of the ventricular triggering period of DDD pacemakers. *Pacing Clin Electrophysiol* 1987; 10:1237–1252.

23. *Chorus II Model 6234, 6244 Dual Chamber Pulse Generator Physician's Manual.* Minnetonka, MN: ELA Medical, 1994.

24. Daubert C, Ritter P, Mabo P, et al. Rate modulation of the AV delay in DDD pacing. In M Santini, M Pistolese, A Alliegro (eds.), *Progress in Clinical Pacing 1990.* New York: Elsevier, 1990, pp 415–430.

25. Janosik DL, Pearson AC, Buckingham TA, et al. The hemodynamic benefit of differential atrioventricular delay intervals for sensed and paced atrial events during physiologic pacing. *J Am Coll Cardiol* 1989;14:499–507.

26. Mehta D, Gilmour S, Ward DE, Camm AJ. Optimal atrioventricular delay at rest and during exercise in patients with dual chamber pacemakers: A non-invasive assessment by continuous wave Doppler. *Br Heart J* 1989;61:161–166.

27. Levine PA, Hayes DL, Wilkoff BL, Ohman AE. *Electrocardiography of Rate-Modulated Pacemaker Rhythms.* Sylmar, CA: Siemens-Pacesetter, 1990.

28. *Relay Models 293-03 and 294-03. Intermedics Cardiac Pulse Generator Physician's Manual.* Angleton, TX: Intermedics, 1992.

29. *The Elite Activity Responsive Dual Chamber Pacemaker with Telemetry (Including DDDR, DDD, DDIR, DDI, DVIR, and*

VVIR). Models 7074, 7075, 7076, and 7077 Technical Manual. Minneapolis: Medtronic, 1991.

30. van Mechelen R, Ruiter J, de Boer H, Hagemeijer F. Pacemaker electrocardiography of rate smoothing during DDD pacing. *Pacing Clin Electrophysiol* 1985;8:684–690.

31. *Meta DDDR 1250H Multiprogrammable Minute Ventilation, Rate Responsive Pulse Generator with Telemetry Physician's Manual.* Englewood, CO: Telectronics Pacing Systems, 1991.

32. *VIGOR™ DDD Models 950 and 955 Pulse Generators Physician's Manual.* St. Paul, MN: Cardiac Pacemakers, 1994.

33. *THERA_{DR} Product Information Manual. Pacemaker Models 7940, 7941, 7942, 7950, 7951, 7952.* Minneapolis: Medtronic, 1994.

34. Lau CP, Tai YT, Fong PC, et al. Atrial arrhythmia management with sensor controlled atrial refractory period and automatic mode switching in patients with minute ventilation sensing dual chamber rate adaptive pacemakers. *Pacing Clin Electrophysiol* 1992;15:1504–1514.

35. *META™ DDDR 1254. User's Guide.* Englewood, CO: Telectronics Pacing Systems, 1993.

36. *VIGOR™ DR Models 1230 and 1235 Adaptive-Rate Pulse Generators Physician's Manual.* St. Paul, MN: Cardiac Pacemakers, 1993.

37. Hayes DL, Higano ST. DDDR pacing: Follow-up and complications. In SS Barold, J Mugica (eds.), *New Perspectives in Cardiac Pacing.* Mount Kisco, NY: Futura, 1991, pp 473–491.

38. Hayes DL, Higano ST, Eisinger G. Electrocardiographic manifestations of a dual-chamber, rate-modulated (DDDR) pacemaker. *Pacing Clin Electrophysiol* 1989;12:555–562.

39. Higano ST, Hayes DL, Eisinger G. Sensor-driven rate smoothing in a DDDR pacemaker. *Pacing Clin Electrophysiol* 1989; 12:922–929.

40. Higano ST, Hayes DL. P wave tracking above the maximum tracking rate in a DDDR pacemaker. *Pacing Clin Electrophysiol* 1989;12:1044–1048.

41. Daubert C, Ritter P, Mabo P, et al. Physiological relationship between AV interval and heart rate in healthy subjects: Applications to dual chamber pacing. *Pacing Clin Electrophysiol* 1986;9:1032–1039.

42. Furman S, Fisher JD. Endless loop tachycardia in an AV universal (DDD) pacemaker. *Pacing Clin Electrophysiol* 1982;5:486–489.

43. Den Dulk K, Lindemans FW, Bar FW, Wellens HJ. Pacemaker related tachycardias. *Pacing Clin Electrophysiol* 1982; 5:476–485.

44. Hayes DL. Endless-loop tachycardia: The problem has been solved? In SS Barold, J Mugica (eds.), *New Perspectives in Cardiac Pacing.* Mount Kisco, NY: Futura, 1988, pp 375–386.

Differential Diagnosis, Evaluation, and Management of Pacing System Malfunction

Paul A. Levine

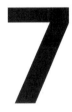

INTRODUCTION

Given the present reliability and longevity of implanted pacemakers,[1] most of the time spent caring for the paced patient will be concerned with evaluating the function of the already implanted pacing system. Part of this time will focus on potential and actual malfunctions. In considering a malfunction, one must be concerned with the entire pacing system, not just the pulse generator. The considerable confusion in the literature regarding the word "pacemaker" can be misleading if one is not aware of it. A more appropriate phrase is "pacing system." This chapter will review the differential diagnosis, evaluation, and management of the common malfunctions of single- and dual-chamber pacing systems.

THE PACING SYSTEM

The pacemaker, or pulse generator, is a device consisting of a power source and the electronic circuitry that controls the system. Used in this limited context, a diagnosis of "pacemaker malfunction" implies that the device is at fault and that the problem can be corrected by either programming or replacing the unit. Problems, however, can also be the result of damage to the lead, a structural or mechanical problem with the lead, or a primary abnormality at the electrode–myocardial interface (which might be best classified as a physiologic, not mechanical, problem[2]), or they can be the result of the pulse generator's being programmed inappropriately for the physiologic requirements of the patient. None of these causes of a pacing system malfunction will be solved by replacing the pulse generator. Increasingly, the term *pacemaker* refers to the entire system, which is composed of the pulse generator, the lead, and the electrode–tissue interface, as well as the interaction among all three components.[3-6] Unless the term "pacemaker malfunction" is explicitly described, it is commonly misunderstood by others as referring to the pulse generator and not the entire system. Hence, in an effort to treat the pacemaker malfunction, correction of the problem is limited to replacement of the pulse generator, when, in actuality, it may be normal.

Given that the term *pacemaker* as used in the literature has two meanings, which may cause confusion, it is strongly recommended that the term *pacemaker* be restricted to the device itself. In this capacity, it would then be synonymous with the term *pulse generator*. A pacemaker, or pulse generator, by itself, is insufficient to stimulate the heart effectively. To accomplish this task, one requires an entire system, which would be composed of the pulse generator, the lead or leads that connect the pulse generator to the heart, and the interface between the pacemaker–lead combination with the patient. In the not-too-distant past, this interface was simply the point of contact between the electrode and the myocardium. This, too, has changed, given the availability of a multiplicity of sensors that may also influence the response of the pacemaker. Thus, when one encounters a malfunction, it should be considered a *pacing system malfunction*. This would promote consideration of all the components of the system and avoid focusing purely on the pulse generator with the potential of missing the true cause of the problem. Although primary malfunctions of pulse generators do occur, they are the least frequent cause of any of the problems likely to be encountered. When presented with a suspected pacing system problem, real-time diagnostic capabilities of the implanted unit, which may include programmed and measured data telemetry, event marker, electrogram telemetry, and event counters, can facilitate the evaluation.

BASELINE DATA

If one is to minimize the chance of misdiagnosing normal function as a malfunction as well as avoid missing a true pacing system malfunction, it is essential to have baseline data on the pacing system. It will also be frequently necessary to utilize the diagnostic features included in many pacemakers today because the surface electrocardiographic recording (ECG) may be insufficient to confirm or differentiate normal function from abnormal.[7-13]

Collection of baseline data concerning the pacing system begins with the decision to implant the pacemaker. These data should include detailed documentation as to the indications for pacing and any studies that impact the specific pacing mode selected. If this has been obtained on an outpatient basis, copies of all pertinent electrocardiograms and other tests should be placed in the hospital chart; otherwise, problems may be encountered with third-party reimbursement and the allegation of an unnecessary procedure. This is perhaps one of the most devastating and time-consuming problems a physician is likely to encounter. Unlike all the other problems discussed in this chapter, it is a purely administrative problem that, unfortunately, cannot be avoided. Preventing such claims and frustrations is both more effective and efficient than having to defend these claims after the fact.

At the time of the implant procedure, the following data[4,14] should be collected: manufacturer, model, and serial numbers of the pulse generator and lead(s), the acute capture and sensing thresholds, and stimulation impedance measurements. These should be obtained with a pacing system analyzer (PSA) set to the pulse width of the permanent pacemaker. With regard to sensing threshold, in addition to recording the amplitude of the endocardial electrogram (EGM), the actual EGM should be recorded with a physiologic recorder or ECG machine as this will provide valuable clues to the adequacy of lead position and provide critical data should future problems develop.[15-17] At the end of the procedure, the programmed parameters of the pacing system are recorded along with lead function measurements and any other data that can be provided by the telemetric capabilities of the implanted device.

After the implant is completed, at least two standard 12-lead ECGs should be obtained. One should show the normal sensing function of the pacing system; namely, it should show whether the device is either inhibited or tracking based upon the programmed mode. This is feasible only if there is a stable native rhythm in one or both chambers. The device should then be programmed so that there will be capture in each chamber so that the morphology of the pacemaker-evoked potentials is documented in each lead of the full 12-lead recording.

When the patient is ambulatory, *overpenetrated* posteroanterior and lateral chest x-rays should be obtained. It is essential that this study be overpenetrated to facilitate visualization of the intracardiac position of the lead(s). An x-ray obtained utilizing the standard technique—which is primarily designed to evaluate the lungs—may not be adequate to document the course and position of the pacing leads within the cardiac silhouette.

Prior to the patient's discharge from the hospital and on each subsequent outpatient pacing system evaluation, precise measurements of demand and magnet rates are obtained with a digital counter, ECG rhythm strips are obtained showing the pacing system function in the demand and magnet modes, and a detailed assessment of the capture and sensing thresholds are obtained within the limits imposed by the programmability of the system. Where measured data concerning lead and battery function as well as event marker, event counter, and electrogram telemetry are able to be provided by the pacemaker–programmer system, these too are obtained and incorporated in the summary of that evaluation.

The above data can be incorporated in the hospital or office chart, placed in a separate pacemaker follow-up chart, or entered into a pacemaker follow-up database computer program, of which there are a number of commercially available systems. Having access to prior records detailing the programmed parameters of the pacemaker and the function of the system will be extremely helpful in identifying a developing problem, often before it becomes clinically overt and causes the patient a problem. Future pacemakers with increased amounts of random access memory will allow the results of this periodic testing to be downloaded into the memory of the pacemaker itself so that the information is immediately available to the physician at the time of subsequent follow-up sessions, even when this evaluation is performed by a physician who may not have access to the hard-copy records.

In the case of a suspected pacing system malfunction, it is essential to obtain sufficient ECG documentation of the problem. Correlation of this information with the clinical examination and symptoms will provide additional guidance as to the urgency of any intervention. Recording and digital artifacts that mimic a malfunction are called pseudomalfunction and must always be included in the differential diagnosis. To minimize the chance of being misled, it is often helpful to record the same events with multiple ECG leads, either simultaneously or sequentially. Careful analysis of the paced rhythm then requires the use of ECG calipers for single-chamber rhythms or trividers, which may facilitate the analysis of dual-chamber rhythms. Trividers, a modified pair of calipers, have three legs instead of two. Legs 1 and 2 can be set to the AV interval; legs 2 and 3 can be set to the atrial escape interval.[18] This chapter is restricted to pacing system malfunctions that are manifested on the ECG. Infection, erosion, venous thrombosis, and other mechanical or soft tissue problems with the pacing system are covered in Chapter 5.

DIFFERENTIAL DIAGNOSIS OF SINGLE-CHAMBER PACING SYSTEM MALFUNCTION

Any malfunction that can occur in a single-chamber pacing system can involve either channel of a dual-chamber system. To promote clarity, this section focuses on the common abnormalities associated with single-chamber systems. The next section will concentrate on dual-chamber systems, which require an understanding of both single-channel malfunctions and the complex interaction of the pacemaker's timing cycles with the native rhythm.

When presented with a paced rhythm, it is first helpful to determine whether pacing stimuli are present. If present, do they capture the appropriate cardiac chamber? If absent, is there a native depolarization that is properly timed to explain the absence? One also needs to look at the native beats in relation to the paced complexes. Are all the native beats sensed correctly? Do they inhibit or trigger the next paced complex? To make this assessment, it is essential to know the programmed parameters of the pacemaker and any unique behavioral characteristics of the particular device or chosen mode.[19,20] A pacing system problem may not be immediately apparent but will be identified using the programming capabilities of the implanted unit combined with telemetered event markers, electrograms, or measured data.

Some pacing system problems are immediately apparent on the basis of examination of the electrocardiographic recording. The malfunction can be persistent or intermittent. One can then identify the basic category of pacing system malfunction. The three major groups are 1) pacing stimuli present with failure to capture, 2) pacing stimuli present with failure to sense, and 3) pacing stimuli absent. Each group will be discussed in more detail.

Pacing stimuli present with failure to capture

To place a malfunction in this group, it is first necessary to be able to identify the pacing stimulus. This is usually obvious in a unipolar pacing system, because the stimuli are physically large (Figure 7.1), but may become a problem with small bipolar outputs (Figure 7.2).[21] Pacing stimuli are electrical transients or nonphysiologic signals of very high frequency. Thus, one also needs to understand how the recording system handles and reproduces these signals. Some systems, particularly ambulatory and in-hospital monitoring units, use special filters to eliminate high-frequency signals to minimize baseline noise on the recording.[22,23] In these cases, the unipolar signal will be markedly attenuated and the bipolar signal may be effectively erased. Sometimes, the signal is simply isoelectric in a given lead. Thus, if a malfunction is suspected, it is essential to record either multiple simultaneous or sequential leads with a system known to accurately reproduce the pacing stimulus artifact. In this case, the technologically older analog recorders are superior to the modern recording systems that digitize the incoming data for transmission to a computer. Other systems have unique high-frequency detection algorithms intended to identify pacing stimuli. However, when any signal of sufficient frequency is detected, a uniform, usually large, amplitude artifact is displayed on the recording precluding differentiation of unipolar from bipolar signals. Even nonpacemaker signals may appear to be a pacing stimulus with these recording systems.

The differential diagnosis of stimuli present with failure to capture is relatively limited. A likely etiology can often be established simply by knowing when the problem was encountered with

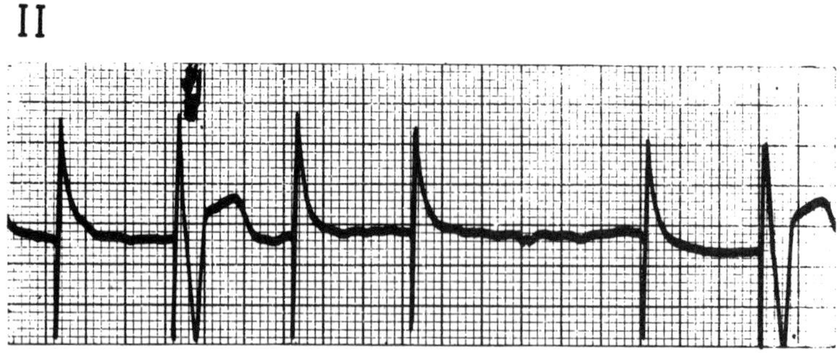

II

Figure 7.1   Pacing stimuli present with intermittent failure to capture. The large unipolar stimuli are readily identified. The gentle downslope following the ineffective pacing stimulus is an RC decay curve. The pause is due to appropriate sensing of a native QRS, which is virtually isoelectric in this lead.

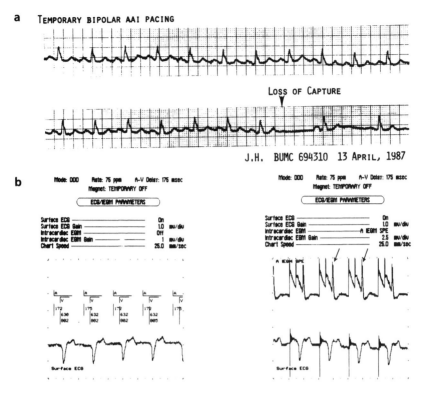

LOSS OF CAPTURE

J.H. BUMC 694310 13 APRIL, 1987

Figure 7.2 (a) Temporary bipolar atrial pacing. The pacing stimulus is so small that it is virtually invisible. Intermittent loss of
capture is noted at the end of the bottom tracing; but even here,
the pacing stimulus remains undetectable, although it is present.
(b) Dual-chamber pacing system with loss of atrial capture and
intact ventricular capture. The surface ECG shown in the left panel
suggests that there is single-chamber ventricular pacing or, because the pacing stimuli are too small to be seen, an idioventricular
rhythm. Simultaneously recorded telemetered event markers identify the paced rhythm as AV sequential even though the stimuli
cannot be seen on the ECG. In the panel on the right, the atrial
output has been programmed to unipolar, resulting in a large,
easily identified pacing stimulus. Still, one cannot confirm atrial
capture based on the surface ECG. The simultaneously obtained
telemetered atrial electrogram obtained by recording between the
ring electrode and the housing of the pulse generator fails to show
an atrial evoked potential but records a large retrograde P wave
following the paced ventricular complex. The retrograde P wave,
although readily seen on the telemetered EGM, is not easily seen
on the surface ECG. In addition, it could not have occurred had
there been atrial capture as the atrial myocardium would have
been physiologically refractory at this time. Hence, there was no
capture associated with the atrial stimulus.

respect to lead implantation. If the loss of capture is occurring within hours or days of the implant, the most likely explanation is lead dislodgment or malposition. Although there may be subtle differences between a *dislodged* and a *malpositioned* lead, these two terms are used interchangeably in this chapter. Loss of capture occurring weeks to months postimplantation is most likely to be due to high capture thresholds resulting from the expected, hence normal, inflammatory reaction that occurs at the electrode–tissue interface during the lead maturation process. If this problem occurs many months to years postimplantation, it is usually due to a mechanical or structural problem with the lead (such as damaged insulation or a conductor fracture) or due to a permanent or transient abnormality in the myocardium itself. Eventually, the battery will deplete such that the actual output, despite its programmed value, will fall below the capture threshold, resulting in loss of capture. Common pacing system abnormalities associated with noncapture are summarized in Table 7.1.

The above differential diagnosis and priority of likelihood is helpful, but it is not sufficient to direct any intervention. Except for lead dislodgment—although unlikely to occur once the system has been demonstrated to be functioning normally for a couple of months postimplantation—other problems have been reported to occur months and even years postimplantation.[24]

Lead dislodgment: Accompanying the loss of capture with an acute lead dislodgment, there will be a change in the morphology of any capture beats that are present, there may be a change in the dipole of the pacing stimulus, and there will be a change in the lead position on a repeat chest x-ray. It is important to obtain the follow-up chest x-ray in an identical position to that used for the baseline study. If the initial study was an anterioposterior view obtained with the patient supine, the follow-up study should be similar. Despite some early reports in the literature to the contrary, neither lead dislodgment nor a simple rise in capture threshold due to tissue reaction at the electrode–myocardial interface will result in a significant change in stimulation impedance, either up or down.[14]

A change in the morphology of the capture beat is often a clue to lead dislodgment, but this is the case only when the entire depolarization is totally controlled by the pacemaker. Changing morphologies due to varying combinations of simultaneous paced and native depolarizations are called fusion beats.[4-6] These are normal and reflect a coincidence of timing. If the paced ventricular

Table 7.1 Differential Diagnosis of Pacing Stimuli Present—Persistent or Intermittent Loss of Capture

Etiology	ECG[a]	Chest X-Ray[b]	Stimulation Impedance	Capture Threshold	Management
Lead dislodgment	Abnormal	Abnormal	Normal	Elevated	Reposition lead
Lead maturation	Normal	Normal	Normal	Elevated	Increase output or trial oral steroids or reposition lead
Late high thresholds	Normal	Normal	Normal	Elevated	Increase output or correct cause or replace lead
Insulation failure	Normal[c]	Normal or conductor deformity	Decreased	Elevated	Replace lead
Conductor fracture	Normal[d]	Abnormal	Increased	Elevated	Replace lead
Battery depletion	Normal	Normal	Normal	Elevated	Replace pulse generator
Functional noncapture	Normal	Normal	Normal	Normal	Decrease rate or decrease refractory period(s) or increase sensitivity

[a] In ECG column, normal refers to a stable morphology of the evoked potential; abnormal refers to a change in the morphology of the evoked potential.
[b] In chest x-ray column, normal refers to stable lead position and no obvious deformity of the conductor coil; abnormal refers to a change in lead position or a deformity of the conductor coil. The insulation is radiolucent and will not be visualized on the x-ray.
[c] The ECG with an insulation failure involving a unipolar lead will show a decrease in the amplitude of the pacing stimulus. An insulation failure involving the outer insulation of a bipolar lead will show an increase in the amplitude of the pacing stimulus. Failure of the internal insulation of a coaxial bipolar lead will show a decrease in stimulus amplitude. This presupposes that all recordings are made with an analog ECG machine.
[d] The ECG with an intermittent conductor fracture may show a varying amplitude pacing stimulus if recorded with an analog ECG machine. See Table 7.5 for a total conductor fracture.

SOURCE: Modified from Levine PA. Pacing system malfunction: Evaluation and management. In PJ Podrid, PR Kowey (eds.), *Cardiac Arrhythmia: Mechanisms, Diagnosis, and Management*. Williams & Wilkins, © 1995. By permission of Williams & Wilkins.

beat is preceded by either a native P wave or an atrial paced beat in the dual-chamber modes, consider fusion beats. Fusion can also occur in the atrium. The morphologic changes in the paced P wave when combined with the native atrial depolarization are more difficult to identify because of the smaller size of the atrial complex.

Correction of a lead dislodgment requires operative intervention to reposition the lead. Prior to this being done, careful attention should be directed to the original chest x-ray, and an adequate heel on the intracardiac portion of the lead should be looked for. Either too little or too much will predispose to dislodgment.[24] One should also review the recorded electrograms from the initial implant, looking for a 2 to 3 mV current of injury pattern (ST-segment elevation). The absence of this degree of current of injury has been correlated with an increased incidence of lead dislodgment; the implication is that the electrode is not making good endocardial contact and is not well engaged within the trabeculae.[15] The only way that one will know this is to record the EGM at the time of the implant; this should be a routine part of the procedure. Although measurement of the amplitude and even slew rate of the EGM with a PSA at the time of implant is also essential, the digital display of the PSA does not provide the additional information concerning ST-segment elevation. At the time of the operative procedure, one should also check the integrity of the anchoring sleeve and its fixation to both the lead and the underlying tissue. If the sleeve is not adequately fixed, it will allow the lead to pull back into the pocket with normal motion of the upper extremity. This has recently been reported as a cause of dislodgment of ICD leads.[25] It is also the most common cause of Twiddler's syndrome, rather than the cause being a patient who manipulated the pulse generator under the skin, although the latter has also occurred as well.[26,27]

One should keep in mind a couple of cautions at the time of lead repositioning. If a likely explanation for the dislodgment was identified prior to the revision, every effort should be made to prevent this from happening again. With respect to repositioning a dislodged lead, a thrombus may have developed around the lead tip, encasing the tines or fins and preventing the lead from being adequately secured at the repeat procedure. Thus, once the lead is thought to be in a good position, the patient should be instructed to take as deep a breath and to cough as vigorously as possible in an effort to assess the mechanical stability of the lead. While the patient is doing these maneuvers, the physician should be stimulating the heart with the PSA set to an output just above threshold while continuously observing both the ECG monitor and fluoroscopic image. Inappropriate motion of the lead on x-ray or loss of capture on the monitor indicates that the lead position is not stable. Given the reason for the repeat intervention, a lead should not be left in a less-than-optimal position in the hope that it will stabilize. If a stable lead position cannot be confirmed, the lead should be removed and replaced with a new lead with either passive or active fixation, depending on the physician's choice.

If the dislodgment is due to Twiddler's syndrome, the most common cause of a late lead dislodgment, the portion of the lead within the pocket should be carefully inspected. If damage to the conductor coil or insulation is noted, the lead should not be reused. If the lead is tightly twisted on itself, it should not be reused because the twisting causes stress within the lead, which may manifest by a structural or mechanical problem months or even years later.

If a dislodgment occurs and the reason is not absolutely apparent that it could be corrected at the second procedure, it would be prudent to remove the dislodged lead and replace it with an active fixation lead. One needs to be aware that use of an active fixation lead does not guarantee chronic stability—dislodgments have also occurred with these leads years postimplantation.[24,28,29]

High thresholds; lead maturation: When the electrode is first inserted, it is making intimate contact with the endocardium. At this time, the capture threshold is often very low, usually less than 1.0 V at a pulse width of 0.5 msec. Two factors combine to induce an inflammatory reaction at the electrode–myocardial interface. One is the mere presence of foreign material in the body. This causes the body to attempt to isolate it. An analogous situation would be an oyster's response to a grain of sand, in which case, the result is a pearl. The second factor, the pressure of the lead–electrode system in contact with the myocardium, induces local trauma, which also elicits an inflammatory reaction. It is this local trauma that is responsible for the current of injury pattern on the acute EGM recording. At the peak of the inflammatory reaction, the electrode is physically displaced from the active excitable myocardium and requires an increased amount of energy to effectively stimulate the heart. The result is a rise in the capture threshold, which is the lowest output setting that consistently results in cardiac depolarization. The increased separation between the electrode and the active myocardial tissue also attenuates the amplitude and the slew rate of the endocardial signal and potentially can result in undersensing. With time, the inflammatory reaction subsides, leaving a thin capsule of fibrous tissue between the electrode and active myocardium. As the distance between the two elements is reduced, the amount of energy required to stimulate the heart decreases, although rarely to levels as low as were recorded at the time of implantation. Sensing also improves.

Sometimes, the inflammatory reaction at the electrode–myocardial interface is excessive, causing the capture threshold to rise above the output of the pacemaker.[30–35] This has been termed *exit block*. If exit block is the reason for intermittent loss of capture, there will be no change in the morphology of any capture beats, nor will there be a change in the radiographic position of the lead. According to the literature, the likelihood of exit block developing cannot be predicted on the basis of the acute capture thresholds because it occurs even when the acute thresholds are excellent. If the implanting physician accepts an electrode position with a high threshold (i.e., $>1.5\,V$), there is an increased likelihood of exit block. The earlier literature reports an incidence of 4 to 5 percent.[28] In recent years no studies have systematically assessed the impact of changes in electrode materials and geometry on the early maturation process. In general, however, chronic capture thresholds and the subacute rise in capture thresholds associated with lead maturation tend to be lower with the newer generation of leads.

Acute management of high thresholds, with or without loss of capture, requires increasing the output of the pacemaker. If this is not feasible, one needs to determine the status of the native underlying rhythm. If it is stable and adequate to physiologically support the patient, one might simply wait for the threshold to fall. If the underlying rhythm is not stable, one will need to insert a temporary pacemaker lead.

Rather than waiting for the expected evolution of the normal maturation process in the presence of high thresholds developing in the weeks to months postimplantation, systemic steroids have been administered in an effort to reduce the inflammatory reaction at the electrode–myocardial interface.[36–41] It was this experience that led to the development of the steroid-eluting electrode, which has been effective in attenuating the inflammatory reaction and its associated early rise in capture and sensing thresholds.[42–44] Indeed, if the threshold does not fall sufficiently to maintain an adequate margin of safety and one elects to reposition the lead, it might be reasonable to replace the lead with one of the steroid-eluting systems. This is also reasonable if there are contraindications to the use of systemic steroids. Steroid-eluting electrodes appear to prevent the acute but transient rise in capture thresholds; their effect on lowering chronic thresholds is less certain. The author has many patients with non–steroid-eluting leads with chronic capture thresholds below 1.0 V. Isolated cases of massive threshold rises have also been encountered with the steroid-eluting leads although the incidence of this system malfunction is probably lower than with non–steroid-eluting leads.[45,46]

During the early postimplantation period, if a threshold rise occurs and one elects to use systemic steroids in an attempt to reverse the phenomenon, a regimen this author has found effective in roughly 50 percent of patients in whom it has been used is 60 mg prednisone per day, often administered in divided doses. In the pediatric population, the dose is 1 mg/kg. Prior to initiating steroids, a detailed measurement of capture threshold is made within the programming capabilities of the system. This measurement is repeated four to five days after the initiation of steroids. If there is no change or if there is a further rise in capture thresholds, the steroids are considered ineffective and are simply discontinued. This is too short a period of time to be concerned with adrenal suppression. If the threshold, however, has decreased by at least two programming steps (pulse width and/or pulse amplitude), it is likely that the steroids are being effective. The dosage is then continued for a month, with biweekly monitoring of capture thresholds. At the end of the month, a slow but progressive tapering schedule is initiated continuing for a minimum of two months. During this period, the patient should be seen on a relatively frequent basis to monitor the response of the capture threshold to the progressive reduction in the steroid dose. If, as the dose is being tapered, the capture threshold starts to rise, the dose should be increased for a couple of weeks and the tapering then resumed at a slower pace. The goal is that the steroids should be able to be discontinued. One should never abruptly discontinue the steroids; an associated rebound effect is likely, with a further rise in the capture threshold. Prior to initiating systemic steroids, the physician must be sure that there are no contraindications to this therapy.

High thresholds; chronic lead: High capture thresholds may develop at any time. Those that are not associated with the acute lead maturation process are not likely to respond to steroids. When this problem is encountered, one should evaluate the patient for transient, and hence reversible, etiologies including electrolyte and acid–base abnormalities such as hyperkalemia and acidemia.[37-39,47-51] Also included are pharmacologic agents such as the antiarrhythmic drugs, of which the 1C agents such as flecainide have developed a particularly poor reputation.[52-60] If a transient cause is identified and that cause can be corrected, the problem can be managed with a transient increase in output or by use of temporary pacing until the situation has resolved.

Permanent rises in capture thresholds may also occur with progressive myocardial fibrosis due to a primary myopathic process or myocardial infarction.[61] If the output programmability of the device is not sufficient to overcome these causes, placement of a new lead will be required. Given that the lead is not infected, explantation is not mandatory. Even if it could be withdrawn, this author would be concerned that the forces required to disengage it from the fibrous tissue anchoring it in place would be sufficient to damage the lead such that it would not be prudent to reuse it.

One must be very cautious about invoking the diagnosis of a high threshold due to a primary myocardial process in the absence of a change in the morphology of the intrinsic P wave or QRS complex. With a stable native complex on the surface ECG, a more likely explanation is a primary problem developing with the lead itself—either a high resistance from a developing conductor fracture, and thus attenuating the amount of energy reaching the heart, or damaged insulation shunting the delivered energy away from the heart. This is another reason not to reuse a chronic lead. Whether the cause of the clinical malfunction is a physiologic problem related to the electrode–tissue interface or a structural abnormality of the lead itself, the effective correction will be the same—replacement of the lead.

If the malfunction were due to a mechanical abnormality developing in the lead, one would expect to see a change in the telemetered or invasively measured stimulation impedance, although this may not always be the case. Normal telemetry values may occur in the presence of an intermittent problem if the lead was functioning properly at the time of the measurements. When the lead impedance is abnormal, a very low impedance value (less than the lowest measurement provided by the system, or <200 ohms) reflects a failure of the insulation, most commonly the inner insulation in a coaxial bipolar lead. A very high lead impedance, either greater than 3000 ohms or above the highest measurement capable of being reported by the implanted system, is consistent with an open circuit. Measurement-to-measurement changes in telemetered lead impedance that are still within the normal range are totally consistent with normal lead function. One report in the literature suggested that changes up to 300 ohms may still be compatible with normal lead function.[62] Further, a change in measured impedances in the absence of a clinical malfunction, such as a massive rise in capture threshold, noncapture, or a sensing problem, may be a telemetry error. Although this might warrant closer follow-up, an isolated abnormality of a telemetry measurement does not mandate operative intervention.

Lead insulation defects: An insulation defect may develop from an intrinsic design and/or manufacturing limitation, as occurred with an early series of polyurethane leads that became subject to an FDA-mandated recall.[63–65] Most insulation problems, however, are due to extrinsic forces applied to the lead either at or following implant that physically damage the lead. In part, this problem is a direct result of the request by the medical community for thinner leads, both unipolar and bipolar. The primary method of reducing the lead's diameter is to reduce the thickness of the insulating material. In-line bipolar coaxial leads are the least forgiving of extrinsic stresses for this very reason. Insulation defects may occur with either silicone rubber or polyurethane,[66,67] that is, independent of the insulating material. Industrywide experience for damaged insulation for all leads, in general, is an incidence of approximately 2.5 percent, but this number is based on a relatively small sample and the incomplete return of lead information at the time of implant and pulse generator replacement.

Extrinsic stresses can result in damage to the insulation and/or a conductor fracture. The two most common stresses occur at either the suture sleeve, where an excessively tight ligature is used to anchor the lead to the underlying fascia, or the point where the lead traverses the plane between the clavicle and first rib on its way to the subclavian vein.[68–76] This has been recently termed the *medial subclavicular musculotendinous complex*[76] but is an increasingly recognized cause of malfunction of both standard pacing and defibrillator leads.

The anchoring sleeve is designed to minimize the chance of dislodgment by minimizing direct stress to the lead from the suture used to secure it to the fascia. However, the sleeve itself is made of silicone rubber. Sufficient force can be applied to the suture such that it overcomes the protective effect of the sleeve and distorts the lead itself, eventually compromising the lead's function. Thus, one wants to use sufficient force to anchor the lead, but not too much, which can damage the lead. If one sees a visible distortion of the conductor coil either at implant or on a follow-up chest x-ray, the ligature around the suture sleeve and lead is too tight.[77,78] Although this was originally considered a benign observation, the late adverse consequences associated with this area of stress have recently been appreciated.[66]

Perhaps the most common method of lead insertion in the United States today is direct access to the subclavian vein using a peel-away lead-introducer kit. Venous access is quick, and the surgical dissection required at the time of implant is minimized. The acute complications associated with this technique are covered in Chapter 5. Increasing numbers of physicians are becoming aware of the potential late complications that may result from this technique.[68–72,74–76] In general, the subclavian venipuncture technique recommends that the needle be directed medially because the venous structures are larger and easier to enter. This is appropriate for temporary lines that will be removed after a few days or weeks. However, for permanent pacing leads, this may result in a late problem if the point of entry between the clavicle and first rib is too medial or the lead traverses either the costoclavicular ligament or subclavius muscle. The normal motion of the arm causes the space between the clavicle and first rib to widen and narrow, much like the jaws of pliers. The lead located in this position can be repeatedly crushed, pinched, or pulled and stretched, resulting in a deformity of the conductor coils, which in turn will predispose to either insulation defects or conductor fractures (Figure 7.3) occurring months to years postimplantation.[74–76] A recent recommendation has been to access the axillary vein rather than the subclavian vein to avoid both the acute and late complications associated with this implant technique.[79–81] There has also been a recommendation to return to the cephalic vein cutdown technique for venous access, which can be accomplished in most patients, even for individuals who require implantation of a dual-chamber system.[82,83] This will totally avoid both the acute and late complications associated with direct subclavian vein access.

Manifestations of a lead insulation defect[13,84–89] are determined, in part, by the location of the defect. In unipolar leads or a defect

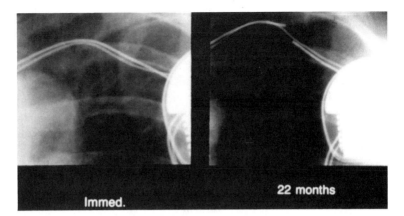

Figure 7.3 Twenty-two months postimplantation of a dual unipolar DDD pacing system, the patient presented with loss of atrial output and no evidence of appropriate sensing. Both silicone rubber insulated unipolar leads had been inserted by a single introducer into the left subclavian vein. The lead fractured at the point where it crossed between the clavicle and first rib, presumably due to the repeated extrinsic trauma associated with the anatomical location of the lead induced by normal arm movements over a period of just under two years.

associated with the proximal conductor of a bipolar lead, there may be extracardiac muscle stimulation due to the electrical current leaking from the defect. Local muscle stimulation in the area of a unipolar pacemaker may also be due to an upside-down pacemaker with the anode or indifferent electrode making direct contact with the underlying muscle. This must be excluded with a chest x-ray before attributing the problem to an insulation defect. The author is also aware of several cases in which the insulating material applied to the pulse generator was damaged, thus allowing for local muscle stimulation with a totally normal lead.

Another manifestation includes changes in the amplitude of the pacing stimulus. This is best identified with an analog ECG recording system. In a unipolar system, there is a shorter path between the exposed conductor and the pulse generator, resulting in attenuation of the pacemaker stimulus amplitude. When the breach involves the outer insulation covering the anodal conductor of a bipolar lead, there will then be two pathways for current flow. One is from the distal tip to the proximal ring electrode; the second is from the distal tip to the proximal conductor, which has been exposed by insulation defect. This will result in a larger "unipolarized" stimulus on the ECG. If the insulation is breached between the distal and proximal conductors of a bipolar lead, the current flow will be short-circuited and little or none of it will ever reach the active electrodes. In this case, the already small bipolar stimulus amplitude will be further attenuated.

In the chronic pacing system, one determines the stimulation threshold by the lowest programmed output that consistently captures the heart. The implication is that all the energy being delivered to the output circuit is reaching the heart. In a lead with an insulation failure, some of that energy is diverted and does not reach the electrode–tissue interface within the heart. Thus, the output at the pulse generator must be increased to allow for this diversion and still result in capture. Because it is not realized that some of the delivered energy does not actually reach the myocardium, the interpretation is that there is a rise in the capture threshold. Although this is correct in one sense—the amount of energy that the pacemaker must deliver is increased as a way to effect capture—it is also incorrect because the amount of energy required to capture at the electrode–myocardial interface is often stable. It is just that the pacemaker must provide increased energy for the critical amount to reach the electrode itself.

Noninvasive telemetry of lead impedance may identify the problem if it is manifest at the time of the interrogation measurements. The lead impedance will fall as the effective surface area of the electrode is increased by the insulation defect. In a voltage-limited output design, as in most present-generation pacemakers, the fall in lead impedance results in an increased battery current drain, which more rapidly depletes the battery. Thus, if an insulation defect is identified in a patient, one must consider the known effects of this defect on the battery when deciding on the optimal procedure. If the pulse generator provides data as to the status of the battery itself—either measured battery voltage (should be 2.7 V or higher) or battery impedance (should be low)—it would be safe to reuse the pulse generator and replace only the lead. If the pulse generator does not have the capability of providing this information, unless this problem has been encountered within a few months to a year postimplantation, the pacemaker should probably be replaced at the same time the lead is replaced.

Sometimes, an intermittent problem is identified on a Holter monitor or is suspected on the basis of symptoms but, when the patient is evaluated in the office, the system is functioning properly. This is particularly likely if the insulation defect occurs between the proximal and distal conductor of a bipolar lead. The defect is not being stressed (and thus unmasked) when the patient is lying quietly on the examination table. The normal elastic recoil of the conductor coils may separate the two wires even if the insulation between them has been breached. A number of maneuvers can be applied to help determine whether a problem exists. While these maneuvers are being performed, the rhythm should be monitored by an ECG machine along with simultaneously telemetered lead impedance measurements, event markers, and/or electrograms (Figure 7.4). One technique that is particularly effective in identifying a problem resulting from a ligature that is too tight around the anchoring sleeve is for the examiner to trace the course of the subcutaneous portion of the lead with his or her fingers while applying pressure at each point. If there is an insulation defect, the two conductor coils will be pushed together, unmasking the problem. Extending the ipsilateral arm as high as possible, as in reaching toward the ceiling or placing the arm behind the back and rotating the shoulder backward, may unmask a problem due to an injury caused by the medial subclavian–muscular complex.

Obtaining a chest x-ray may reveal a problem, although the insulation defect will not be seen because the insulating material is radiolucent. One might see a deformity of the conductor coil (Figure 7.5) or a very medial entry into the vein, allowing one to infer the diagnosis when these observations are combined with the clinical and telemetry data. However, a radiographic abnormality in the absence of independent corroboration of a system malfunction would be insufficient grounds to recommend an operative intervention.

Open circuit: The most common cause of an open circuit is a conductor fracture. The second, but more embarrassing, cause is a failure to adequately tighten the set screw in the terminal pin connector block of the pulse generator (Figure 7.6). The latter is due primarily to lack of attention to detail at the time of implantation and is easily corrected by tightening the set screw. Unfortunately, this requires an operative intervention to accomplish. More difficult to manage are lead fractures, which were particularly common in the early days of cardiac pacing, when conductors were composed of a single coiled filament. The repetitive flexion eventually weakened the conductor, resulting in a fracture. This could be accelerated by added stresses to the lead from either a tight anchoring ligature or angulation of the lead around a fibrous band.

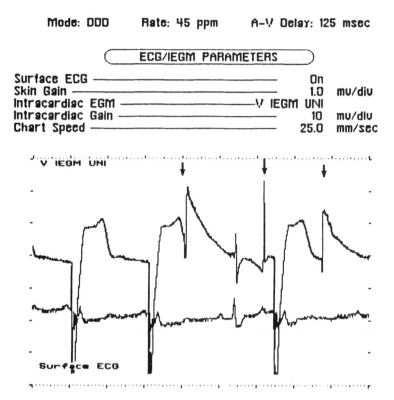

Mode: DDD   Rate: 45 ppm   A-V Delay: 125 msec

ECG/IEGM PARAMETERS

Surface ECG ————————————— On
Skin Gain ————————————— 1.0   mv/div
Intracardiac EGM ————————V IEGM UNI
Intracardiac Gain ————————— 10   mv/div
Chart Speed ————————————— 25.0   mm/sec

V IEGM UNI

Surface ECG

Figure 7.4   Repeated ventricular oversensing with resultant inhibition was demonstrated in this dual bipolar DDD pacing system. Measured data telemetry reported a ventricular lead impedance of < 250 ohms; the baseline had been 645 ohms. Telemetry of the ventricular electrogram while simultaneously recording a surface ECG demonstrates nonphysiologic large electrical transients occurring at a time when the pacemaker is being inhibited, indicating that the pacemaker is sensing these signals. The ventricular sensitivity had been reduced in an attempt to minimize this oversensing problem. However, the nonphysiologic transients were approximately 20 mV, larger than the least sensitive setting of the pacemaker, and the oversensing continued. However, the reduced sensitivity resulted in undersensing of the native R waves, resulting in competition. The nonphysiologic electrical transients were treated as PVCs by the pacemaker and activated the PVC algorithm, extending the refractory period and resulting in intermittent functional atrial undersensing.

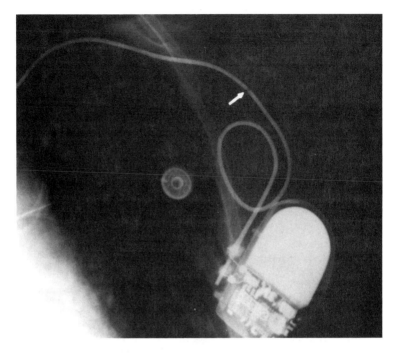

Figure 7.5 In-line bipolar coaxial lead with an indentation (identified by an arrow) created by a tight ligature around the lead. This has been called a pseudofracture and was previously considered to be of little clinical consequence. It has since been learned that the excessively tight ligature predisposes to both conductor fractures and insulation defects.

The incidence of fractures markedly decreased with the introduction of multiple filaments and improved alloys that were more flexible than the earlier wires as well as having redundancy, which further protects the patient. In recent years, there has been an increased incidence of conductor fractures due to the repeated chronic trauma to the lead following direct access to the subclavian vein using the introducer technique. The incidence of this problem, although increasing, remains low and is less than that of insulation defects.

There are two common clinical manifestations of an open circuit. With a total open circuit, no energy will traverse the gap between the two portions of the lead and there will be a failure of output on the ECG and loss of capture. This is included in the class of malfunction associated with an absent pacing stimulus. If the two

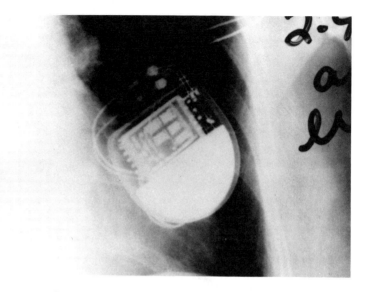

Figure 7.6 The patient in whom this x-ray was obtained presented with two problems: local pectoral muscle stimulation and intermittent no output on the ventricular channel. The x-ray demonstrates that the pacemaker is upside down in the pocket. Many unipolar and polarity programmable pacemakers have a unidirectional insulating boot applied at the time of manufacture. When situated in the pocket properly, the anode will be against the subcutaneous tissue and not the skeletal muscle. On an x-ray, this will be indicated by the leads exiting the connector block in a clockwise direction although this rule-of-thumb will become invalid with the manufacture of pulse generators specifically designed to be located in the left pectoral fossae. The leads in this patient exit in a counterclockwise direction. In addition, the terminal pin of the top lead can be seen to extend through the set-screw connector block. This is not the case with the bottom or ventricular lead. It is not seated in the connector properly, resulting in an open circuit.

ends of the conductor are making any contact at all, the resistance to current flow will be increased. This increase will, in turn, attenuate the amount of current and energy reaching the heart, but a stimulus will be present. If the effective energy reaching the heart is subthreshold, there will be loss of capture.[90–92] Although a physical break in the conductor is the most common cause of an open circuit and usually is not manifest until months to years postimplantation, there are two circumstances when an open circuit can occur at the time of implantation. One is a failure to tighten the set screw and the lead pulls out of the set-screw connector block (see Figure 7.6). The other involves a small unipolar pacemaker used as a replacement for an earlier generation larger model pacemaker. If there is air trapped within the pocket, this may serve as an insulator separating the indifferent electrode on the case of the pacemaker from the patient's tissues.[93,94]

A partially open circuit may also result in pauses but is caused by oversensing associated with make–break contact between the ends of the conductor coil or between the terminal pin and an inadequately tightened set-screw within the connector block. This can result in nonphysiologic electrical transients that are sensed by the pacemaker and cause pauses from oversensing.

Diagnosis of an open circuit may be facilitated by taking advantage of the diagnostic capabilities incorporated in many present generation pacemakers. Event marker telemetry will confirm an output pulse even if one is not visible on the ECG. This is a real possibility due to the recording limitations with bipolar systems.[21] Telemetry of measured data for lead impedance will demonstrate a significant rise (Figure 7.7)[7,95] if the problem is manifest at the time of measurement. A total open circuit will have an infinitely high impedance if the insulation remains intact. However, if there is a concomitant break in the insulation, as may occur if the lead is totally transected, the impedance may be normal or only minimally elevated because the conductor will be exposed to the tissue via the severed insulation.

An x-ray will often show the conductor fracture, particularly with unipolar leads. One may have to rotate the patient and take multiple views to eliminate overlapping portions of the lead in a given plane that might obscure the fracture. Sometimes this is easier to accomplish in a catheterization laboratory using fluoroscopy while rotating either the x-ray tube or the patient. In-line bipolar coaxial leads are the most difficult with regard to radiographic identification of a conductor fracture. Unless there is total disruption of both conductors at the same place, the intact proximal or distal conductor may mask the defect in the other conductor.

If the fracture is located in the subcutaneous portion of a unipolar lead and the insulating material is silicone rubber, the lead can be repaired by splicing the fractured ends. If the insulating material is polyurethane, no attempt at repair should be undertaken because no adhesive is available to repair the insulation after splicing the conductor. In-line bipolar coaxial leads also cannot be repaired in the clinical setting. Thus, in most lead fractures, the

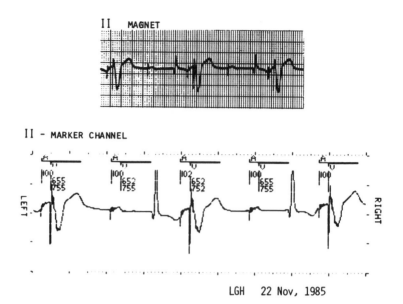

II MAGNET

II - MARKER CHANNEL

LEFT

RIGHT

LGH   22 Nov, 1985

Figure 7.7(a)   No intermittent output on the ventricular channel was noted at routine follow-up. This malfunction persisted with application of a magnet, which should result in asynchronous (DOO) function. When the ECG is recorded simultaneously with telemetered event markers, although no stimulus is present on the surface ECG, the pacemaker is indicating that it has released a ventricular output each time. (From Levine, PA. The complementary role of electrogram, event marker and measured data telemetry in the assessment of pacing system function. *J Electrophysiol* 1987;1:404–416. Reprinted with permission.)

···························· MEASURED DATA ····························

PACEMAKER RATE .... 70.0 PPM

MAGNET RATE .... 80.1 PPM

CHANNEL MEASUREMENTS:

	VENTRICLE	ATRIUM	
PULSE VOLTAGE	5.3	5.0	VOLTS
PULSE CURRENT	.1	10.6	MAMPS
PULSE ENERGY	0	26	μJOULES
PULSE CHARGE	0	5	μCOULOMBS
LEAD IMPEDANCE	1990	472	OHMS

Figure 7.7(b)   Measured data telemetry indicates that the ventricular lead impedance is intermittently 1990 ohms. This is the highest number that the Pacesetter AFP™ system will report and is consistent with an open circuit. The pulse current, pulse energy, and pulse charge are minimal, which is compatible with this assessment.

malfunctioning lead will be abandoned in situ and replaced with a new lead. The terminal pin of the abandoned lead should be covered with an insulating cap and then anchored to the underlying tissue so that the lead is not pulled into the vascular system when no longer connected to the pulse generator.

Recording artifact: One always needs to be cognizant of recording artifacts. The first-generation digital ECG machines could generate large-amplitude signals from a bipolar stimulus, mimicking the pattern of a unipolar signal, thus suggesting an insulation defect. There may also be beat-to-beat variation in the amplitude of the pacing stimulus, all due to the digitizing process (Figure 7.8). Unlike analog recording systems that continuously sample the electrical potentials, a digital system takes discrete measurements 250 times a second or instantaneously every 4 msec. This is adequate for the standard ECG, but it is not sufficient to record the pacing stimulus, which is usually a negative pulse of less than 1.0 msec duration followed by a recharge pulse of lower amplitude, greater duration, and opposite polarity. Thus, the sampling phenom-

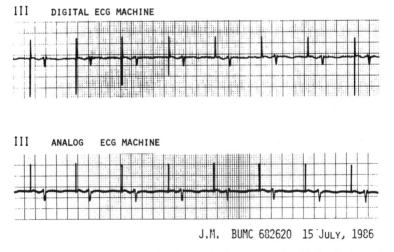

J.M. BUMC 682620 15 July, 1986

Figure 7.8 A lead III ECG rhythm strip is recorded with both digital (top) and analog (bottom) ECG machines. The digitizing process causes a marked beat-to-beat fluctuation in the amplitude of the bipolar pacing stimulus. This is an artifact of the recording system. The same surface ECG lead recorded with an analog system has a uniform amplitude pacing stimulus, although it is more difficult to see; it is faint because it is recorded with a heat stylus rather than an ink pen.

357

enon may miss the pacemaker pulse entirely, detect the large negative signal, or detect a small positive signal, creating dramatic fluctuations in both polarity and amplitude of the pacemaker pulse.

To minimize the resultant confusion that occurred in the clinical community, at least two of the major ECG manufacturers (Hewlett-Packard and Marquette) developed "pacemaker pulse detectors." The newer systems treat any high-frequency electrical transient as a pacemaker pulse for which they generate a relatively uniform amplitude signal on the ECG. If there are other causes of infrequent electrical transients, the ECG may look as if there is a pacemaker stimulus when the patient does not even have a pacemaker. In other cases, it magnifies a signal of very low amplitude associated with the Vario function of both the Elema and Telectronics pacemakers, mimicking an unstable runaway situation (Figure 7.9). Another example of pseudorunaway occurs with the new impedance-based, rate-modulated pacemakers such as the Telectronics Meta™ VVIR and DDDR systems because these low-amplitude signals, difficult to detect with a standard analog ECG, are magnified by some of the digital systems. This also renders the ECG itself difficult to interpret, and differentiating unipolar from bipolar pacing becomes virtually impossible. Even some pacemaker programmer printers suffer from the same limitation (Figure 7.10).

Functional noncapture: When a pacing stimulus occurs in the physiologic refractory period of a native depolarization, it will not capture. This is not a primary capture malfunction and should not be classified as such. This may be due to a primary problem of failure to sense or to functional undersensing. Functional undersensing is associated with the basic timing design of the system. It was particularly common in the committed AV sequential (DVI) pacing systems associated with pseudo-pseudofusion beats and sandwich complexes. The atrial stimulus occurred in the refractory period of the native atrial depolarization that conducted to the ventricle. The ventricular output then coincided with the refractory period of the ventricular depolarization. Thus, in an absolutely normally functioning pacing system, there was functional failure to capture on both the atrial and ventricular channels (Figure 7.11). The use of the term *functional noncapture* indicates that the myocardium is not capable of being depolarized at that time. This should not be considered a primary capture malfunction. The common causes of functional noncapture are listed in Table 7.2.

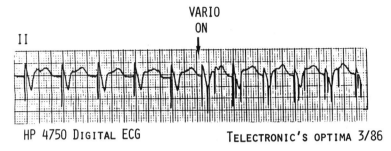

VARIO
ON

II

HP 4750 DIGITAL ECG   TELECTRONIC'S OPTIMA 3/86

Figure 7.9 To eliminate the marked fluctuation in the amplitude and polarity of the pacing stimulus when recorded with the digital ECG system, some manufacturers have introduced additional recording artifacts that may also be misinterpreted. Hewlett-Packard redesigned their Pagewriter II™ model 4750 system to generate a uniform amplitude spike in response to any identified high-frequency transient. In this example, the Vario feature of a Telectronics Optima™ pacemaker was activated. When Vario is engaged, pacing occurs at 120 ppm for 16 cycles with a progressive decrease in the pulse voltage on each subsequent paced beat until 0 V is reached. To fine-tune each voltage reduction, the pacemaker "dumps" small pulses of energy out of the can. The ECG machine detected each of these small, otherwise invisible, pulses of energy and generated a large stimulus, making it look as if there were a problem. In addition, this particular pacemaker was bipolar and the large stimuli would raise concerns of a lead insulation defect if one did not know about this recording artifact. This design makes ECG interpretation of the impedance-based rate-modulated pacing systems extremely difficult as the entire recording become obscured by "stimulus" artifacts.

Table 7.2   Common Causes of Functional Noncapture

Single chamber
   True undersensing
   Long refractory period
Dual chamber
   Atrial undersensing
   Committed DVI
   Blanking period
   Safety pacing
   PVARP extension algorithms post-PVC
   Long PVARP and high base rate

DVI = atrioventricular sequential pacing; PVARP = postventricular atrial refractory period; PVC = preventricular contraction.

II

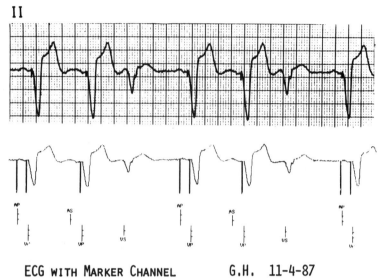

ECG WITH MARKER CHANNEL   G.H. 11-4-87
SYMBIOS7006 - DDD

Figure 7.10   The Medtronic 9710 programmer–printer system also generates a uniform amplitude stimulus regardless of whether the system is bipolar or unipolar. Normal DDD function is demonstrated on the top tracing with the expected diminutive stimuli associated with the bipolar Symbios 7006™ system. However, the Medtronic programmer–printer system recording the same rhythm generates large stimuli. The notations below the rhythm strip are the Medtronic event markers, termed Marker Channel™.

Pacing stimuli present with failure to sense

The ability of the pacing system to sense a native depolarization depends on a multiplicity of factors. A number of special circuits are incorporated in the sense amplifier of the pacemaker to enable it to recognize native signals while ignoring inappropriate signals. Ideally, the pacemaker should sense a low-amplitude QRS complex while ignoring both T waves, which are very low frequency and low amplitude signals, and myopotentials, which are higher frequency signals but also of a relatively low amplitude. In trying to walk the proverbial tightrope between sensing a low-amplitude appropriate signal and a higher amplitude inappropriate signal, there may be occasional signals that should be sensed but are not sensed due to a mismatch between the engineering specifications of the sense amplifier and the frequency characteristics of the native signal. Although this is not a true device malfunction because the

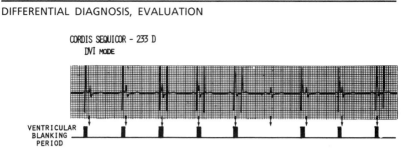

CORDIS SEQUICOR - 233 D
DVI MODE

VENTRICULAR
BLANKING
PERIOD

Figure 7.11 Functional undersensing on both the atrial and ventricular channels and functional noncapture are all shown in this rhythm strip from a normally functioning Cordis Sequicor™ pacemaker programmed to the DVI mode. In the DVI mode, there is no atrial sensing. Thus, the failure to sense endogenous atrial activity is not a malfunction. The failure of the atrial stimulus to capture is not unexpected, given that it is being delivered during the PR interval at a time when the atrial myocardium is physiologically refractory. Associated with the atrial stimulus is a ventricular blanking period to minimize the chance of crosstalk. If the intrinsic deflection of the native R wave coincides with the blanking period, it will not be sensed. Thus, the failure to sense the native R wave is in accord with the design of the system. Rather than being a true malfunction, it represents functional undersensing. Similarly, the release of the ventricular stimulus occurs at the end of the AV interval because the R wave was not sensed due to the blanking period. This allows the stimulus to be delivered when the ventricular myocardium is physiologically refractory. Hence, one would not expect capture. This is termed *functional noncapture.* Thus this tracing—which demonstrates atrial "undersensing," intermittent ventricular "undersensing," atrial "noncapture," and ventricular "noncapture"—actually reflects totally normal pacing system function and not a true malfunction. (From Levine PA, Mace RC. *Pacing Therapy—A Guide to Cardiac Pacing for Optimum Hemodynamic Benefit.* Mount Kisco, NY: Futura, 1983. Reprinted with permission.)

device is functioning properly in accord with its design specifications, it is one that cannot be appreciated in the clinical setting and may require replacement of the pulse generator with a different model or one from a different manufacturer. Basically, the design of the sense amplifier requires a series of tradeoffs. If it were too sensitive, it would respond to any signal that came along, thus leading to inappropriate inhibition or triggering, depending on the programmed mode. If it were too insensitive, the pacing system would no longer respond to physiologically inappropriate signals and the system might also fail to recognize appropriate signals. The failure to respond to a physiologically appropriate signal occurring during the alert period of the timing cycle is termed *undersensing.*

Table 7.3 Differential Diagnosis of Pacing Stimuli Present—Intermittent or Persistent Failure to Sense

Etiology	Diagnostic Evaluation*	Management*
Lead dislodgment	12-lead ECG with pacing; chest x-ray	Reposition lead
Endocardial signal too small	Telemetered EGM; sensing threshold assessment	Increase sensitivity or change sensing configuration or replace lead
Temporary change in EGM	Identification of new medication or electrolyte or acid–base imbalance	Discontinue medication or correct metabolic problem or change sensing configuration or increase sensitivity
Permanent change in EGM	New MI or cardiomyopathy; telemetered electrogram; sensing threshold	Increase sensitivity or change sensing configuration or replace lead
Ectopic beats	Telemetered EGM; Holter or ECG monitoring	Increase sensitivity or change sensing configuration or replace lead
Insulation failure	Fall in lead impedance by more than 300 ohms; telemetered EGM	Change sensing configuration until lead can be replaced
Functional undersensing	Careful assessment of pacing intervals	Decrease refractory period(s)

*Some suggested options may not be available with a given pulse generator. Only definitive management options are listed. In each case, increasing the sensitivity may correct the problem but, as with a primary lead failure, this may be a temporizing measure only.
SOURCE: Modified from Levine PA. Pacing system malfunction: Evaluation and management. In PJ Podrid, PR Kowey (eds.), *Cardiac Arrhythmia: Mechanisms, Diagnosis, and Management.* Williams & Wilkins, © 1995. By permission of Williams & Wilkins.

The differential diagnosis of undersensing along with the diagnostic tests and management options is detailed in Table 7.3.

One of the responsibilities of the implantation procedure is to determine whether the endocardial electrogram will be of sufficient amplitude and slew rate so that it can be sensed.[14,96–101] Sometimes, at the time of implantation, the patient's rhythm is under the control of a temporary pacemaker and there is no native signal to assess. Should this be encountered, it is strongly advised that a bipolar pacing system with extensive sensitivity and polarity programmability be implanted. This will allow the pacemaker to be programmed either to very sensitive settings should a native rhythm return, while minimizing the likelihood of oversensing problems, or to a different sensing configuration, which may restore normal sensing if native beats that are not sensed at the original parameters should occur. At other times, although the dominant native signal is more than adequate, ectopic beats, either ventricular- or atrial-conducted with aberration, occur at a later date; because of the variation in the sequence of ventricular activation, they are too small to be recognized by the pacemaker as an appropriate signal, which results in undersensing. Thus, for a reason similar to that proposed for lead selection in a pacemaker-dependent patient who does not have a stable rhythm at the time of implant, a system with extensive programmability should be considered for anyone in whom ectopy is likely to develop.

Specific mention is warranted concerning the feasibility of using the telemetered or recorded EGM in place of the PSA-measured signal at the time of implant or the noninvasively determined sensing threshold postimplantation.[102,103] Although these signals provide valuable information, they are not identical to the input signal after it has been processed by the pacemaker's sense amplifier. For example, the sense amplifier in the telemetry circuit of the Pacesetter units employs filters that approximate the American Heart Association standard for ECG recordings. This provides a signal with which physicians are familiar (Figure 7.12), but one that will differ markedly from that processed and amplified by the pacemaker's sensing circuit. Noninvasive assessment of the sensing threshold requires that the sensitivity of the pacemaker be progressively decreased until sensing fails. The sensing threshold is the least sensitive setting at which normal sensing still occurs. The sensing threshold should not be obtained by measuring the peak-to-peak amplitude of the telemetered EGM because, although there is usually a close correlation, there may also be dramatic differences

ATRIAL AND VENTRICULAR ELECTROGRAMS

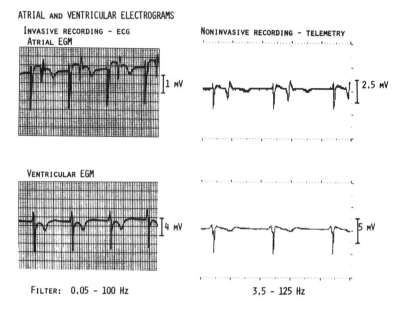

Figure 7.12 Atrial and ventricular unipolar electrograms were recorded at the time of lead placement using a standard ECG machine. The atrial and ventricular electrograms were then telemetered from the implanted AFP™ immediately at the end of the procedure. Other than losing some of the low-frequency components within the ST-T wave section of the complex, the signals are virtually identical. The telemetry sense amplifier is intentionally designed to approximate the American Heart Association standards for ECG recordings. It is thus different from the pacemaker's sense amplifier, and for this reason measuring the amplitude of telemetered EGM may not correlate well with the sensing threshold.

between the two measurements. If large T waves are visible on the telemetered EGM, one knows that the telemetry circuit utilizes a different filter than the sensing circuit (Figure 7.12).

Change in native signal: Another etiology of undersensing—the failure to sense a physiologically appropriate signal—is that the signal has changed.[104–106] The change in the signal may be permanent, as with a myocardial infarction or a primary myopathic process. It also may result from a change in the sequence of depolarization, as with development of a bundle branch block.

The changes listed above are permanent changes in the signal, but similar changes may occur on a temporary basis. Hyperkalemia results in a widening of the QRS complex and an attenuation of the P wave on the surface ECG. Similar changes will be occurring with the electrogram, which will result in undersensing on the ventricular or atrial channel, respectively. Pharmacologic therapy, particularly the antiarrhythmic agents that alter Phase 0 of the cardiac action potential, can change the intrinsic properties of the signal contributing to undersensing. In patients who present with an undersensing problem, it is imperative to check the patient's medications, particularly for any agents that may have been recently started. If possible, these agents should be discontinued before considering an operative intervention to replace or reposition the lead. One should also check the patient's serum electrolytes and arterial blood gases and correct any identified abnormalities before considering interventions other than programming to a more sensitive setting.

Inappropriate programmed sensitivity: An embarrassing cause of undersensing is an inappropriately programmed sensitivity. Confusion about the terms *high* and *low* sensitivity may result in incorrect programming. When an undersensing problem is encountered, one should increase the sensitivity or program the pacemaker to a higher sensitivity so that the system will recognize and respond to lower amplitude signals. Sensitivity is denoted in the programming parameters as the amplitude of the signal that can be sensed. A sensitivity of 1 mV would be more sensitive (higher sensitivity) than 2 mV. Similarly, if there is an oversensing problem and one wants to decrease or reduce the sensitivity, it means that the pacemaker will be less responsive, in which case the incoming signal must be larger than the amplitude chosen for the pacemaker to recognize it as an appropriate signal. Thus, a sensitivity of 4 mV, although a higher number, is really a lower sensitivity than 2 mV. Patients have been referred to the author for pulse generator replacement or lead repositioning for an undersensing problem even after the physician reported programming a "high" sensitivity when, in actuality, the physician had programmed a higher number, which was actually a lower sensitivity. These problems are easy to treat assuming that the pacemaker has sufficient sensitivity programmability.

Lead insulation defect: Lead insulation defects were discussed in the previous section on stimuli present with loss of capture. The insulation defect, if outside the heart, will attenuate the incoming signal. The signal will be an electrical average between the true electrode inside the heart and the false "electrode"—the exposed conductor coiled under the insulation defect. If the pacemaker has the ability to telemeter the EGM and there is a baseline recording available, one can compare the two signals.[13,84] If there is no change in the surface ECG manifestations of the native depolarization but there is a change in the endocardial electrogram, one should suspect an insulation defect. Other findings include a decrease in stimulation impedance, increase in battery current drain, rise in capture threshold, change in pulse artifact amplitude if recorded with an analog system, and possible extracardiac muscle stimulation. These findings are all corroboratory, supporting that the likely cause of the sensing failure is a breach in the insulation. One can temporize by increasing the sensitivity of the system, but definitive correction will require repair or replacement of the lead.

Lead dislodgment: Although lead dislodgment usually results in loss of capture, it is also frequently accompanied by undersensing. The electrode may no longer be in contact with the myocardium, or it may have been totally displaced from the appropriate cardiac chamber. In any case, the incoming signal will be different from and usually smaller than that recorded at implant, resulting in sensing failure. Correction requires repositioning the dislodged lead, although here, too, increasing the sensitivity may restore normal sensing function until the lead can be repositioned.

Lead maturation: The inflammatory reaction that occurs at the electrode–myocardial interface physically separates the electrode from active functional myocardium. This will attenuate the amplitude of the signal. The signal has been reported to decrease by as much as 20 to 40 percent when compared to the electrogram amplitude recorded at implantation. It also attenuates the slew rate, which may be the major reason for sensing failure because the input signal to the pacemaker now falls outside the engineering specifications that define the EGM for the proper sensing.

Treatment requires increasing the sensitivity of the pacemaker while initiating the other suggestions provided earlier for high capture thresholds associated with lead maturation.

Component malfunction: Problems may occur with the sense amplifier of the pacemaker, resulting in an undersensing problem. There is no good way to assess this noninvasively. Problems with the sense amplifier can certainly be suspected if the telemetered EGM is of large amplitude and good slew rate given the fact that the telemetry and sensing amplifier of most units with this capability are different. Similar observations can be made at the time of operative intervention. If the recorded EGM is large with a good slew rate (>1 V/sec) and the PSA-reported signal amplitude is large, one should suspect that the cause of the problem was intrinsic to the pulse generator. In the overall differential diagnosis of this problem, this is the least common cause of undersensing.

Functional undersensing: Functional undersensing is a failure to sense an appropriate physiologic signal with resultant competition but the undersensing is caused by the normal design of the pacemaker. With respect to single-chamber pacing systems, this most commonly occurs with native beats occurring very early in the cardiac cycle after the last paced or sensed complex. The pacemaker, just like the heart, has a refractory period. This is an interval after pacing or sensing during which the pacemaker is incapable of responding to a native depolarization. Thus, if a true native complex occurs during the refractory period, the pacemaker ignores it and behaves as if it had never occurred.

If too many signals are seen in a very short period of time, the likelihood is that this is electrical noise rather than true physiologic signals. This is termed *electromagnetic interference* (EMI). The presence of EMI precludes the pacemaker's differentiating electrical noise from an intrinsic rhythm; rather than inhibiting the pacemaker when the patient might be asystolic, the pacemaker reverts to asynchronous function, termed *noise mode operation.*[107–110]

With respect to dual-chamber designs, any period of refractoriness not specifically following a native or paced signal in the respective chamber can result in undersensing. A well-known example includes committed DVI pacing with atrial nonsensing (see Figure 7.11) and forced ventricular nonsensing during the AV delay. This occurs because the ventricular channel is rendered refractory following release of the atrial output pulse.[111,112] In an early generation of dual-chamber pacing, the VAT mode, atrial sensing triggered ventricular pacing but there was no ventricular sensing. This, too, is an example of functional undersensing, now the forced competition occurs on the ventricular channel.[113] Both DVI and VAT pacing are considered anachronisms by present-day standards even though they were state-of-the-art when first introduced.

Another timing circuit that may lead to functional undersensing is the ventricular blanking period in the current generation of dual-chamber pacing systems.[111,114] This circuit is designed to prevent the oversensing problem of crosstalk with the resultant ventricular output inhibition following the atrial output pulse. Although the ventricular blanking period may be as short as 12 msec, the intrinsic deflection of the sensed EGM is shorter than that, and blanking-period-induced undersensing may occur. All the above, although less than clinically desirable, are compatible with the design features of the respective pacemakers and thus reflect normal pacing system function. These examples might be best described as *functional undersensing* to differentiate them from a true malfunction (Table 7.4).

Pacing stimuli absent with failure to capture

The next major category of pacing system malfunction occurs when the stimulus is truly absent (Figure 7.13). One must be certain that this is not an artifact of a diminutive bipolar pacing stimulus further obscured by being isoelectric in a given lead (Figure 7.14). Hence, one should record multiple leads simultaneously or sequentially. Indeed, this might be the one indication for which to use a digital ECG machine that recreates a uniform amplitude stimulus in response to any high-frequency transient. Then one will at least be able to confirm that the stimulus artifact is really absent. The differential diagnosis of pacing stimuli absent is summarized in Table 7.5.

Table 7.4   Common Causes of Functional Undersensing in Single- and Dual-Chamber Pacing Systems

Single chamber
   Long refractory periods
   Noise mode
   Triggered mode
Dual chamber
   Blanking period
   Safety pacing
   Committed DVI pacing
   PVARP extension post-PVC
   Ventricular oversensing
   Long PVARP and high base rate

DVI = atrioventricular sequential pacing; PVARP = postventricular atrial refractory period; PVC = preventricular contraction.

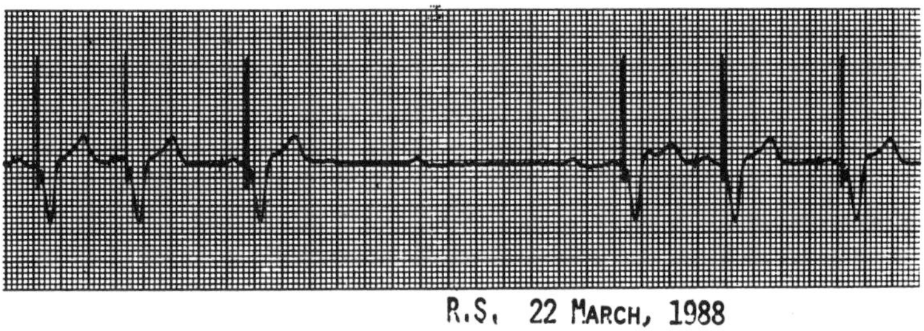

R.S. 22 MARCH, 1988

Figure 7.13 Pacing system malfunction, pacing artifact absent. Intermittent pauses occur without a visible pacing artifact. The ventricular stimulus was retouched for clarity. The atrial stimulus in this DDD system is a diminutive signal in this lead. Neither atrial nor ventricular stimuli are present during the pause.

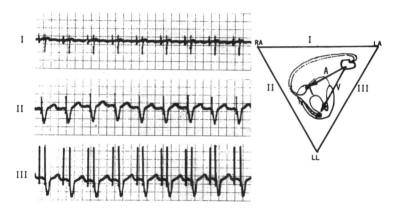

Figure 7.14 In assessing the presence or absence of pacing stimuli and even native complexes, it is imperative to examine multiple leads, recorded either simultaneously or sequentially. Leads I, II, and III are recorded sequentially from a patient with a dual unipolar DDD pacing system. The pulse generator was located in the left pectoral fossa. The basic dipole of the pacing stimuli is parallel to lead III, resulting in the expected large unipolar signals. In lead II, the atrial stimulus is virtually perpendicular to the lead, and thus no stimulus is recorded. In fact, had only lead II been monitored, the rhythm would have been interpreted as P wave synchronous ventricular pacing. In lead I, two pacing stimuli are readily visible, but the ventricular evoked potential is virtually isoelectric. Had this been the only lead monitored, one might have mistakenly made the diagnosis of ventricular noncapture. The multiple leads confirm AV sequential pacing with normal capture. To the right of the rhythm strips, a schematic of the pacing system is diagrammed within Einthoven's triangle. RA = right arm, LA = left arm, IL = left leg of the standard ECG leads.

369

Table 7.5 Differential Diagnosis of Pauses—Pacing Stimuli Absent

Etiology	Diagnostic Evaluation	Management
Oversensing	Magnet—pauses eliminated	Reduce sensitivity or program to bipolar sensing configuration
	Confirm with provocative maneuvers	Replace with bipolar system if unipolar
	Event marker telemetry	Replace lead
	Electrogram telemetry	
	Lead impedance—variable	
Open circuit	Lead impedance—high	
	Magnet—pauses persist	
Loose set screw	Chest x-ray—terminal pin not seated properly	Reoperate to secure set screw
Air in pocket	Chest x-ray—lateral may visualize air in pocket	Aspirate air
	Usually replacement procedure with new pacemaker smaller than original	Apply pressure dressing
Conductor fracture	Chest x-ray—conductor coil discontinuity	Replace lead
Internal insulation failure	Lead impedance low (<250 ohms)	Program to unipolar output configuration until lead can be replaced
	Magnet—pauses persist	
	Chest x-ray—normal or conductor coil deformity	
Component malfunction	Magnet—pauses persist	Replace pulse generator
	Telemetry—inconsistencies in measured data	Operative reassessment of lead function before attributing problem to pulse generator
Hysteresis	Native rate slower than paced rate	Reprogram if no longer appropriate
	Pauses follow only sensed beats	Reassurance as normal function
	Interrogation of programmed parameters	

Oversensing: *Oversensing* is the sensing of either a nonphysiologic or a physiologically inappropriate signal. This is particularly common in unipolar pacing systems programmed to a high sensitivity. In this case, the sensing of skeletal muscle potentials is the prime example able to confirm that the stimulus artifact is really absent.[115–120] Bipolar sensing has a greater signal-to-noise ratio, which makes oversensing far less common in the bipolar mode,[121,122] but oversensing can still occur. Strong electrical fields, as with arc welding equipment or radar installations, can be sensed.[123,124] Bipolar sensing is relatively immune to the usual myopotential oversensing, but both it and unipolar systems may detect diaphragmatic muscle potentials.[125,126] Native signals that can be sensed by either bipolar or unipolar sensing configurations are T waves and afterpotentials. Although there are reports of concealed ventricular ectopy causing pacemaker inhibition, this is theoretical and has never been unequivocally confirmed.[127,128]

A cause of oversensing within a normally functioning lead may be found with some active fixation endocardial leads that have both an electrically active collar and a fixation helix. An additional requirement is that the helix has some side-to-side motion within the collar. When the two electrically active metal components come into contact, a nonphysiologic electrical transient is created. This signal may be relatively massive, in which case it will not be amenable to programming a reduced sensitivity even though this is usually effective for the more physiologic signals such as myopotentials.[129] There is one report in the literature of correcting this problem by programming the sensing mode to a unique polarity configuration termed a *special unipolar* sensing configuration.[130] This is feasible only with some bipolar systems capable of sensing between the proximal ring electrode and the housing of the pulse generator while the electrical transient is generated solely via the distal conductor due to contact between the helix and the tip electrode.

Similar to the generation of nonphysiologic signals in the normally functioning coaxial bipolar leads, a break in the integrity of the inner insulation of an in-line bipolar lead can result in similar nonphysiologic electrical transients that will be sensed and cause inhibition or triggering, depending on the programmed parameters of the pacemaker and the lead in which this is occurring. The nonphysiologic transient is caused by the distal and proximal conductors making contact. As both conductors are integral to the generation of the false signal, the oversensing will persist in both

371

the bipolar and each unipolar sensing configuration. When recorded via telemetered EGMs, these signals are often massive (>20 mV), precluding elimination of the oversensing by a simple reduction in sensitivity (see Figure 7.4). The only option for a totally pacemaker-dependent patient, who does not have an adequate native escape rhythm and who does not have ectopy, is to program the pacemaker to the asynchronous mode (AOO, VOO, or DOO). This should be a temporary measure, however, used only until the problem can be definitively corrected by lead replacement. The testing procedures described earlier to identify a breach in the inner insulation of a bipolar coaxial lead should be employed while simultaneously recording both the surface ECG and either the telemetered EGMs or event markers.

When presented with recurrent pauses, one can quickly differentiate oversensing from the other causes of the absence of pacing artifact by applying a magnet to the pacemaker. The magnet will cause the pacemaker to revert to asynchronous function. If the pauses are eliminated, the problem is that of oversensing. However, this bedside technique will not identify the source of the signal being sensed. To determine the source of the oversensing, it is sometimes necessary to record the surface ECG while the patient is in the environment in which the reported symptoms occur. It may be necessary to have the patient perform provocative maneuvers as were described earlier in the section on lead evaluation. One could also have the patient do upper extremity isometric exercises, tensing the pectoral muscles, or do situps to tense the abdominal muscles in the case of an abdominal implant.[117] The patient should be asked to take very deep breaths if diaphragmatic oversensing is suspected.[125,126]

In the case of oversensing of usual physiologic signals such as myopotentials or T waves, programming the pacemaker to a less sensitive setting will usually correct the problem. This is feasible only if the native signal for which sensing is desired is sufficiently large to allow it to continue to be appropriately sensed. If reducing the sensitivity will result in undersensing of appropriate signals, one might program the pacemaker to the triggered mode (Figure 7.15). This will result in a stimulus being triggered rather than being inhibited by oversensing. This may lead to brief periods of more rapid, irregular pacing rather than the absence of pacing. The author has found this to be an effective technique with unipolar atrial pacing systems where a reduction of the sensitivity to 4 or 5 mV would result in functional AOO pacing. Oversensing should

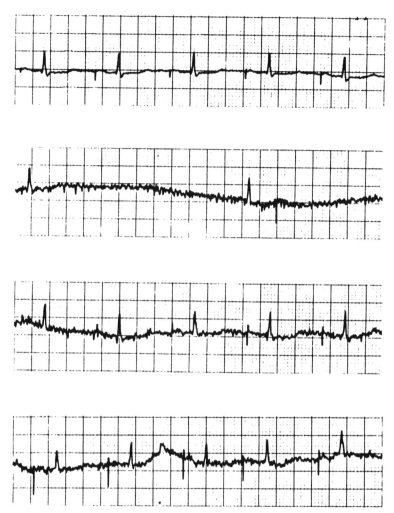

Figure 7.15 A series of four rhythm strips obtained from a patient with a unipolar atrial pacing system. The top tracing shows normal atrial pacing. The second shows marked inhibition associated with isometric upper extremity exercises. Although oversensing could be eliminated by reducing the sensitivity (third tracing), this resulted in atrial undersensing. The bottom tracing demonstrates the pacing system function with the pacemaker programmed to the triggered mode. Now there is appropriate sensing of native P waves, but when oversensing occurs, an atrial stimulus is triggered, resulting in a slightly irregular and more rapid rate while avoiding the marked inhibition seen in the AAI mode when the sensitivity was programmed to allow sensing of the endogenous atrial activity.

be anticipated at the time of implantation and can usually, but not always, be prevented by the choice of a bipolar system. In the case of T-wave or afterpotential oversensing, increasing the refractory period will often correct the problem.

Open circuit: Second to oversensing as a cause of persistent or intermittent pauses associated with the absence of a pacing stimulus is an open circuit. Event marker telemetry will indicate that the pacemaker released a pulse. A simultaneously recorded ECG will be necessary to demonstrate that this output pulse never reached the heart, as no stimulus is recorded. Measured data telemetry will report an infinitely high stimulation impedance. Because most systems can report the impedance only as high as some preset top limit, either the top limit number or the simple notation "high" will be reported. The key is that this is a dramatic change from the baseline recordings. With an open circuit, there is no current drain associated with the programmed output; thus, the battery current drain, if able to be provided by the measured data, will decrease from baseline. Some systems, such as the Elema Dialog™ and Sensolog™ products, can provide lead impedance measurements on a beat-by-beat basis. Others, such as the Pacesetter AFP™, Phoenix II™, Paragon™, and Synchrony™ systems, the Medtronic Pasys™, Elite™, Legend™, and Thera™ systems, and the Intermedics Cosmos™, Nova™, and Relay™ series of devices, make individual measurements on a single output pulse. Thus, repeated interrogations are necessary to identify an intermittent problem.

Application of a magnet to the pacemaker will not eliminate the pauses because, as far as the pacemaker is concerned, it is already generating the output pulse. The problem is that this stimulus is unable to be delivered to the electrode–myocardium interface.

An open circuit has a number of possible causes. The most common is a conductor fracture. Investigation of this possibility is discussed earlier in this chapter. The second is a failure to tighten the set screw adequately. There are a number of potential explanations for this failure. One is simple inattention to detail as the critical portion of the procedure—namely, lead placement—is completed and the implanting team begins to relax. An inadequately tightened set screw will not be recognized in the patient who has an adequate native rhythm at the end of the procedure, and the pacemaker is then assumed to be appropriately inhibited. The problem is often recognized only when the patient is being monitored during the postimplant period and develops the transient bradycardia that was the reason for the pacemaker implantation.

Another time a set screw might be poorly secured is when the Allen wrench is not easily disengaged from the set screw after the screw is tightened. When this happens, there is a natural tendency to turn the Allen wrench in the opposite (counterclockwise) direction; although the set screw may have been initially secured, it is then unscrewed ever so slightly as the wrench is freed, which may be sufficient for the lead to be pulled out of the connector block opening the circuit.

As a last step after securing the lead terminal pin in the set-screw connector block, the physician should give a gentle tug on the lead to be certain that it is secure. This may be misleading with an in-line coaxial bipolar lead—one set screw may be secure and the other not—but only one screw is needed to prevent the lead from being withdrawn with gentle traction; both need to be secured to ensure appropriate pacing. In those systems that have bipolar–unipolar output configuration programmability, the distal set screw should always be secured first, following which a gentle tug should be applied to the lead. If the proximal set screw is not adequately tightened, the pacemaker can be programmed to a unipolar output configuration, avoiding the need for a repeat operative procedure. However, one should be aware of the theoretical problems associated with this approach. Tugging on the lead before both set screws are tightened may pull the terminal pin connector of the in-line coaxial bipolar lead apart if the tug is too vigorous. To avoid this problem completely, both set screws should be secured before tugging on the lead. Some pulse generators utilizing an L connector have only a single set screw directed to the distal contact while the proximal contact is made by way of a spring within the connector block. In the future, it may be possible to totally eliminate set screws to ensure a stable and secure contact.

Open circuits have been encountered with in-line coaxial bipolar leads even when both set screws have been appropriately tightened. This is a function of differences between designs of the various 3.2-mm terminal pin leads. There is the Medtronic design, the Cordis design, and VS-1 and IS-1 configurations (see Chapter 2). As the tolerances are very close, there may be a lead–pulse-generator mismatch when one manufacturer's pulse generator is used with another manufacturer's lead. In this case, the proximal set screw can actually tighten down on the insulation and not on the proximal terminal pin.

A very uncommon cause of an open circuit has been reported with unipolar pacing systems when the pocket is too large and air is trapped within the pocket. The air serves as an insulating barrier to current flow. Treatment requires aspiration of the air and a pressure dressing to minimize its reaccumulation.[93,94]

Pulse generator component malfunction: This is very rare and probably the least frequent etiology of a pacing system malfunction. When a systematic design problem predisposes to a particular problem, most manufacturers inform the physicians by way of a safety alert or technical memorandum. Depending on the severity of the potential problem, the manufacturer may initiate recall of the product or recall may be required by the Food and Drug Administration (FDA) after it reviews the available data reported from the field as well as by the manufacturer. The diagnostic evaluation of a suspected component malfunction includes magnet application, which is unlikely to restore an output. Where measured data telemetry is available, it might provide clues, such as inconsistent measurements or being unable to access this information. For example, a high lead impedance suggesting an open circuit but without the expected concomitant decrease in the battery current drain might be obtained. Or a battery current drain that far exceeds that commonly seen at similar output and rate settings might be found. One needs to be aware of what is normal for the implanted pacemaker. If this information is not known, the manufacturer should be contacted.

Where measured data telemetry is not available or is not obtainable, careful intraoperative measurements should be made. The clinical problem will not be corrected by replacing the pulse generator if the problem is really due to a conductor fracture or a short circuit between the inner and outer conductors of a bipolar lead. If the assessment is that the pulse generator is at fault, it should be returned to the manufacturer along with a summary of the clinical observations and copies of representative ECG rhythm strips, interrogation printouts, and any other available data. The device should be returned even if another manufacturer's pulse generator is used as the replacement device because this is the only way in which the manufacturer has a chance of identifying a potentially serious problem that might be a concern with other units of this same family of device. The manufacturer is required by law to report all malfunctions and its analysis of the returned device to the FDA.

Misinterpretation of normal function: Common causes of pauses associated with normal function include the presence of hysteresis, the device being programmed to a lower rate than recalled by the physician, the output being intentionally programmed to 0 V, or the mode being programmed to "off" (which is feasible in some units). In each case, the device would be functioning properly even though the initial rhythms may be misinterpreted as a malfunction. All these causes can be readily identified by interrogating the pacemaker as to its programmed parameters. The pacemaker can be reprogrammed to restore capture.

Recording artifacts: Recording artifacts may mimic a pacing system malfunction. Most commonly, this involves a transient disconnection of the monitoring lead, resulting in a loss of the recorded signal. This becomes clear when there is simultaneous failure of the native rhythm as well as the paced rhythm or when there is a depolarization without a repolarization and vice versa. Management involves correcting the recording systems and reassuring the patient and support staff who may have initially called the problem to the physician's attention. Another valuable technique is to assess the patient when the purported rhythm or pacing system failure is occurring. If the problem is real, the patient should be symptomatic. But if the patient is well and simultaneously has a good pulse when the ECG says there is no heartbeat at all, the problem is clearly extrinsic to the patient–pacemaker system.

Intermittent or persistent recurrence of symptoms

When a patient who has a pacemaker calls the physician's office complaining of a recurrence of symptoms or the development of new symptoms, it is both natural and appropriate to be concerned that there may be a problem with the system. All the previously discussed pacing system malfunctions need to be considered within the limits of the capabilities of the pacemaker. If, on evaluation, the pacing system is shown to be functioning normally, one needs to consider the possibility that either it is programmed inappropriately for the patient's physiologic needs (pacemaker syndrome) or the symptoms are due to a condition independent of the pacing system. Pacemaker syndrome, discussed in Chapter 3, is particularly common with single-chamber VVI and VVIR pacing when the atrium is intact.[114,131-138] Pacemaker syndrome may also occur in dual-chamber pacing systems when there is loss of atrial capture or sensing or an inappropriately programmed paced and sensed AV delay. Identification of pacemaker syndrome requires correlating the patient's symptoms with periods of pacing. Pacemaker syndrome can then be further confirmed by demonstrating a fall in systolic blood pressure and pulse pressure with pacing as compared to the native rhythm or the presence of cannon A waves in the jugular veins during periods of pacing. Although this is adequate to establish the diagnosis, it is often not sufficient to justify a repeat intervention to the various organizations that will be paying for a second operative procedure and also for an entirely new pacemaker. It is thus helpful to document the hemodynamic limitations imposed by the electrically normal pacing system with techniques that allow hard-copy recordings. If there is sustained retrograde conduction, an ECG rhythm strip showing this should be included in the medical record. In addition to the ECG, some tests that have been particularly helpful and can be easily accomplished on an outpatient basis include oculopneumoplethysmography[139] and echo-Doppler techniques.[140,141] The OPG-Gee™ provides a printout that will show the central retinal artery pressure, which is a direct reflection of cerebral perfusion pressure. Fluctuations with a decrease in pressure during periods of pacing confirm the hemodynamic embarrassment and establish a diagnosis of pacemaker syndrome. Using the echo-Doppler technique, one can look at changes in stroke volume output with random AV synchrony. Selected panels from each of these studies should be copied and included in the hospital medical record; the document will be reviewed by the insurance company or Medicare intermediaries at some time following the procedure. The medical record should be accompanied by an explanation of the studies and how the observations explain the patient's symptoms.

If the concern is that the patient's symptoms are related to chronotropic incompetence and a failure of the pacemaker rate to accelerate appropriately, it is also important to prove that increasing the paced rate will be effective in alleviating the symptoms before a normally functioning non–rate-modulated pacemaker is replaced with a sensor-controlled device. This is easily accomplished with back-to-back exercise tests, allowing a rest period between the two studies. The first study is performed with the pacemaker in its non–rate-modulated mode. A gentle protocol such as the Naughton, Modified Bruce, or Chronotropic Assessment Exercise Protocol should be used. When the patient has recovered, the second exercise test is performed with the pacemaker programmed to the triggered mode using a temporary pacemaker connected to skin leads to provide concomitant chest wall stimulation, which the implanted device will sense and fire in accord with the triggered mode design. One can also use repeated programming increments of the rate to increase the rate during the exercise test. The duration of exercise, the length of time it takes for the patient to recover, and a clinical assessment of the patient's response to the two studies are compared to determine whether changing the non–rate-modulated pacemaker to a rate-responsive unit will be beneficial to the patient in terms of improved exercise capacity.

DUAL-CHAMBER PACING SYSTEM MALFUNCTION

There are four major classes of dual-chamber pacing system malfunction.[142] The first involves all the abnormalities previously discussed as occurring with single-chamber pacing systems. The abnormalities in this case occur on one or both of the two channels of the dual-chamber system. Although this may sometimes be obvious, there are situations in which the problem will not be readily apparent because of the interaction of the paced rhythm with the native conduction system while the patient remains asymptomatic. The second class consists of the unique rhythms that can occur only with a dual-chamber system, such as crosstalk and endless-loop tachycardia (ELT) or pacemaker-mediated tachycardia (PMT). PMTs are no longer found only with dual-chamber pacing systems. The third class of problems is the advent of sensor technology that has led to the recognition of some "single-chamber PMTs," which may occur when the sensor is responding to a physiologically inappropriate signal, which, in turn, drives the pacemaker. The fourth class of problems is primarily due to a lack of understanding of the system and not appreciating the unique behavioral eccentricities of a pacemaker when it is functioning within its design specifications.[143,144] Each of these problems is discussed below.

Pacing stimulus present with loss of capture

Ventricular loss of capture: Ventricular loss of capture will sometimes be obvious—as in the patient with high-grade AV block who loses capture on the ventricular channel—but it may be very difficult to identify if there is intact AV nodal conduction. One will then see AV pacing with the ventricular stimulus coinciding with the native QRS such that it appears to capture, particularly if the duration of the native R wave is increased, as with a bundle branch block (Figure 7.16). If the R wave is of normal duration, it will appear as if the patient is having repeated fusion complexes, when actually there is intact native conduction with simultaneous loss of capture. At the time of routine evaluation, one should either increase or decrease the AV interval to confirm that capture is intact. One can also program the pacemaker to a nonsynchronous mode so that the pacing function is dissociated from intrinsic atrial or ventricular activity.

Atrial loss of capture: On the atrial channel, particularly with unipolar pacing, the atrial evoked potential may be obscured by the large atrial stimulus even though it is present. By the same token, more than one 12-lead ECG has been interpreted as normal AV sequential pacing when there was loss of atrial capture. If ventriculoatrial conduction is present, as reflected by a retrograde P wave in the ST-T wave of the pace ventricular beat, there must have been loss of atrial capture. Sometimes, however, the retrograde P wave is hidden within the T wave or is so small on the surface ECG that it is simply not seen. In this situation, access to atrial electrogram telemetry may prove to be very helpful (see Figure 7.2b). Neither EGM nor event marker telemetry will presently allow confirmation of atrial capture in most systems. The telemetered event markers simply confirm that the pulse generator released a stimulus, not that it captured while the pacemaker's

Figure 7.16 (a) This tracing was interpreted as normal P wave synchronous ventricular pacing with the ventricular stimulus coinciding with the onset of a slightly widened R wave. However, on subsequent evaluation when the AV interval was shortened, the PR interval appeared stable and there was no change in the morphology of the ventricular complex, raising concerns about loss of capture. When the output was increased, it became apparent that there was a loss of ventricular capture at the lower output and the coincidence of the pacing stimulus with the conducted R wave had misled the monitoring staff. (b) A noninvasive capture threshold test. The AV interval had been shortened to ensure ventricular capture if it were present. When the output is reduced from 5.0 to 4.0 V, there is loss of ventricular capture with a resumption of normal AV conduction. The dramatic change in QRS morphology is apparent from these tracings.

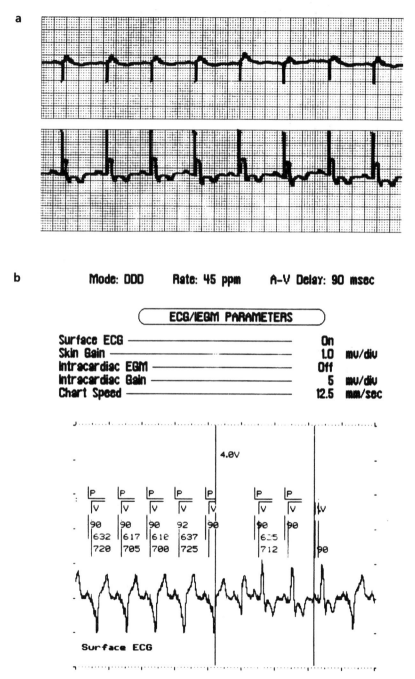

a

b

Mode: DDD   Rate: 45 ppm   A-V Delay: 90 msec

ECG/IEGM PARAMETERS

Surface ECG	On	
Skin Gain	1.0	mv/div
Intracardiac EGM	Off	
Intracardiac Gain	5	mv/div
Chart Speed	12.5	mm/sec

output saturated the telemetry amplifier, rendering it ineffective for demonstrating capture for a variable duration after delivery of the pacing stimulus. By the time the telemetry amplifier has recovered, the evoked potential will have been completed.[10] In systems with output and sensing configuration programmability, unipolar pacing via the distal tip electrode and EGM telemetry via the special unipolar configuration (proximal ring electrode to housing of pulse generator) may show the evoked potential as a reversal of the RC decay curve occurring within 10 to 20 msec of the stimulus (Figures 7.2b and 7.17).[145]

Because most presently implanted pulse generators do not have this capability, one will need to use the programmable options offered by the pulse generator.[146–148] Altering the AV interval will show no change in paced ventricular QRS morphology in the absence of atrial capture. If atrial capture was intact but the evoked

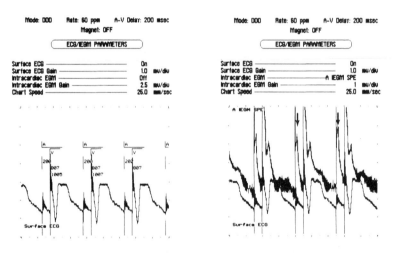

Figure 7.17 When atrial capture cannot be confirmed on the surface ECG, it sometimes helps to look at the intracardiac signal. This is feasible only if one can record the signal from a site remote from the pacing stimulus. If the same electrode that paces is used to obtain the EGM, the multivolt output will overwhelm and saturate the telemetry amplifier. In the example on the left, the output configuration is unipolar between the tip electrode and the housing of the pulse generator. The electrogram is the special unipolar between the ring electrode and the case of the pacemaker. A discrete evoked potential is visible approximately 20 msec after the pacing stimulus, thus confirming capture. See Figure 7.2 (b) for the appearance of loss of capture and retrograde conduction.

potential was isoelectric, a change in the paced QRS morphology may occur with alterations in the programmed AV delay as long as there is some AV conduction. The changing AV interval will result in an increased or decreased amount of ventricular fusion. Programming to the AAI mode or functional AAI mode by reducing the ventricular output to a subthreshold level (this has been called the AVI or ADD mode,[146,147] depending on whether the basic mode was DVI or DDD, respectively) will readily unmask atrial noncapture. However, this would not be safe to do in the presence of complete heart block even if atrial capture were intact. In that setting, increase the rate to above the native atrial rate. If there is capture, the sinus mechanism will be suppressed and there will be a stable AV sequential paced rhythm (Figure 7.18). If atrial capture is absent, one will see AV pacing complexes alternating with

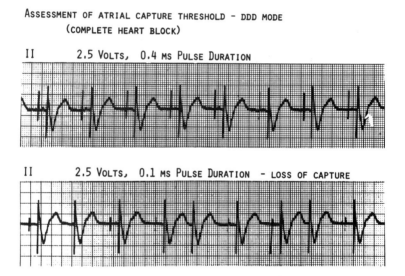

ASSESSMENT OF ATRIAL CAPTURE THRESHOLD – DDD MODE
(COMPLETE HEART BLOCK)

II   2.5 VOLTS,   0.4 MS PULSE DURATION

II   2.5 VOLTS,   0.1 MS PULSE DURATION   – LOSS OF CAPTURE

Figure 7.18 To assess atrial capture in the patient with complete heart block, increase the atrial rate above the native sinus rate. This will result in AV sequential pacing (top). As long as atrial capture is intact, the faster paced rate will overdrive-suppress the sinus mechanism. When loss of atrial capture occurs as the atrial output is intentionally reduced, the sinus mechanism will escape; when it falls in an atrial alert period, it will be sensed, triggering a ventricular output resulting in an irregular rhythm. There will be ventricular pacing at all times, thus always protecting the patient. (From Levine PA. Confirmation of atrial capture and determination of atrial capture thresholds in DDD pacing systems. *Clin Prog Pacing Electrophysiol* 1984;2:465–473. Reprinted with permission.)

PV complexes as the sinus P wave occurs during the atrial alert period.[147] Finally, in some cases an esophageal lead can be used to record an atrial electrogram to document atrial capture or noncapture.[145]

Dual-chamber pacing with sensing malfunction

Undersensing: Loss of sensing is not critical when there is an inadequate native rhythm with consistent stimulation in the respective chamber. In addition, there is no good way to assess sensing capability when the native rate is too slow. However, loss of atrial sensing when there is an intact sinus rhythm may be more difficult to recognize in the dual-chamber system than in the single-chamber pacing system. For example, in the setting of a sufficiently rapid sinus rate, loss of atrial sensing in the DDD mode when there is intact AV nodal conduction will result in functional DVI pacing with total pacing system inhibition. The potential loss of atrial sensing will not become apparent unless the physician programs the pacemaker to an unphysiologically short AV interval. This should demonstrate P-wave synchronous ventricular pacing; however, with atrial undersensing, total pacing system inhibition would continue. The P wave was not being sensed and thus was not tracked while the conducted R wave inhibited the pacemaker and reset the timing cycles. The availability of event marker telemetry will quickly identify that there is loss of sensing (Figure 7.19). Where loss of sensing is intermittent and AV conduction is otherwise intact but at a longer PR interval than the PV interval, one will see PV pacing alternating with PR pacing.

Atrial undersensing may occur in two settings postimplantation even when a good EGM was obtained at the time of pacemaker implantation. A decrease in the amplitude of the atrial EGM has been demonstrated in both animals and humans during exercise.[149-151] Thus atrial undersensing might occur at the higher sinus rates; yet at rest, the atrial sensing threshold mass demonstrates a good margin of safety for proper sensing with respect to the programmed sensitivity parameter. In addition, there may be a transient decrease in the amplitude of the atrial EGM occurring during the early electrode-maturation phase following implantation. An incidence of 7.5 percent of atrial undersensing associated with lead maturation has been reported in the literature.[152] Usually, this undersensing problem will spontaneously resolve or can be managed by increasing the programmed sensitivity of the pulse genera-

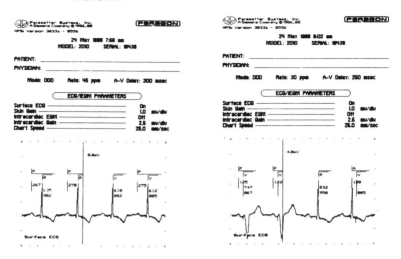

Figure 7.19 Side-by-side sensing threshold tests are performed taking advantage of the telemetered event markers. This is particularly helpful with the ventricular sensing test because the ECG does not change (the pacemaker is inhibited); but when sensing fails, the small bipolar ventricular stimulus falls into the native R wave and is obscured. The event markers clearly differentiate normal sensing from the lack of sensing (left). The AV interval was shortened so that the ventricular output would also serve as a marker for atrial sensing. The event marker labeled P clearly identifies atrial sensing. When the sensitivity is reduced to 4.0 mV, the P wave is no longer sensed, resulting in the absence of a P event marker. The second complex in this section of the recording is functional DVI-type pacing with an atrial pseudo-pseudofusion beat. The intrinsic deflection of the native R wave then occurs during crosstalk detection window, resulting in safety pacing with an abbreviated AV interval of 120 msec.

tor. Permanent undersensing occurs in about 1 percent of patients. Restoration of appropriate sensing would require operative intervention to reposition or replace the atrial lead. Given that most cases of atrial undersensing that occur in the first days or weeks postimplantation will resolve spontaneously, it would be prudent to observe the patient for a period of weeks to months with the pacemaker programmed to a more sensitive setting before a decision is made to require a repeat operative procedure.

On the ventricular channel, the ventricular stimulus may repeatedly fall within the native QRS, resulting in either a fusion or a pseudofusion complex. This may be normal because one cannot determine where the intrinsic deflection (ID) that is sensed by the pacemaker occurs within the cardiac depolarization represented by the surface QRS complex. If the ID occurs late within the QRS, then the above behavior is normal. If it occurs before the AV interval timer has completed, the R wave should have been sensed and the above represents a malfunction. Unlike atrial undersensing, event marker telemetry will not facilitate this assessment with the pacemaker in the DDD mode. To evaluate ventricular sensing, one can increase the AV interval but only if intrinsic conduction is present and occurs within the programmed AV delay. If the ventricular stimulus occurs after the QRS complex has ended, there is definitive evidence of ventricular undersensing. One could also program the pacemaker to a nonsynchronized mode— for example, VVI—at which time ventricular undersensing will become readily apparent.

Oversensing: Oversensing in a single-chamber pacing system results in either inhibition or triggering, depending on the programmed mode of the pacemaker. In a dual-chamber system, there will also be inhibition or triggering; but in this case it will depend on which channel the oversensing occurs. If oversensing occurs on the ventricular channel, both the atrial and ventricular outputs will be inhibited and the timing cycles reset. If the ventricular sensitivity is reduced to minimize oversensing, there will be a predilection to oversensing on the atrial channel. This will result in termination of the atrial escape interval and initiation of a sensed AV interval. This has been termed *oversensing drive* with salvos of ventricular pacing occurring at or near the maximum tracking rate (Figure 7.20).

When evaluating a dual-chamber system, particularly the DDD mode, one cannot simply assume that an asymptomatic patient with a stable rhythm on the surface ECG represents normal pacing system function. As long as the patient has a rhythm, native or otherwise, there is no urgency. But for the patient whose need for the pacemaker is intermittent, as with hypersensitive carotid sinus syndrome or Stokes-Adams syncope secondary to intermittent complete heart block, it would be potentially dangerous to miss a problem because of the superficial appearance of normality. The patient will remain asymptomatic until the episode requiring pacing system support occurs, at which time the lack of proper pacing system performance may allow the recurrence of symptoms.

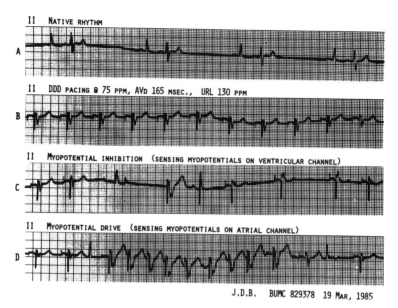

II NATIVE RHYTHM

A

II DDD PACING @ 75 PPM, AVD 165 MSEC., URL 130 PPM

B

II MYOPOTENTIAL INHIBITION (SENSING MYOPOTENTIALS ON VENTRICULAR CHANNEL)

C

II MYOPOTENTIAL DRIVE (SENSING MYOPOTENTIALS ON ATRIAL CHANNEL)

D

J.D.B. BUMC 829378 19 MAR, 1985

Figure 7.20 In a dual-chamber pacing system, oversensing occurring on the atrial and ventricular channels results in dramatically different rhythms. The top tracing (A) is the patient's native rhythm prior to implantation of the pacemaker. In (B), his rhythm is totally controlled by the pacemaker. (C) demonstrates ventricular oversensing, in this case of myopotentials; the pacemaker is inhibited and the rate slows below the programmed lower rate limit. When there is atrial oversensing, as shown in (D), the sensed P triggers a ventricular output. This has been called myopotential drive; it results in brief periods of ventricular pacing at or near the maximum tracking rate. (From Levine PA. Normal and abnormal rhythms associated with dual-chamber pacemakers. *Cardiol Clin* 1985;3:595–616. Reprinted with permission.)

Unique dual-chamber rhythms

Crosstalk: Crosstalk is the sensing of the far-field signal in the opposite chamber, causing the pacemaker to either inhibit or trigger an output depending on its design. Crosstalk has been reported with single-chamber atrial pacing systems in which the far-field QRS is sensed inhibiting and resetting the basic pacing interval.[153,154] Lengthening the atrial refractory period to preclude far-field sensing will correct this problem. Crosstalk has also been reported in the now obsolete VAT mode when there was atrial sensing of a far-field ventricular ectopic beat triggering a ventricular output on

387

top of the T wave of the ectopic beat.[155,156] Crosstalk, however, most commonly refers to ventricular sensing of the far-field atrial stimulus in a DVI, DDI, or DDD pacing system. Sensing this stimulus will result in inhibition of the ventricular output and resetting of the atrial escape interval. This is not dangerous to the patient who has intact AV conduction, and in this setting, it has even been proposed that crosstalk can be intentionally used to achieve a very rapid atrial paced rate for diagnostic or therapeutic purposes.[157] However, in the presence of concomitant AV block, crosstalk can be catastrophic, resulting in ventricular asystole (Figure 7.21).[158,159]

Crosstalk was first reported in the noncommitted DVI systems, which were able to fully isolate the atrial and ventricular output circuits internal to the pacemaker in addition to bipolar leads, which further minimized far-field sensing.[160] The advent of dual unipolar DVI systems was an absolute guarantee of crosstalk, which would have rendered this mode unsafe. To prevent crosstalk, the ventricular refractory period was initiated simultaneously with release of the atrial output pulse.[161,162] This resulted in

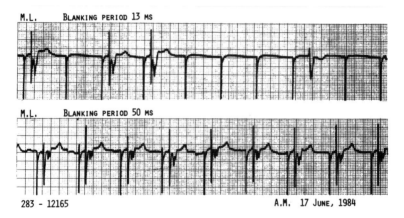

Figure 7.21 (top) Classic crosstalk-mediated ventricular output inhibition. This was intentionally induced by programming a short ventricular blanking period, high atrial output, and high ventricular sensitivity. This patient had high-grade AV block, which is the worst setting for crosstalk. The hallmark of crosstalk in a ventricular-based timing system is that the AA interval equals the sum of the atrial escape interval and ventricular blanking period. (bottom) In an atrial-based timing system, it may be difficult to differentiate crosstalk from an open circuit. Crosstalk, in this example, was eliminated by increasing the blanking period.

committed DVI pacing, which was associated with a multiplicity of confusing rhythms having both functional atrial and ventricular undersensing and noncapture, all of which were technically normal. However, this design was successful in absolutely preventing crosstalk. In an effort to eliminate the confusing and potentially adverse rhythms associated with committed pacing, technologic advances included changes in the atrial pulse configuration using a rapid-recharge ("super-fast") pulse to minimize residual polarization effects along with the ability to totally but transiently disengage the ventricular sense amplifier coincident with completion of the atrial escape interval. This brief period of inability to sense is termed a *blanking period*. It varies from 12 to 125 msec and is programmable in some units.

The advent of a blanking period, although generally effective, did not absolutely prevent crosstalk. The ability to program very short blanking periods, very high atrial outputs (up to 10 V and 1.6 msec pulse widths), and very high ventricular sensitivities (up to 0.5 mV) each predisposed to crosstalk; and the combination of two or more of these factors virtually guaranteed crosstalk in some devices. As an added insurance policy, special circuits were added to the ventricular timing system to prevent the undesirable consequences associated with crosstalk. Following the blanking period, a special detection or sensing window was added on the ventricular channel. This window varied in duration from 51 msec to 150 msec. A signal sensed during this interval will be treated by the pacemaker as if it were crosstalk but rather than inhibiting the ventricular output, a ventricular output will be triggered at an abbreviated AV interval (Figure 7.22).[163] Because it was shorter than the programmed AV interval, Intermedics called this abbreviated AV interval Nonphysiologic AV Delay™, Medtronic called this feature Safety Pacing™, and Pacesetter termed it Safety Standby Pacing™. Crosstalk continues to be uncommon but episodes of safety pacing are relatively common. Commonly, safety pacing occurs when an atrial stimulus coincides with a late-cycle PVC. There then appears to be ventricular undersensing, with a ventricular output signal falling in the ST segment of the ectopic beat. If one measures this AV interval, the shortening from the programmed AV interval will identify this as a triggered output due to normal ventricular sensing. Knowledge of this phenomenon allows one to conclude that the ectopic beat was sensed during the crosstalk detection window.

Although the blanking period is far superior to committed

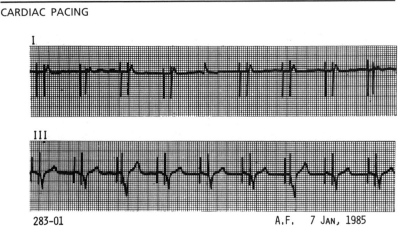

I

III

283-01   A.F.   7 Jan, 1985

Figure 7.22 Crosstalk that occurs in the presence of a special crosstalk detection window triggers a ventricular output pulse rather than inhibiting it. This usually occurs at a shorter than programmed AV interval. Intermittent AV-interval shortening is seen in the two tracings. This reflects episodes of crosstalk triggering a ventricular output pulse. In the top tracing, for example, the second and ninth beats show AV-interval shortening.

pacing, any interval of refractoriness can result in functional undersensing. In some cases, the ventricular blanking period can be programmed as short as 13 msec. However, no matter how short the blanking period, the intrinsic deflection of the native QRS complex is even narrower. Thus, there is the potential that a native QRS complex may not be sensed if it coincides with the atrial output pulse and the associated ventricular blanking period. This results in a phenomenon termed *blanking period undersensing*, which is an example of functional undersensing. This is further complicated by the fact that all the present dual-chamber systems have AV-interval programmability. Unlike in the committed DVI systems, in which the AV interval was 155 msec or shorter, long AV in-tervals in conjunction with blanking period undersensing have a potentially greater chance of the released ventricular output coinciding with the vulnerable period of a native ventricular ectopic beat (Figures 7.11 and 7.23).

Crosstalk with either ventricular output inhibition or pacing at an abbreviated AV interval is a pacing system malfunction due to ventricular oversensing of a far-field atrial stimulus. However, the same timing circuits designed to prevent or minimize the potentially adverse consequences of crosstalk can result in rhythms that

390

BLANKING PERIOD INDUCED UNDERSENSING

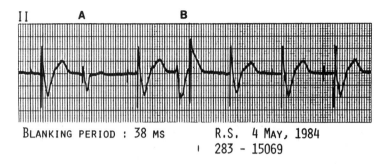

BLANKING PERIOD : 38 MS   R.S. 4 MAY, 1984
                                 ı 283 - 15069

Figure 7.23 Any period of refractoriness can result in a native complex not being sensed. The downside of the blanking period is that late-cycle ventricular ectopic beats may not be sensed, resulting in competition. This is a form of functional undersensing. In this example, the atrial stimulus coincided with the onset of the PVC labeled A, but the intrinsic deflection occurred outside the blanking period, and so the PVC was properly sensed and inhibited the pacemaker's ventricular output. The atrial stimulus is released within the early portion of the PVC, labeled B; its intrinsic deflection coincides with the blanking period, and so it is not seen. Thus at the end of the programmed AV interval, a ventricular stimulus is released. There is both functional undersensing and functional noncapture when this happens. (From Levine PA. Normal and abnormal rhythms associated with dual-chamber pacemakers. *Cardiol Clin* 1985;3:595–616. Reprinted with permission.)

demonstrate functional undersensing, which may be real, as in the case of blanking periods, or only apparent, as in the case of the crosstalk detection window. It needs to be stressed that the commonly encountered rhythms that are a consequence of the protective circuitry intended to minimize the adverse consequences associated with true crosstalk reflect totally normal pacing system function. This may result in functional undersensing that allows release of a ventricular stimulus at a time when the myocardium is physiologically refractory. Thus, the ventricular stimulus will also be ineffective. This is functional noncapture (see Tables 7.2 and 7.4).

Endless-loop (pacemaker-mediated) tachycardias: In the DDD mode, the normally functioning pacemaker is supposed to sense atrial activity and trigger a ventricular output in response to the native P wave. However, there is an assumption on the part of the clinical staff caring for the patient that the pacemaker does not share. This is that the sensed atrial activity should be sinus. The DDD pacemaker in a patient who develops atrial fibrillation or flutter may track the pathologic atrial signals (e.g., flutter or fibrillatory waves). This will drive the ventricular channel of the pacemaker at or near its maximum tracking rate (MTR).[164,165] Similarly, atrial oversensing, such as myopotentials, can drive the ventricular output at or near its MTR. Each of these rhythms is a form of a pacemaker-mediated tachycardia (PMT), which is a paced tachycardia that is sustained by the continued active participation of the pacemaker in the rhythm. A PMT is not the same as a pacemaker-induced tachycardia, in which the pacemaker induces a tachycardia by intentional or unintentional (undersensing) competition, but once the tachycardia has begun, the pacemaker is inhibited and no longer plays an active role in the rhythm.

The first PMTs that became widely recognized in the literature were not due to tracking atrial fibrillation or atrial flutter or oversensing on the atrial channel. Instead, they were due to sensing retrograde atrial activity arising from a premature ventricular contraction (PVC). This sets up a repetitive sequence of the sensed retrograde P wave triggering a ventricular output at the end of the maximum tracking rate interval. The delay created by waiting for the MTR to complete before the ventricular stimulus was released allowed the atrium and AV node to physiologically recover. The depolarization resulting from a ventricular paced beat is then again able to conduct in a retrograde direction. This next retrograde P wave is sensed, triggering another ventricular output, and resulting in a sustained PMT.[166–170] Because this resembled the endless loop that can be seen in computers, Furman and associates labeled this rhythm an endless-loop tachycardia (ELT) to differentiate it from the other forms of PMT.[171,172] The majority of PMTs in the literature are of the endless-loop variety, running either at (Figure 7.24) or below the programmed maximum tracking rate.[173,174] In the following discussion, PMT and ELT are used interchangeably.

Even in paced patients who have the ability to conduct retrograde, PMT is not seen on a routine basis. The normal depolarization of the atrium, and possibly the AV node, immediately prior to the ventricular depolarization, as with appropriate AV synchrony, renders these structures physiologically refractory at a time when ventricular activation occurs. Thus, although the patient must have the appropriate substrate for an ELT to occur, this is not sufficient. There needs to be a trigger, some event that results in AV dissociation and allows retrograde conduction to occur follow-

INITIATION AND TERMINATION OF AN ENDLESS-LOOP TACHYCARDIA

II   DDD MODE, ATRIAL OUTPUT SUBTHRESHOLD, PVARP 150 MSEC

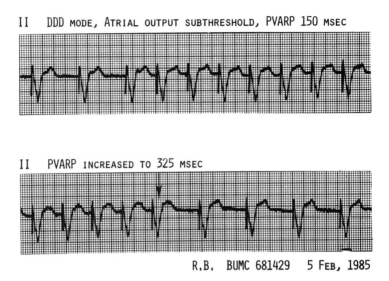

II   PVARP INCREASED TO 325 MSEC

R.B.   BUMC 681429   5 FEB, 1985

Figure 7.24   Pacemaker-mediated tachycardias may be initiated by any event that results in AV dissociation. This episode was triggered by reducing the atrial output to a subthreshold level and reducing the PVARP so that it was shorter than the retrograde VA interval. The endless-loop tachycardia was then terminated by increasing the PVARP.

ing either a native or paced ventricular beat. PVCs, because these occur so commonly in most individuals, are the usual trigger. ELTs can also be initiated by atrial undersensing, atrial oversensing, loss of atrial capture, or magnet application to the pacemaker—basically by any event that results in even one cycle of relative AV dissociation.

Once initiated, an endless-loop pacemaker-mediated tachycardia will continue unless there is spontaneous VA block. The likelihood of spontaneous VA block is increased if the pacemaker is programmed to a very high maximum tracking rate, taking advantage of endogenous fatigue of the AV node.[175,176] A high tracking rate, however, needs to be specifically assessed before being programmed on a permanent basis because retrograde conduction may be superior to anterograde conduction in some individuals.[166]

Reports in the literature indicate that anterograde P waves tend to be larger than retrograde P waves.[177–180] Thus, if there is sufficient sensitivity programmability, one might be able to walk

393

the tightrope between sensing appropriate antegrade P waves and not responding to retrograde P waves. The potential limitation of sensitivity programmability is that the sinus P wave also decreases in amplitude as the rate increases. In this case, one may have undersensing with loss of appropriate atrial tracking when it is needed the most—namely, at higher rates.[150,151] Also, the relative amplitudes of the anterograde and retrograde atrial electrograms (AEGMs) need to be assessed, because although the anterograde AEGM is usually larger than the retrograde AEGM, exceptions will occur that eliminate this as a treatment option.[166]

A variety of special PVC detection circuits automatically lengthen the refractory period in response to a sensed PVC.[181,182] One needs to be aware that there is a subtle difference between the pacemaker's definition of a PVC and that of the clinician. The pacemaker defines a PVC as a sensed R wave that is not preceded by sensed or paced atrial activity. Thus an atrial premature beat that coincides with the PVARP will not be sensed, but if the atrial premature beat is conducted, the R wave will be treated as a PVC. Similarly, myopotential oversensing on the ventricular channel will be treated as repeated PVCs. These events are more accurately called premature ventricular events (PVEs) and not PVCs.[183] By the same token, a true late-cycle PVC that is preceded by an atrial output pulse will not be called a PVC by the pacemaker. Nevertheless, the pacemaker is correct in most instances when it labels a beat as being a PVC. In the setting of a PVC, some pacemakers will automatically extend the postventricular atrial refractory period to prevent the pacemaker from sensing a retrograde P wave, but will allow a short PVARP at other times, thus enabling high maximal tracking rates.

A number of adverse rhythms have been associated with automatic extension of the atrial refractory period, leading to sustained pacemaker inhibition with first-degree AV block and a PR interval significantly longer than the programmed PV interval.[183,184] This situation is created by a P wave coinciding with the PVARP and hence not being sensed. However, the P wave is conducted and the sensed R wave is treated as a PVC by the pacemaker, extending the PVARP and again precluding sensing of the next P wave. Although disconcerting when encountered, it is not dangerous because the patient has an intact native rhythm. PV pacing is restored following one nonconducted P wave.

However, PVCs are not the only initiating event for an endless-loop pacemaker-mediated tachycardia. As such, the special atrial refractory period extensions associated with sensed PVCs are, at best, a secondary line of protection. In fact, they may not prevent a PMT at all. If there is a P wave occurring toward the end of the extended PVARP, it will not be sensed. The atrial output pulse, which is released at the end of the atrial escape interval, may demonstrate functional noncapture if it coincides with the physiologic refractory period of the atrium initiated by the retrograde atrial depolarization. By the time the subsequent ventricular paced beat is released, the atrium and AV node have physiologically recovered and allowed retrograde conduction to occur. The PVARP automatically returns to its previous shorter setting because there is an atrial output pulse prior to the ventricular paced complex. The retrograde P wave can be sensed initiating the PMT at this time. The PMT was not prevented; it was simply postponed for one cycle.[166]

The only way to prevent an endless-loop tachycardia absolutely is to program a PVARP that is longer than the retrograde conduction interval.[170] Although this may limit the maximum atrial rate that can be sensed, it is not usually a problem in most paced patients, who are older and do not require very high maximal tracking rates. With some present-generation pacemakers, the automatic shortening of the PV interval as the sinus rate increases, a phenomenon termed *rate-responsive AV delay*, may allow a relatively longer PVARP yet still program a higher maximal tracking rate.

In patients who need a relatively high maximal tracking rate—and hence a short PVARP—and who are prone to PMTs, the addition of a special algorithm that recognizes and terminates the PMT protects the patient against sustained periods of an endless-loop tachycardia.[184,185] A number of tachycardia identification and termination algorithms are now incorporated in commercially released pacemakers. Intermedics was the first to introduce such an algorithm. In the first-generation algorithm, the tachycardia had to run at the programmed maximal tracking rate for 15 cycles. The ventricular output was then dropped after the sixteenth sensed P wave. The tachycardia, if due to a true PMT, was terminated. In their second generation, these algorithms block a ventricular output after only six cycles. Pacesetter has taken a slightly different approach. After 10 cycles, it extends the PVARP on the tenth beat, which will prevent sensing of the retrograde P wave and terminate the tachycardia. However, if the tachycardia is due to an endogenous atrial rhythm coinciding with the maximum tracking rate, both systems will have repetitive pauses with these algorithms.

In an attempt to minimize the system responding to a physiologic tachycardia, new algorithms that automatically adjust the PV interval in response to a sensed tachycardia and then measure the resultant VP interval have been introduced.[173] This was first incorporated in the ELA Chorus™ dual-chamber pacemakers with further modification now being included in other systems. After a period of sustained rapid pacing, the pacemaker automatically changes the PV interval. If the tachycardia is due to a native atrial rhythm, the VP interval will then shorten by the same amount the PV interval is lengthened. In this case, the tachycardia termination algorithm will not be activated. If the VP interval remains stable, the logic in the pacemaker then classifies this as an ELT and activates its tachycardia termination algorithm.

ELTs can also run at rates slower than the maximal tracking rate. This occurs when the sum of the VA and AV intervals is greater than the maximal tracking rate interval. This is called a balanced ELT.[173,174] If the definition of a PMT requires that the tachycardia rate be at the MTR, a balanced ELT will never be recognized by this algorithm. Additional tachycardia algorithms incorporated in some present-generation devices allow programming a rate definition of a PMT as being lower than the MTR or enable the automatic scanning to differentiate a physiologic from pacemaker-mediated tachycardia any time the PV rate exceeds a preset minimum, most commonly 100 ppm. Either approach allows identification of balanced ELTs with appropriate intervention on the part of the implanted pacing system.

ALTERATIONS IN PACEMAKER TIMING CYCLES

The first generation of single-chamber pacemakers were termed *fixed-rate devices*. Not only were they not capable of sensing but they were locked into a rate that was preset by the manufacturer. The only time the rate would change was associated with battery depletion. That was 35 years ago. Since then, there are many stimuli that may cause the pacing rate to change. These stimuli include magnet application, battery depletion, atrial sensing–ventricular tracking (VDD, DDD) systems, and responses to a variety of nonatrial triggers or sensors.[182–189] Malfunction of a device component may also cause a rate change, but this is perhaps the least common of all the options. In addition, one must be cautious when interpreting an ECG because alterations in recording speed may appear to be a rate change that, if not appreciated, can result in a misdiagnosis of pacing system malfunction[190,191] when the pacemaker is, in fact, normal.

Differentiating the above possibilities requires a knowledge of the basic performance of the pacing system, the programmed parameters of the device, and a clinical assessment of the patient. For example, in the case of a recording artifact with alterations in paper speed, the pseudo-rate change will be associated with concomitant changes in the QRS and QT intervals. Such changes are not physiologic. At the "faster" rates, the QRS and QT intervals will be shortened. At the slower rates, they will be lengthened to a degree that is not physiologic.

A VVIR pacemaker programmed to the rate-modulated mode would be expected to have variations in its rate. However, if the rate-modulated parameters were disabled, the rate should be stable. In dual-chamber systems, one should carefully examine the paced ventricular complex for a preceding visible P wave. When endogenous atrial activity is not seen, the ability to telemeter the AEGM will enable the physician to readily determine whether the pacemaker is tracking appropriate physiologic atrial signals or is oversensing. One might also encounter AV sequential pacing at a rate faster than the programmed base rate in the presence of the DVIR, DDIR, or DDDR modes. Thus, knowledge of the programmed parameters of the pacing system is essential before attempting a detailed interpretation of the observed rhythm— and certainly before subjecting the patient to an operative intervention for a presumed diagnosis of pacing system malfunction. One also needs to be aware of pacemaker eccentricities, phenomena specific to each model of pacemaker and independent of the generic mode.

PACEMAKER ECCENTRICITIES

A pacemaker eccentricity is a unique behavior of the pacemaker that would be unexpected based on a knowledge of the pacing mode but that is normal for that model of pacemaker. The behavior of each manufacturer's device in responding to magnet application is often unique.[188] Although the industry lacks standardization, one usually knows that a magnet has been applied to the pacemaker, thus minimizing concern. The author has fallen into the trap of being shown a tracing with a magnet applied to the pacemaker but not being told this and jumping to the initial—but premature and incorrect—conclusion that there was a major problem. A clue that a magnet has been applied in dual-chamber systems is that there is loss of both atrial and ventricular sensing, assuming that a native rhythm is present, a possible but unlikely scenario.

System eccentricities that occur during normal demand function are the most confusing. Virtually every pacemaker has one or more behavioral quirks. Space here allows neither a comprehensive listing of all such phenomena nor a description of their mechanism. Some eccentricities that are no longer of clinical consequence because they have been corrected or eliminated from the manufacturers' present generation devices include the AV disable feature and autonomous pacemaker tachycardia associated with the Versatrax™ series,[192,193] the uplink telemetry hold,[194] and atrial output inhibition due to an upper rate limit circuit[195,196] on the atrial channel in the Symbios™ series of pacemakers from Medtronic. The first-generation DDD pacemaker from Telectronics, the Autima I™, had a blanking period associated with atrial sensing.[197] Persistence of a blanking period at the end of the atrial escape interval in the DDI mode of AFP™ and Genisis™ from Pacesetter, and this same mode in Sorin DDD™ pacemakers, led to unexpected ventricular competition from technologically normal blanking period undersensing.[198,199] A number of units have the ability to induce cross-stimulation.[200] Cross-stimulation is the unexpected direct stimulation of one cardiac chamber by an output pulse to the other chamber. This is caused by a crossover in delivered output from one channel to the opposite channel internal to the pacemaker due to the close proximity of the circuits. In the case of dual unipolar systems, the atrial and ventricular output circuits share a common pathway, and the indifferent electrode or the housing of the pulse generator facilitates this phenomenon.

All the above were unintentional functional aberrations and have been corrected in subsequent iterations of these devices or in later models from the manufacturer. In addition, there are intentional device eccentricities, such as the various automatic atrial refractory period extensions that follow a PVC and the rhythms that might result from them. Another intentional eccentricity is safety pacing with pseudo-undersensing of a late-cycle PVC. Unless all these rhythms are appreciated as reflecting normal pacing system behavior for a given device, they may be misinterpreted as indicative of a pacemaker malfunction. Such misinterpretation could lead to an incorrect decision to replace the pacemaker and/

or lead. This has occurred, much to the consternation of both the physician and the patient, when the analysis from the manufacturer is "normal device function" and thus there is no warranty credit. More difficulty arises when third-party payors deny payment or send the patient a letter indicating that the procedure was unnecessary. In most cases, the patient is not at jeopardy from the observed "unexpected" pacemaker behavior. Thus, when a pacing system behavior that is not readily understood is encountered, the manufacturer should be contacted before any specific invasive interventions are undertaken. Each manufacturer maintains a technical support service and a 24-hour telephone number.

PACEMAKER DIAGNOSTICS

Given the multiplicity of confusing rhythms, in which clinically stable rhythms may reflect a true pacing system malfunction but an apparent bizarre and unexpected behavior that would otherwise be interpreted as a malfunction may actually reflect normal system function, increasing numbers of manufacturers are including various aids within the pacemaker to assist the physician in evaluating the system. These include both real-time diagnostic aids as well as system-overview capabilities. Many real-time diagnostic capabilities have been discussed in this chapter, but they are reviewed further at this time.

Measured data

Measured data is the ability of the pacemaker to provide data regarding battery status, with specific measurements such as battery voltage, current drain, and internal impedance. A decrease in the battery voltage has recently been identified as an appropriate marker to identify the point at which there is an increase in the frequency of pacemaker surveillance for signs of battery depletion.[201] This may allow a marked reduction and expense associated with frequent routine transtelephonic monitoring at an arbitrary time following implantation of the pacemaker.

Measured data also includes measurements of pulse voltage, charge, current, energy, and stimulation impedance. Lead or stimulation impedance measurements may be particularly helpful in identifying an open circuit, which will be associated with a very high impedance (see Figure 7.7) or a breach of the internal insulation of a bipolar coaxial lead, in which case, the impedance will be very low.[202–209] One should be cautious with respect to this information. A measurement that is significantly changed from previous results should be reconfirmed to eliminate the concern about a telemetry error. If the patient is manifesting a problem with the pacing system, such as oversensing, undersensing, or noncapture, these measurements may identify the likely etiology. However, in the absence of a clinical problem, a diligent search should be undertaken for an intermittent problem, perhaps in association with an increased frequency of surveillance, but operative intervention is not absolutely required as long as the patient is doing well. This will also provide time to contact the technical support services offered by the manufacturers to obtain additional guidance or assistance if it is needed.

The limitation of the measured data is that measurements are made when the programmer forces the pacemaker to deliver one or more stimuli. This is essential for the measurements to be obtained. However, if the problem that has been identified is intermittent, the measurements read normal when there is truly a problem with the lead or pulse generator. This requires a high index of suspicion and repeated measurements, perhaps even while the patient is subjected to provocative maneuvers, in an effort to unmask a problem.

Event markers

Event markers have been shown in multiple figures in this chapter. These comprise timing information telemetered from the pacemaker to the programmer and are displayed on a screen or printed. Basically, these markers, which have also been called Marker Channel™ annotated event markers and main timing events, are a report of what the pacemaker is doing. Unique notations or marks are generated for paced and sensed events, in some cases, events occurring during the refractory period (termed *sensed* but no longer used) as well as an indication of refractory period duration.[210–215]

In isolation, event markers have limited value. They are an extremely powerful tool when combined with the simultaneously recorded electrocardiogram. Pauses can be identified as due to oversensing or an open circuit, as shown in Figure 7.7. With diminutive bipolar output pulses that may not be visible on the standard electrocardiogram, telemetered event markers will identify whether the P wave or QRS complex is paced or sensed.

The major limitation of event markers is that they simply report what the pacemaker is doing. If an output pulse is released, the markers show this, whether there is an open circuit and the impulse never reaches the heart (see Figure 7.7) or there is noncapture (see Figure 7.16). To appropriately interpret the event markers, one must also be able to observe the standard ECG and correlate the behavior of the pacemaker with the actual events that are occurring in the patient.

Electrograms

The electrogram is the signal occurring inside the heart that triggers the pacemaker's sensing circuit. It is often a much larger signal than that recorded on the surface of the body by an electrocardiogram.[97-100] The ability to examine the endocardial electrogram (EGM) is very helpful in identifying false signals that are being sensed (oversensing), as shown in Figure 7.4, or in confirming the presence of signals that are not readily identified on the surface ECG, as in Figures 7.2 and 7.17.

Some physicians have recommended using the telemetered electrogram as a way of performing a sensing threshold evaluation.[216,217] This is inappropriate. Some systems do not provide a calibration scale; others utilize a different set of filters in the telemetry amplifier compared with those used in the sense amplifier. In these settings, although there may generally be a close correlation between the amplitude of the telemetered electrogram, there may also be marked discrepancies due to the different filters. The filters in the amplifier of the sensing circuit tend to focus on one portion of the frequency spectrum in an effort to minimize or eliminate T waves, which have low frequency, and high-frequency signals such as myopotentials. Electrogram telemetry circuits tend to use a wider bandpass and do not eliminate some of the other signals.[102] The presence of a relatively prominent repolarization wave on the electrogram indicates that the telemetry circuit utilizes filters that differ from those in the sensing circuit, as shown by Figure 7.25.

Electrograms may also provide clues as to why there is a sensing problem or why the noninvasively measured sensing threshold is obtained by progressively reducing the sensitivity until intermittent or persistent failure to sense is demonstrated.[218-227] This, however, requires the additional capability of adjusting both the gain and the sweep speed of the signal once it has been frozen. When displayed at a relatively slow recording speed, a complex may look very good with a large amplitude; however, when the signal is displayed at a faster sweep speed, it may be shown to be

401

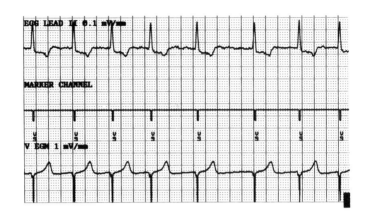

Figure 7.25 Telemetered ventricular electrogram from a Medtronic Thera™ shown with a simultaneously recorded surface ECG and telemetered event markers with the pacemaker programmed to the VVI mode. Note the relatively prominent T wave on the EGM, which is the bottom tracing.

splintered and/or have segments that are composed of predominantly low-frequency components, with the actual rapid intrinsic deflection being of relatively low amplitude. An example is shown in Figure 7.26.

Thus, the ability to examine the electrogram provides additional insights and understanding about the overall pacing system performance, but the electrogram should never be a substitute for the noninvasively assessed sensing threshold.

Measured data, event markers, and electrogram telemetry are all considered real-time data. Depending on the findings, these data may provide valuable clues to a pacing system abnormality that had been identified on a standard ECG or ambulatory electrocardiographic monitor. However, if the problem is intermittent, the real-time data may be entirely normal, in which case, a more extensive evaluation will be required. Further, the real-time diagnostics may identify a developing pacing system problem but one that has not yet resulted in any adverse consequences for the patient. Additional evaluation or even intervention might be warranted, depending on the specific clinical setting. Any data acquired using the diagnostic

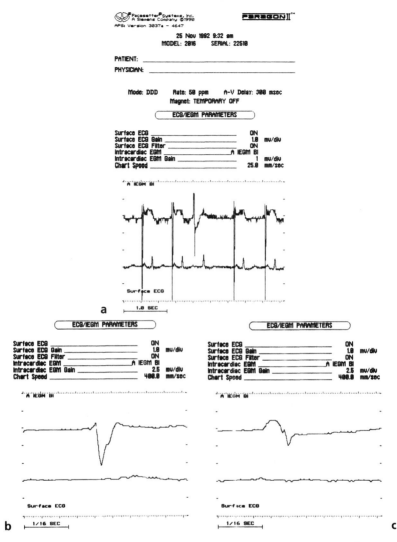

Figure 7.26 (a) Bipolar atrial electrogram with a simultaneously recorded surface ECG. There is an isolated atrial premature beat that appears to be at least 3 mV in amplitude but, when the sensing threshold was assessed, there was intermittent failure to sense at 1 mV. The sensing threshold for the sinus P wave was greater than 5 mV. (b) Increase in the sweep speed to 400 mm/sec and a reduction in the gain to 2.5 mV/division. This atrial electrogram represents the sinus P wave and it corresponds to the noninvasively measured sensing threshold. (c) Increase in the sweep speed to 400 mm/sec and a reduction in the gain to 2.5 mV/division. This atrial electrogram represents the atrial premature beat. Much of the amplitude noted when the sweep speed was 25 mm/sec was comprised of very low frequency components. The complex is also splintered with a slew rate significantly lower than the sinus complex, accounting for the intermittent undersensing at a 1 mV sensitivity.

403

capabilities of the implanted pacemaker that impact the physician's ability to care for the patient or serve as justification for further studies or even intervention should be included as a permanent part of the medical record.

Event counters

Event counters provide information about the function of the pacing system over a period of time. That period is based on the sampling rate of the counters and the amount of random access memory that is dedicated to this task. Event counters have also been called diagnostic data, pacemaker Holter, and data logging. This feature may provide an overview of the behavior of the pacing system with respect to specific events or activation of various algorithms, an overview of the general behavior of the system, or a report of the pacing system with respect to time. Each manufacturer has its own set of unique labels for the specific counters in its various products, but, generically, there are three separate capabilities.[228-238]

Total system performance counters: These are counters that report the total number of events within each pacing state (AV, AR, PV, PR), sometimes with a further separation as to rate distribution within each pacing state. Many systems will also report the number of premature ventricular sensed events. These are native R waves that are sensed but are not preceded by a sensed or paced atrial event. Although many of these are true PVCs, they may also reflect episodes of ventricular oversensing, accelerated junctional rhythms, or atrial undersensing with intact AV nodal conduction. Hence the term PVE to distinguish these events from PVC, which has a precise clinical implication. The data collected by the total system performance counter may be displayed in a tabular format with columns of numbers or bars or as a histogram showing heart-rate distribution (Figure 7.27).

The potential value to the medical staff caring for the patient is that these counters provide an overview of the behavior of the pacing system since the last evaluation. The interpretation of these counters requires a knowledge of the patient's clinical status and the integrity of capture and sensing within the pacing system. For example, if the system reports that all the complexes were paced in the ventricle, either AV or PV, it is a report of the pacemaker's behavior. Loss of atrial or ventricular capture could not be ascertained from these counters, and a true pacing system

Pacesetter®
©1994
APS: Proto 3283q – 95/04/19 16:24

Synchrony°II

5 Jul 1995 1:06 pm
MODEL: 2022   SERIAL: 30427

PATIENT: _____

PHYSICIAN: _____

2:1 Block Rate at 165 ppm

(─────── EVENT HISTOGRAM ───────)

Total Time Sampled 192d 22h 24m 9s
Sampling Rate EVERY EVENT

Mode	DDD
Sensor	PASSIVE
Rate	50 ppm
Max Track	155 ppm
Maximum Sensor Rate	120 ppm
A-V Delay	175 msec
Rate Resp. A-V Delay	ENABLE

Note: The above values were obtained
when the histogram was interrogated.

Rate ppm	PV	PR	AV	AR	PVE
		Event Counts			
0-60	4,889,431	100	2,573,813	26	99
61-67	3,549,033	203	0	0	1,432
68-75	3,698,771	996	0	0	9,994
76-85	1,197,727	4,734	0	0	40,715
86-100	144,623	7,018	0	0	99,224
101-119	18,209	2,234	0	0	53,542
120-149	30,344	297	0	0	2,670
> 149	0	16	0	0	427
Total:	13,528,138	15,598	2,573,813	26	208,103

Total Event Count: 16,325,678

Percent Paced in Atrium	16%
Percent Paced in Ventricle	99%
Total Time at Max Track Rate	0d 0h 46m 55s

Percent of Total Time

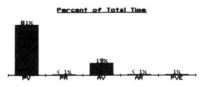

Figure 7.27(a)   Total system performance counter (Event Histogram) from a Pacesetter Synchrony II pulse generator. The sampling rate is every event and data are presented for 192 days, 22 hours, 24 minutes, and 9 seconds. The pacemaker was implanted for complete heart block. The PVEs reflect true isolated PVCs, which seem like a large number, but occurs because of the long duration of monitoring. There is also a subsystem performance counter included in these data, as the pacing system functioned at the programmed maximal tracking rate for a total of 46 minutes, 55 seconds.

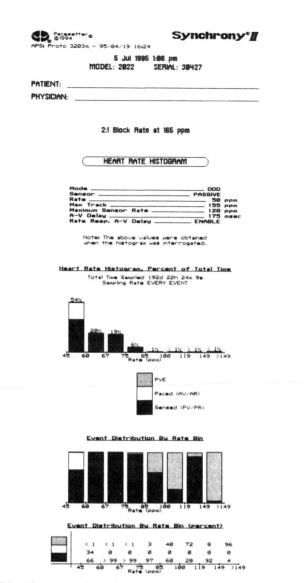

Figure 7.27(b)   The same data shown in 7.27a reformatted into a Heart Rate Histogram showing the percentage of rates at each bin further identified with respect to atrial sensed (native) or atrial paced (rates above the base rate would reflect sensor drive but the sensor, in this case, was disengaged). It becomes apparent from this format that very few of the native atrial events rise above a rate of 85 ppm, which is compatible with chronotropic incompetence, given that the programmed maximal tracking rate was allowed to increase to 155 ppm. Also, the shaded bars in the Event Distribution graph represent the proportion of PVEs within each rate bin. They occur, primarily at the higher rates reflecting a shorter coupling interval, but they are still relatively few in total number.

problem might go unrecognized if one relied only on the counters.

If the pacing system is functioning properly with respect to capture and sensing, the total system performance counters provide insight as to chronotropic function based on the distribution of sensed atrial activity, the response of the sensor, the percentage of time the sensor is controlling the pacemaker, and the status of AV nodal conduction based on the percentage of PR and AR complexes compared with the percentage of PV and AV complexes. Frequent PVEs at a low rate may be a marker for intermittent atrial undersensing with intact AV nodal conduction or for accelerated junctional rhythms; a large number of PVEs at a high rate may reflect true ventricular ectopic beats. The data provided by all the event counters need to be correlated with the clinician's knowledge of the patient.

Subsystem performance counters: Subsystem performance counters track and report the behavior of specific algorithms or features of the pacing system. These include, but are not limited to, sensor-indicated rates, number of times the PMT algorithm was activated, the amount of time spent at the programmed maximal tracking rate, the number of automatic mode switch episodes, the peak filtered atrial rates that triggered the mode-switch episodes or occurred above a predefined rate, and the total number of atrial events or the total number of ventricular events. The value of these counters is that they separate specific events from the overall total system performance counter and provide information with respect to the frequency with which that algorithm or feature was utilized.

These counters may be displayed as a summary total, a table of events, a histogram, or a more detailed presentation of each event, depending on the design of the specific counter and the information that is stored. An example of a subsystem performance counter is shown in Figure 7.28.

Time-based system performance counters: A limitation of both the total and subsystem performance counters when the data are displayed in either a cumulative table or histogram format is that specific events will be lost within the overall mass of data. A third counter capability places each of the individual events in the specific sequence of their occurrence. These are classified as time-based system performance counters. They have many names, including "rolling trend" and "event record." Some data may be

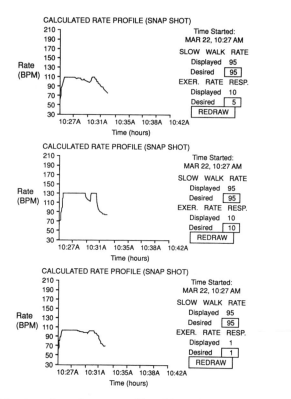

Figure 7.28 A series of rate profiles from the Intermedics Relay DDDR pacing system. The patient performs a walk while the system collects the sensor data. These data are collected by the programmer. The physician is then able to enter new sensor parameters into the programmer and the system automatically calculates the expected heart-rate response based on the new settings combined with the raw sensor signal. The physician can then choose the sensor parameters that will provide the best response for the patient. This is an example of a subsystem performance counter. It reports only sensor performance without regard to the intrinsic heart rate or other pacemaker algorithms.

stored with a specific data and time stamp, and other data are a continuous display acquired during the preceding hours or days. In the continuous display, as new data are added, the oldest is deleted. Thus, when these data are retrieved by the physician, they provide a detailed report of the behavior of the entire pacing system or of one feature of the pacing system with respect to the time just preceding the evaluation. If the rate increased, whether this is caused by sensor drive or a spontaneous rhythm, the patient is

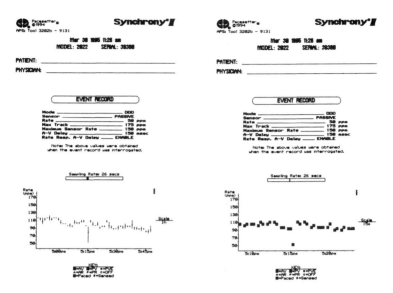

Figure 7.29 A pair of panels from the Event Record from a Pacesetter Synchrony II pulse generator. This is a time-based system performance counter monitoring the actual pacing system behavior at a sampling rate of 26 seconds. The indication for pacing was complete heart block. The sensor was passive (disengaged). The office evaluation of the pacing system was normal, but the Event Record recorded intermittent drops in the rate as shown by the vertical line extending down to a low rate in the panel on the left. The scale was expanded (right panel) showing each paced event, and there is one cycle of AV pacing in the midst of a stable sinus rhythm with PV pacing. On further evaluation, this was intermittent atrial undersensing.

likely to remember what was occurring at the time, which will allow the physician to correlate the behavior of the pacing system with the patient's activities and symptoms, as shown in Figure 7.29.

There are two subsets to the time-based system performance counter. One is that specific events such as activation of a unique algorithm trigger storage of that event for retrieval at a later date. These are often associated with a time and date stamp. These, however, will not recognize a symptomatic event that does not also invoke one of the special algorithms in the device. With the continuous recording, the patient may be able to activate a marker to identify the event, but with earlier systems, the patient had to go to the physician's office or pacemaker clinic in a timely manner to enable these data to be retrieved before they were overwritten. An

409

increase in random access memory capacity has seen the introduction of Patient Triggered Event Records™. This system allows the patient to not only mark a symptomatic event by placing a magnet over the pacemaker for at least 0.5 seconds, but also store the event in a memory bin that will not be erased until the data are retrieved by the physician using the programmer for the implanted system, even if this is not until months later. In addition, the pacemaker will apply a time and date stamp to the event. For example, a patient may experience an episode of palpitations while traveling and mark and store the data totally within the pacemaker. The physician can retrieve the data at a later date. The limitation with the current technology is that although it provides a report of the paced behavior with respect to pacing and sensing as well as a rate distribution, it does not provide a representation of the actual rhythm that may have occurred at that time. Thus, the same limitations associated with event markers apply to these data and to all the data reported by the various event counters; the report of a output pulse does not mean that capture was intact or that a sensed event was a true P or R wave rather than oversensing or some other problem.

Although having only one counter available offers valuable information that may help the physician manage the patient and program the pacemaker, there may be significant gaps in the evaluation. The various event counters providing an overview of the behavior of the entire system since the last evaluation, the performance of the specific algorithms or features, and a time-based system performance counter complement one another. The goal is that all counters will be available simultaneously without the physician's having to intentionally select one rather than another. The ability to provide this capability will depend on the memory capacity of the individual pacemaker.

SUMMARY

As mentioned at the beginning of this chapter, it is important to maintain appropriate records containing all the baseline data and results of the periodic detailed evaluations of the pacing system. These records provide the substrate on which to assess a new observation or information. One should also take advantage of the diagnostic capabilities incorporated into many present-generation pacemakers. These features include programmed parameter interrogation, lead and battery function telemetry, event marker and electrogram telemetry, and event counters for native and paced events, including sensor performance and other unique algorithms. Examples of many of these capabilities have been used to illustrate the various conditions described throughout this chapter. Although the same information can usually be obtained by other means, doing so may be time-consuming and more complicated. The goal of any therapy is not only that it be effective but that it also be able to be evaluated and fine-tuned efficiently and accurately in the office environment for the benefit of the patient.

When a true pacing system malfunction is encountered, the full differential diagnosis should be considered. This includes primary problems arising with the pulse generator, the lead(s), and the patient, as well as the interaction between these three components. It is embarrassing, expensive, and potentially dangerous to subject the patient to an operative procedure to replace a normally functioning pacemaker when the observed "problem" could have been easily corrected by programming the pacemaker. Thus, any prior data that are available should be reviewed, the programmed parameters of the pacing system should be obtained, and all available diagnostic features of the given device should be utilized before arriving at a final decision and plan. To do less than this will, all too often, result in an incorrect diagnosis—to the detriment of the patient, the physician, and the overall health-care economy.

REFERENCES

1. Song SL. The Bilitch report: Performance of implantable cardiac rhythm management devices. *PACE* 1994;17:692–704.
2. Furman S, Benedek ZM, Andrews CA, et al. Long-term follow-up of pacemaker lead system. *PACE* 1995;18:271–285.
3. Furman S. Cardiac pacing and pacemakers VI. Analysis of pacemaker malfunction. *Am Heart J* 1977;94:378–386.
4. Mond HG. *The Cardiac Pacemaker, Function and Malfunction.* New York: Grune & Stratton, 1983.
5. Castellanos A, Lemberg L. Pacemaker arrhythmias and electrocardiographic recognition of pacemakers. *Circulation* 1973;47:1382–1391.
6. Barold SS. *Modern Cardiac Pacing.* Mount Kisco, NY: Futura, 1983.

7. Levine PA. The complementary role of electrogram, event marker and measured data telemetry in the assessment of pacing system function. *J Electrophysiol* 1987;1:404–416.
8. Kruse I, Markowitz T, Ryden L. Timing markers showing pacemaker behavior to aid in the follow-up of a physiologic pacemaker. *PACE* 1983;6:801–805.
9. Olson WH, McConnell MV, Sah RL, et al. Pacemaker diagnostic diagrams. *PACE* 1985;8:691–700.
10. Levine PA, Sholder J, Duncan JL. Clinical benefits of telemetered electrograms in assessment of DDD function. *PACE* 1984;7:1170–1177.
11. Sholder J, Levine PA, Mann BM, et al. Bidirectional telemetry and interrogation in cardiac pacing. In SS Barold, J Mugica (eds.), *The Third Decade of Cardiac Pacing, Advances in Technology and Clinical Application.* Mount Kisco, NY: Futura, 1982; pp 145–171.
12. Levine PA. Confirmation of atrial capture and determination of atrial capture thresholds in DDD pacing systems. *Clin Prog Pacing Electrophysiol* 1984;2:465–473.
13. Van Beek GJ, Den Dulk K, Lindemans FW, et al. Detection of insulation failure by gradual reduction in noninvasively measured electrogram amplitudes. *PACE* 1986;9:772–775.
14. Ohm OJ, Breivik K, Hammer EA, et al. Intraoperative electrical measurements during pacemaker implantation. *Clin Prog Pacing Electrophysiol* 1984;2:1–23.
15. Parsonnet V, Bilitch M, Furman S, et al. Early malfunction of transvenous pacemaker electrodes: A three-center study. *Circulation* 1979;60:590–596.
16. Gordon AJ, Vaqueiro MD, Barold SS. Endocardial electrograms from pacemaker catheters. *Circulation* 1968;38:82–89.
17. Arnold AG. Predictive value of ST segment elevation in cardiac pacing. *Br Heart J* 1980;44:416–418.
18. Long R. Technical Memo on Trividers. Sylmar, CA: Pacesetter Systems Inc., 1986.
19. Levine PA, Schuller H, Lindgren A. *Pacemaker ECG—An Introduction and Approach to Interpretation.* Solna, Sweden: Siemens-Pacesetter, 1986.
20. Schuller H, Fahraeus T. *Pacemaker EKG—A Clinical Approach.* Solna, Sweden: Siemens-Elema AB Pacemaker Division, 1980.
21. Levine PA. Electrocardiography of bipolar single and dual-chamber pacing systems. *Herzschrittmacher* 1988;8:86–90.

22. Sheffield LT, Berson AL, Bragg-Remschel D, et al. AHA special report: Recommendation for standards of instrumentation and practice in the use of ambulatory electrocardiography. *Circulation* 1985;71:626A–636A.

23. Cherry R, Sactuary C, Kennedy HL. The question of frequency response. *Amb Electrocardiol* 1977;1:13–14.

24. Hecht SR, Berdoff RL. Radiographic recognition of pacemaker lead complications. *Clinical Progress in Electrophysiology and Pacing* 1986;4:189–198.

25. Schwartzman D, Nallamouthu N, Callans DJ, et al. Postoperative lead-related complications in patients with nonthoracotomy defibrillation lead systems. *J Amer Coll Cardiol* 1995;26:776–786.

26. Meyer JA, Fruehan CT, Delmonico JE. The pacemaker Twiddler's syndrome: A further note. *J Thorac Cardiovasc Surg* 1974;67:903–907.

27. Veltri EP, Mower MM, Reid PR. Twiddler's syndrome: A new twist. *PACE* 1984;7:1004–1009.

28. Furman S, Pannizzo F, Campo I. Comparison of active and passive adhering leads for endocardial pacing. *PACE* 1979; 2:417–427.

29. Lal RB, Avery RD. Aggressive pacemaker Twiddler's syndrome: Dislodgement of an active fixation ventricular pacing electrode. *Chest* 1990;97:756–757.

30. Trautwein W. Electrophysiological aspects of cardiac stimulation. In M Schaldach, S Furman (eds.), *Advances in Pacemaker Technology*. New York: Springer-Verlag, 1975; pp 11–23.

31. Siddons H, Sowton E. Threshold for stimulation. In: *Cardiac pacemakers*. Springfield, IL: Charles C Thomas, 1967; pp 145–174.

32. Davies JG, Sowton E. Electrical threshold of the human heart. *Br Heart J* 1966;28:231–239.

33. Furman S, Hurzeler P, Mehra R. Cardiac pacing and pacemakers IV. Threshold of cardiac stimulation. *Am Heart J* 1977;94:115–124.

34. Ohm OJ, Breivik K, Anderssen KS. Strength–duration curves in cardiac pacing. In C Meere (ed.), *Proceedings of the Sixth World Symposium on Cardiac Pacing*. Montreal, 1979; Chapter 20–2.

35. Irnich W. The chronaxie time and its practical importance. *PACE* 1980;3:292–301.

36. Preston TA, Judge RD, Lucchesi BR, et al. Myocardial threshold in patients with artificial pacemakers. *Am J Cardiol* 1966;18:83–89.

37. Preston TA, Fletcher RD, Lucchesi BR, et al. Changes in myocardial threshold. Physiologic and pharmacologic factors in patients with implanted pacemakers. *Am Heart J* 1967; 74:235–242.

38. Sowton E, Barr I. Physiologic changes in threshold. *Am NY Acad Sci* 1969;167:679–685.

39. Preston TA, Judge RD. Alteration of pacemaker threshold by drug and physiologic factors. *Ann NY Acad Sci* 1969;167:686–692.

40. Beanlands DS, Akyurekli Y, Keon WJ. Prednisone in the management of exit block. In C Meere (ed.), *Proceedings of the Sixth World Symposium on Cardiac Pacing.* Montreal, 1979; Chapter 18–3.

41. Nagatomo Y, Ogawa T, Kumagae H, et al. Pacing failure due to markedly increased stimulation threshold two years after implantation: Successful management with oral prednisolone, a case report. *PACE* 1989;12:1034–1037.

42. Kruse IM, Terpstra B. Acute and long-term atrial and ventricular stimulation thresholds with a steroid-eluting electrode. *PACE* 1985;8:45–49.

43. Mond H, Stokes K, Helland J, et al. The porous titanium steroid-eluting electrode: A double-blind study assessing the stimulation threshold effects of steroid. *PACE* 1988;11:214–219.

44. Klein HH, Steinberger J, Knake W. Stimulation characteristics of a steroid-eluting electrode compared with three conventional electrodes. *PACE* 1990;13:134–137.

45. Crossley GH, Reynolds D, Kay GN, et al. Treatment of patients with prior exit block using a novel steroid-eluting active fixation lead. *PACE* 1994;17:2042–2046.

46. O'Reilly MV, Murnaghan DP, Williams MD. Transvenous pacemaker failure induced by hyperkalemia. *JAMA* 1974; 228:336–337.

47. Hughes JC Jr, Tyers GFO, Torman HA. Effects of acid–base imbalance on myocardial pacing thresholds. *J Thorac Cardiovasc Surg* 1975;69:743–746.

48. Schlesinger Z, Rosenberg T, Stryjer D, et al. Exit block in myxedema treated effectively with thyroid hormone therapy. *PACE* 1980;3:737–739.

49. Lee D, Greenspan K, Edmands RE, Fisch C. The effect of electrolyte alteration on stimulus requirement of cardiac pacemakers. *Circulation* 1968;38:VI–124.
50. O'Reilly MV, Murnaghan DP, Williams MB. Op. Cit. 1974.
51. Gettes LS, Shabetai R, Downs TA, et al. Effect of changes in potassium and calcium concentrations on diastolic threshold and strength–interval relationships of the human heart. *Ann NY Acad Sci* 1969;167:693–705.
52. Hellestrand KJ, Burnett PJ, Milne JR, et al. Effect of the antiarrhythmic agent flecainide acetate on acute and chronic pacing thresholds. *PACE* 1983;6:892–899.
53. Levick CE, Mizgala HF, Kerr CR. Failure to pace following high dose anti-arrhythmic therapy—reversal with isoproterenol. *PACE* 1984;7:252–256.
54. Nielsen AP, Griffin JC, Herre JM, et al. Effect of amiodarone on acute and chronic pacing thresholds. *PACE* 1984;7: 462.
55. Dohrmann ML, Godschlager N. Metabolic and pharmacologic effects on myocardial stimulation threshold in patients with cardiac pacemakers. In SS Barold (ed.), *Modern Cardiac Pacing*. Mount Kisco, NY: Futura, 1985; pp 161–170.
56. Montefoschi N, Boccadamo R. Propafenone-induced acute variation of chronic atrial pacing threshold: A case report. *PACE* 1990;13:480–483.
57. Salel AF, Seagren SC, Pool PE. Effects of encainide on the function of implanted pacemakers. *PACE* 1989;12:1439–1444.
58. Guarnieri T, Datorre SD, Bondke H, et al. Increased pacing threshold after an automatic defibrillatory shock in dogs; effects of class I and class II antiarrhythmic drugs. *PACE* 1988;11:1324–1330.
59. Hayes DL. Effect of drugs and devices on permanent pacemakers. *Cardiology* 1991;8:70–75.
60. Adornato E, Monea P, Pennisi V, et al. Influence of flecainide on cardiac pacing threshold with different electrodes. *Eur JCPE* 1992;2:255–258.
61. Szabo Z, Solti F. The significance of the tissue reaction around the electrode on the late myocardial threshold. In M Schaldach, S Furman (eds.), *Advances in Pacemaker Technology*. New York: Springer-Verlag, 1975; pp 273–287.

62. Ben-Zur UM, Platt SB, Gross JN, et al. Direct and telemetered lead impedance. *PACE* 1994;17:2004–2007.
63. Byrd CL, McArthur W, Stokes K, et al. Implant experience with unipolar polyurethane pacing leads. *PACE* 1983;6:868–882.
64. Raymond RD, Nanian KB. Insulation failure with bipolar polyurethane pacing leads. *PACE* 1984;7:378–380.
65. Hayes DL, Holmes DR Jr, Merideth J, et al. Bipolar tined polyurethane ventricular leads: A four-year experience. *PACE* 1985;8:192–196.
66. Sholder J, Duncan J, Helland J. Clinical and technical considerations of bipolar coaxial pacing leads. *Technical Memorandum No. 17.* Sylmar, CA: Pacesetter Systems Inc., July 1991.
67. Stokes K, Stephenson N. The implantable cardiac pacing lead—Just a simple wire? In SS Barold, J Mugica (eds.), *The Third Decade of Cardiac Pacing: Advances in Technology and Clinical Applications.* Mount Kisco, NY: Futura, 1982; pp 365–416.
68. Stokes K, Staffenson D, Lessar J, et al. A possible new complication of subclavian stick: Conductor fracture. *PACE* 1987;10:748.
69. Anonymous. Subclavian puncture procedure may result in lead conductor fracture. *Medtronic News* 1986–1987 (Winter):27.
70. Suzuki Y, Fujimori S, Sakai M, et al. A case of pacemaker lead fracture associated with thoracic outlet syndrome. *PACE* 1988;11:326–330.
71. Arakawa M, Kambara K, Ito HA, et al. Intermittent oversensing due to internal insulation damage of temperature sensing rate responsive pacemaker lead in subclavian venipuncture method. *PACE* 1989;12:1312–1316.
72. Fyke FE. Simultaneous insulation deterioration associated with side-by-side subclavian placement of two polyurethane leads. *PACE* 1988;11:1571–1574.
73. Kranz J, Crystal DK, Wagner CL, et al. Thoracic outlet compression syndrome: The first rib. *Northwest Med* 1969; 68:646–650.
74. Jacobs DM, Fink AS, Miller RP, et al. Anatomical and morphologic evaluation of pacemaker lead compression. *PACE* 1993;16:434–444.
75. Magney JE, Flynn DM, Parsons JA, et al. Anatomical mechanisms explaining damage to pacemaker leads, defibrillator

leads and failure of central venous catheters adjacent to the sternoclavicular joint. *PACE* 1993;16:445–457.

76. Magney JE, Parsons JA, Flynn DM, et al. Pacemaker and defibrillator lead entrapment: Case studies. *PACE* 1995; 18:1509–1517.

77. Witte A. Pseudo-fracture of pacemaker lead due to securing suture: A case report. *PACE* 1981;4:716–718.

78. Dunlap TE, Popak KD, Sorkin RP. Radiographic pseudofracture of the Medtronic bipolar polyurethane pacing lead. *Am Heart J* 1983;106:167–168.

79. Byrd CL. Safe introducer technique. *PACE* 1990;13: 501.

80. Magney JE, Staplin DH, Flynn DM, et al. A new approach to percutaneous subclavian venipuncture to avoid lead fracture or central venous catheter occlusion. *PACE* 1993;16:2133–2142.

81. Nickalls RWD. A new percutaneous intraclavicular approach to the axillary vein. *Anesthesia* 1987;42:151–154.

82. Furman S. Venous cutdown for pacemaker implantation. *Ann Thorac Surg* 1986;41:438–439.

83. Ong LS, Barold SS, Lederman M, et al. Cephalic vein guidewire technique for implantation of permanent pacemakers. *Am Heart J* 1987;114:753–756.

84. Levine PA. Clinical manifestations of lead insulation defects. *J Electrophysiol* 1987;1:144–155.

85. Ekbom K, Nilsson BY, Edhag O. Rhythmic shoulder girdle muscle contractions as a complication in pacemaker treatment. *Chest* 1974;66:599–601.

86. Kruse IM, Mark J, Ryden L. Mechanical wear of pacemaker lead insulation: A cause of loss of pacing. *PACE* 1980;3:159–161.

87. Van Gelder LM, El Gamal MIH. False inhibition of an atrial demand pacemaker caused by insulation defect in a polyurethane lead. *PACE* 1983;6:834–839.

88. Sanford CF. Self-inhibition of an AV sequential demand pulse generator due to polyurethane lead insulation disruption. *PACE* 1983;6:840–844.

89. Widlansky S, Zipes DP. Suppression of a ventricular inhibited bipolar pacemaker by skeletal muscle activity. *J Electrocardiol* 1974;7:371–373.

90. Salem DN, Bornstein A, Levine PA, et al. Fracture of pac-

ing electrode mimicking failure of pulse generator. *Chest* 1978;74:673–674.

91. Coumel P, Mugica J, Barold SS. Demand pacemaker arrhythmias caused by intermittent incomplete electrode fracture. *Am J Cardiol* 1975;36:105–109.

92. Barold SS, Scovil J, Ong LS, et al. Periodic pacemaker spike attenuation with preservation of capture: An unusual electrocardiographic manifestation of partial pacing electrode fracture. *PACE* 1978;1:375–380.

93. Lasala AF, Fieldman A, Diana DJ, et al. Gas pocket causing pacemaker malfunction. *PACE* 1979;2:183–185.

94. Kreis DJ, LiCalzi L, Shaw RK. Air entrapment as a cause of transient cardiac pacemaker malfunction. *PACE* 1979;2:641–643.

95. Levine PA, Schuller H, Lindgren A. Pacemaker ECG utilization of pulse generator telemetry—A benefit of space age technology. Solna, Sweden: Siemens-Elema AB Pacemaker Division, 1988.

96. Levine PA. *Why Programmability? Indications for and Clinical Utility of Multiparameter Programmable Pacemakers.* Sylmar, CA: Pacesetter Systems Inc., 1981.

97. Furman S, Hurzeler P, DeCaprio V. Cardiac pacing and pacemakers III: Sensing the cardiac electrogram. *Am Heart J* 1977;93:794–801.

98. Ohm OJ. The interdependence between electrogram, total electrode impedance and pacemaker input impedance necessary to obtain adequate functioning demand pacemakers. *PACE* 1979;2:465–485.

99. Evans GL, Glasser SP. Intracardiac electrocardiography as a guide to pacemaker positioning. *JAMA* 1971;216:483–485.

100. Levine PA, Klein MD. Discrepant electrocardiographic and pulse analyzer endocardial potentials, a possible source of pacemaker sensing failure. In C Meere (ed.), *Proceedings of the Sixth World Symposium on Cardiac Pacing.* Montreal, 1979, Chapter 34–16.

101. Kleinert M, Elmqvist H, Strandberg H. Spectral properties of atrial and ventricular endocardial signals. *PACE* 1979;2:11–19.

102. Levine PA, Podrid PJ, Klein MD, et al. Pacemaker sensing: Comparison of signal amplitudes determined by electrogram telemetry and noninvasively measured sensing thresholds. *PACE* 1989;12:672.

103. Hauser RG, Edwards LN, Giuffree VF. Limitations of pacemaker system analyzers for the evaluation of implantable pulse generators. *PACE* 1981;4:650–657.
104. Ohm OJ. Demand failures occurring during permanent pacing in patients with serious heart disease. *PACE* 1980;3:44–55.
105. Griffin JC, Finke WL. Analysis of the endocardial electrogram morphology of isolated ventricular beats. *PACE* 1983;6:315.
106. Barold SS, Gaidula JJ. Failure of demand pacemaker from low-voltage bipolar ventricular electrograms. *JAMA* 1971; 215:923–926.
107. Barold SS, Falkoff MD, Ong LS, et al. Interference in cardiac pacemakers: Exogenous sources. In N El Sherif, P Samet (eds.), *Cardiac Pacing and Electrophysiology* (3rd ed.). Philadelphia: WB Saunders, 1991; pp 608–632.
108. Irnich W. Interference in pacemakers. *PACE* 1984;7:1021–1048.
109. Falkoff MD, Ong LS, Heinle RA, et al. The noise sampling period: A new cause of apparent sensing malfunction of demand pacemakers. *PACE* 1978;1:250–253.
110. Strathmore NF. Interference in cardiac pacemakers. In K Ellenbogen, GN Kay, BL Wilkoff (eds.), *Clinical Cardiac Pacing*. Philadelphia: WB Saunders, 1995; pp 770–779.
111. Levine PA, Seltzer JP. Fusion, pseudofusion, pseudopseudofusion and confusion: Normal rhythms associated with atrioventricular sequential "DVI" pacing. *Clin Prog Pacing Electrophysiol* 1983;1:70–83.
112. Barold SS, Falkoff MD, Ong LS, et al. Characterization of pacemaker arrhythmias due to normally functioning AV demand (DVI) pulse generators. *PACE* 1980;3:712–723.
113. Bathen J, Gundersen J, Forfang K. Tachycardias related to atrial synchronous ventricular pacing. *PACE* 1982;5:471–475.
114. Levine PA, Mace RC. *Pacing Therapy—A Guide to Cardiac Pacing for Optimum Hemodynamic Benefit.* Mount Kisco, NY: Futura, 1983.
115. Fetter J, Bobeldyk GL, Engman FJ. The clinical incidence and significance of myopotential sensing with unipolar pacemakers. *PACE* 1984;7:871–881.
116. Ohm OJ, Morkrid L, Hammer E. Amplitude–frequency characteristics of myopotentials and endocardial potentials as

seen by a pacemaker system. *Scand J Thorac Cardiovasc Surg Supp* 1978;22:41–46.

117. Levine PA, Caplan CH, Klein MD, et al. Myopotential inhibition of unipolar lithium pacemakers. *Chest* 1982; 82:461–465.

118. Halperin JL, Camunas JL, Stern EH, et al. Myopotential interference with DDD pacemakers: Endocardial electrographic telemetry in the diagnosis of pacemaker-related arrhythmias. *Am J Cardiol* 1984;54:97–102.

119. Williams DO, Thomas DJ. Muscle potentials simulating pacemaker malfunction. *Br Heart J* 1976;38:1096–1097.

120. Ohm OJ, Bruland H, Pedersen OM, et al. Interference effect of myopotentials on function of unipolar demand pacemakers. *Br Heart J* 1974;36:77–84.

121. Gabry MD, Behrens M, Andrews C, et al. Comparison of myopotential interference in unipolar–bipolar programmable DDD pacemakers. *PACE* 1987;10:1322–1330.

122. Breivik K, Ohm OJ, Engedal H. Long-term comparison of unipolar and bipolar pacing and sensing using a new multi-programmable pacemaker system. *PACE* 1983;6:592–600.

123. Warnowicz-Papp MA. The pacemaker patient and the electromagnetic environment. *Clin Prog Pacing Electrophysiol* 1983;1:166–176.

124. Sager DP. Current facts on pacemaker electromagnetic interference and their application to clinical care. *Heart Lung* 1987;16:211–221.

125. Peter T, Harper R, Sloman G. Inhibition of demand pacemakers caused by potentials associated with inspiration. *Br Heart J* 1976;38:211–212.

126. Barold SS, Ong LS, Falkoff MD, et al. Inhibition of bipolar demand pacemaker by diaphragmatic myopotentials. *Circulation* 1977;56:679–683.

127. Levine PA, Pirzada FA. Pacemaker oversensing: A possible example of concealed ventricular extrasystoles. *PACE* 1981;4:199–203.

128. Massumi RA, Mason DT, Amsterdam EA, et al. Apparent malfunction of demand pacemaker caused by non-propagated (concealed) ventricular extrasystoles. *Chest* 1972;61:426.

129. Sarmiento JJ. Clinical utility of telemetered intracardiac electrograms in diagnosing a design-dependent lead malfunction. *PACE* 1990;13:188–195.

130. Nalos PC, Nytray W. Benefits of intracardiac electrograms

and programmable sensing polarity in preventing pacemaker inhibition due to spurious screw-in lead signals. *PACE* 1990;13:1101–1104.

131. Ausubel K, Furman D. The pacemaker syndrome. *Ann Intern Med* 1985;103:420–429.

132. Nishimura RA, Gersh BJ, Holmes DR, et al. Outcome of dual-chamber pacing for the pacemaker syndrome. *Mayo Clin Proc* 1983;58:452–456.

133. Love JC, Haffajee CI, Alpert JS. Reversibility of hypotension and shock by atrial or atrioventricular sequential pacing in patients with right ventricular infarction. *Am Heart J* 1984;108:5–13.

134. Toivonen LK, Pohjola-Sintonen S. Vasodilator therapy— Induced pacemaker syndrome. *Chest* 1987;91:919–920.

135. Den Dulk K, Lindemans FW, Brugada P, et al. Pacemaker syndrome with AAI rate variable pacing: Importance of atrioventricular conduction properties, medication and pacemaker programmability. *PACE* 1988;11:1226–1233.

136. Parsonnet V, Myers M, Perry GY. Paradoxical paroxysmal nocturnal congestive heart failure as a severe manifestation of the pacemaker syndrome. *Am J Cardiol* 1990;65:683–685.

137. Ellenbogen KA, Thames MD, Mohanty PK. New insights into pacemaker syndrome gained from hemodynamic, humoral and vascular responses during ventriculoatrial pacing. *Am J Cardiol* 1990;65:53–59.

138. Heldman D, Mulvihill D, Nguyen H, et al. True incidence of pacemaker syndrome. *PACE* 1990;13:526.

139. Gee W. Ocular pneumoplethysmography in cardiac pacing. *PACE* 1983;6:1268–1272.

140. Rediker DE, Eagle KA, Homma S, et al. Clinical and hemodynamic comparison of VVI versus DDD pacing in patients with DDD pacemakers. *Am J Cardiol* 1988;61:323–329.

141. Stewart WJ, Dicola VC, Harthorne JW, et al. Doppler ultrasound measurement of cardiac output in patients with physiologic pacemakers. *Am J Cardiol* 1984;54:308–312.

142. Levine PA. Normal and abnormal rhythms associated with dual-chamber pacemakers. *Cardiol Clin* 1985;3:595–616.

143. Levine PA, Seltzer JP. Runaway or normal pacing? Two cases of normal rate responsive (DDD) pacing. *Clin Prog Pacing Electrophysiol* 1983;1:177–183.

144. Levine PA, Seltzer JP. AV universal (DDD) pacing and atrial fibrillation. *Clin Prog Pacing Electrophysiol* 1983;1:275–281.

145. Levine PA, Schuller H, Lindgren A. *Pacemaker ECG—An Introduction and Approach to Interpretation.* Solna, Sweden: Siemens-Pacesetter, 1986.

146. Levine PA, Brodsky SJ, Seltzer JP. Assessment of atrial capture in committed atrioventricular sequential (DVI) pacing systems. *PACE* 1983;6:616–623.

147. Levine PA. Confirmation of atrial capture and determination of atrial capture thresholds in DDD pacing systems. *Clin Prog Pacing Electrophysiol* 1984;2:465–473.

148. Van Mechelen R, Vandekerckhove Y. Atrial capture and dual chamber pacing. *PACE* 1986;9:21–25.

149. Van Mechelen R, Hart CT, De Boer H. Failure to sense P waves during DDD pacing. *PACE* 1986;9:498–502.

150. Bricker JT, Ward KA, Zinner A, Gillette PC. Decrease in canine endocardial and epicardial electrogram voltage with exercise: Implications for pacemaker sensing. *PACE* 1988;11:460–464.

151. Frohlig G, Schwerdt H, Schieffer H, et al. Atrial signal variations and pacemaker malsensing during exercise: A study in the time and frequency domain. *J Am Coll Cardiol* 1988;11:806–813.

152. Byrd CL, Schwarts SJ, Gonzales M, et al. DDD pacemakers maximize hemodynamic benefits and minimize complications for most patients. *PACE* 1988;11:1911–1916.

153. Moss AJ, Rivers RJ Jr, Kramer DH. Permanent pervenous atrial pacing from the coronary vein: Long-term follow-up. *Circulation* 1979;59:222–225.

154. Moss AJ. Therapeutic uses of permanent pervenous atrial pacemakers: A review. *J Electrocardiol* 1975;8:373–390.

155. Adelman AG, Lopez JF. Arrhythmias associated with the synchronous pacemaker. *Am Heart J* 1967;74:632–641.

156. Castellanos A, Lemberg L. Disorders of rhythm appearing after implantation of synchronized pacemakers. *Br Heart J* 1964;26:747–754.

157. Levine PA, Venditti FJ, Podrid PJ, et al. Therapeutic and diagnostic benefits of intentional crosstalk-mediated ventricular output inhibition. *PACE* 1988;11:1194–1201.

158. Sweesy MW, Batey RL, Forney RC. Crosstalk during bipolar pacing. *PACE* 1988;11:1512–1516.

159. Batey FL, Calabria DA, Sweesy MW, et al. Crosstalk and blanking periods in a dual chamber pacemaker. *Clin Prog Pacing Electrophysiol* 1985;3:314–318.

160. Furman S, Reicher-Reiss H, Escher DJW. Atrioventricular sequential pacing and pacemakers. *Chest* 1973;63:783–789.
161. Levine PA, Seltzer JP. Op. Cit. 1983.
162. Barold SS, Falkoff MD, Ong LS, et al. Interpretation of electrocardiograms produced by a new unipolar multiprogrammable "committed" AV sequential demand (DVI) pacemaker. *PACE* 1981;4:692–708.
163. Barold SS, Belott PH. Behavior of the ventricular triggering period of DDD pacemakers. *PACE* 1987;10:1237–1252.
164. Levine PA, Seltzer JP. AV universal (DDD) pacing and atrial fibrillation. *Clin Prog Pacing Electrophysiol* 1983;1:275–281.
165. Greenspan AJ, Greenberg RM, Frank WS. Tracking of atrial flutter by DDD pacing, another form of pacemaker mediated tachycardia. *PACE* 1984;7:955–960.
166. Levine PA, Selznick L. *Prospective Management of the Patient with Retrograde Ventriculoatrial Conduction: Prevention and Management of Pacemaker-Mediated Endless-Loop Tachycardias.* Sylmar, CA: Pacesetter Systems, Inc., 1990.
167. Luceri RM, Castellanos A, Zaman L, et al. The arrhythmias of dual-chamber cardiac pacemakers and their management. *Ann Intern Med* 1983;99:354–359.
168. Den Dulk K, Lindemans FW, Bar FW, et al. Pacemaker-related tachycardias. *PACE* 1982;5:476–485.
169. Rubin JW, Frank MJ, Boineau JP, et al. Current physiologic pacemakers: A serious problem with a new device. *Am J Cardiol* 1983;52:88–91.
170. Levine PA. Postventricular atrial refractory periods and pacemaker mediated tachycardias. *Clin Prog Pacing Electrophysiol* 1983;1:394–401.
171. Furman S, Fisher JD. Endless-loop tachycardia in an AV universal (DDD) pacemaker. *PACE* 1982;5:486–489.
172. Oseran D, Ausubel K, Klementowicz PT, et al. Spontaneous endless-loop tachycardia. *PACE* 1986;9:379–386.
173. Limousin M, Bonnett JL. A multi-centric study of 1816 endless loop tachycardia (ELT) response. *PACE* 1990;13:555.
174. Ausubel K, Gabry MD, Klementowicz PT, et al. Pacemaker-mediated endless-loop tachycardia at rates below the upper rate limit. *Am J Cardiol* 1988;61:465–467.
175. Denes P, Wu D, Dhingra R, et al. The effects of cycle length on cardiac refractory periods in man. *Circulation* 1974;49:32–41.

176. Amikam S, Furman S. Programmed upper-rate-limit-dependent endless loop tachycardia. *Chest* 1984;85:286–288.
177. McAlister HF, Klementowicz PT, Calderon EM, et al. Atrial electrogram analysis: Antegrade versus retrograde. *PACE* 1988;11:1703–1707.
178. Klementowicz PT, Furman S. Selective atrial sensing in dual-chamber pacemakers eliminates endless-loop tachycardias. *J Am Coll Cardiol* 1986;7:590–594.
179. Pannizzo F, Amikam S, Bagwell P, et al. Discrimination of antegrade and retrograde atrial depolarization by electrogram analysis. *Am Heart J* 1986;112:780–786.
180. Bernheim C, Markewitz A, Kemkes BM. Can reprogramming of atrial sensitivity avoid endless-loop tachycardia? *PACE* 1986;9:293.
181. Haffajee C, Murphy J, Gold R, et al. Automatic extension vs. programmability of the atrial refractory period in the prevention of pacemaker mediated tachycardia. *PACE* 1985;8:A–56.
182. Den Dulk K, Hamersa M, Wellens HJJ. Role of an adaptable atrial refractory period for DDD pacemakers. *PACE* 1987;10:425.
183. Levine PA, Lindenberg BS. Diagnostic data: An aid to the follow-up and assessment of the pacing system. *J Electrophysiol* 1987;1:396–403.
184. Satler JF, Rackley CE, Pearle DL, et al. Inhibition of a physiologic pacing system due to its anti-pacemaker-mediated tachycardia mode. *PACE* 1985;8:806–810.
185. Van Gelder LM, El Gamal MIH, Sanders RS. Tachycardia-termination algorithm: A valuable feature for interruption of pacemaker mediated tachycardia. *PACE* 1984;7:283–287.
186. Duncan JL, Clark MF. Prevention and termination of pacemaker-mediated tachycardia in a new DDD pacing system (Siemens Pacesetter Model 2010T). *PACE* 1988;11:1679–1683.
187. Levine PA, Seltzer JP. Runaway or normal pacing? Two cases of normal rate responsive (VDD) pacing. *Clin Prog Pacing Electrophysiol* 1983;1:177–183.
188. Levine PA. Magnet rates and recommended replacement time indicators of lithium pacemakers. *Clin Prog Pacing Electrophysiol* 1986;4:608–618.
189. Levine PA, Hayes DL, Wilkoff BL, Ohman A. *Electrocardiography of Rate-Modulated Pacemaker Rhythms.* Sylmar, CA: Pacesetter Systems Inc., 1990.

190. Levine PA. Pacemaker pseudomalfunction. *PACE* 1981;4: 563–565.

191. Mond HG. Sloman JG. The malfunctioning pacemaker system. *PACE* 1981;4:49–60.

192. Seltzer JP, Levine PA, Watson WS. Patient-initiated autonomous pacemaker tachycardia. *PACE* 1984;7:961–969.

193. Van Gelder LM, El Gamal MIH. Myopotential interference-inducing pacemaker tachycardia in a DVI programmed pacemaker. *PACE* 1984;7:970–972.

194. Lindenberg BS, Hagan CA, Levine PA. Design-dependent loss of telemetry: Uplink telemetry hold. *PACE* 1989;12: 823–826.

195. Levine PA, Lindenberg BS. Upper-rate-limit circuit-induced rate slowing. *PACE* 1987;10:310–314.

196. Barold SS. Missing atrial stimulus during DDD pacing. *PACE* 1995;18:1711–1712.

197. Levine PA, Lindenberg BS, Mace RC. Analysis of AV universal (DDD) pacemaker rhythms. *Clin Prog Pacing Electrophysiol* 1984;2:54–73.

198. Bertuso J, Kapoor A, Schafer J. A case of ventricular undersensing in the DDI mode: Cause and correction. *PACE* 1986;9:685–689.

199. Erlbacher JA, Stelzer P. Inappropriate ventricular blanking in a DDI pacemaker. *PACE* 1986;9:519–521.

200. Levine PA, Rihanek BD, Sanders R, et al. Cross-stimulation: The unexpected stimulation of the unpaced chamber. *PACE* 1985;8:600–606.

201. Freedman RA, Marks ML, Chapman P. Telemetered pacemaker battery voltage preceding generator elective replacement time: Use of guide utilization of magnet checks. *PACE* 1995;18:863.

202. Sholder JA, Levine PA, Mann BM, et al. Bidirectional telemetry and interrogation in cardiac pacing. In SS Barold, J Mugica (eds.), *The Third Decade of Cardiac Pacing: Advances in Technology and Clinical Applications.* Mount Kisco, NY: Futura, 1982; pp 145–166.

203. Tanaka S, Nanba T, Harada A, et al. Clinical experience with telemetry pacing systems and long-term follow-up: Clinical aspects of lead impedance and battery life. *PACE* 1983;6:A–30.

204. Castallenet M, Garza J, Shaners SP, et al. Telemetry of

programmed and measured data in pacing system evaluation and follow-up. *J Electrophysiol* 1987;1:360–375.

205. Clarke M, Allen A. Early detection of lead insulation breakdown. *PACE* 1985;8:775.

206. Winokur P, Falkenberg E, Gerrard G. Lead resistance telemetry: Insulation failure prognosticator. *PACE* 1985;8:A–85.

207. Schmindinger H, Mayer H, Kaliman J, et al. Early detection of lead complications by telemetric measurements of lead impedance. *PACE* 1985;8:A–23.

208. Levine PA, Sanders R, Markowitz HT. Pacemaker diagnostics: Measured data, event marker, electrogram and event counter telemetry. In K Ellenbogen, GN Kay, BL Wilkoff (eds.), *Clinical Cardiac Pacing*. Philadelphia: WB Saunders, 1995; pp 639–655.

209. Levine PA, Schuller H, Lindgren A. *Pacemaker ECG: Utilization of Pulse Generator Telemetry*. Solna, Sweden: Siemens-Elema AB Pacemaker Division, 1988.

210. Kruse I, Markowitz HT, Ryden L. Timing markers showing pacemaker behavior to aid in the follow-up of a physiologic pacemaker. *PACE* 1983;6:801–805.

211. Olson W, McConnell M, Sah R, et al. Pacemaker diagnostic diagrams. *PACE* 1985;8:691–700.

212. Furman S. The ECG interpretation channel (editorial). *PACE* 1990;13:225–226.

213. Levine PA. Pacemaker diagnostic diagrams (letter). *PACE* 1986;9:250.

214. Olson W, Goldreyer BA, Goldreyer BN. Computer-generated diagnostic diagrams for pacemaker rhythm analysis and pacing system evaluation. *J Electrophysiol* 1987;1:367–387.

215. Levine PA. The complementary role of electrogram, event marker and measured data in the assessment of pacing system function. *J Electrophysiol* 1987;1:404–416.

216. Strathmore NF, Mond HG. Noninvasive monitoring and testing of pacemaker function. *PACE* 1987;10:1359–1370.

217. Goldschalger N. After the implant: Principles of follow-up, Intel Reports. *Cardiac Pacing Electrophysiol* 1991;10:1–4.

218. Levine PA, Sholder J, Duncan JL. Clinical benefits of telemetered electrograms in the assessment of DDD function. *PACE* 1984;7:1170–1177.

219. Clarke M, Allen A. Use of telemetered electrograms in the

assessment of normal pacing system function. *J Electrophysiol* 1987;1:388–395.

220. Edery T. Clinical applications of pacemaker-telemetered intracardiac electrograms. *Technical Concept Paper.* Minneapolis: Medtronic Inc., 1991.

221. Hughes HC, Furman S, Brownlee RR, et al. Simultaneous atrial and ventricular electrogram transmission via a specialized single-lead system. *PACE* 1984;7:1195–1201.

222. Sarmiento JJ. Clinical utility of telemetered intracardiac electrograms in diagnosing a design-dependent lead malfunction. *PACE* 1990;13:188–195.

223. Luceri RM, Castellanos A, Thurer RJ. Telemetry of intracardiac electrograms: Applications in spontaneous and induced arrhythmias. *J Electrophysiol* 1987;1:414–424.

224. Pirolo JS, Tweddel JS, Brunt EM, et al. Influence of activation origin: Lead number and lead configuration on the noninvasive electrophysiologic detection of cardiac allograft rejection. *Circulation* 1991;84:III-344–III-354.

225. Nalos PC, Nytray W. Op. Cit. 1990.

226. Marco DD, Gallagher D. Noninvasive measurement of retrograde conduction times in pacemaker patients. *J Electrophysiol* 1987;1:388–394.

227. Gladstoe PJ, Duxbury GB, Berman ND. Arrhythmia diagnosis by electrogram telemetry: Involvement of dual-chamber pacemaker. *Chest* 1987;91:115–116.

228. Sanders R, Martin R, Frumin H, et al. Data storage and retrieval by implantable pacemakers for diagnostic purposes. *PACE* 1984;7:1228–1233.

229. Levine PA, Lindenberg BS. Diagnostic data: An aid to the follow-up and assessment of the pacing system. *J Electrophysiol* 1987;1:396–403.

230. Levine PA. *Utility and Clinical Benefits of Extensive Event Counter Telemetry in the Follow-up and Management of the Rate-Modulated Pacemaker Patient.* Sylmar, CA: Pacesetter Systems Inc., 1992.

231. Newman D, Dorian P, Downar E, et al. Use of telemetry functions in the assessment of implanted antitachycardia device efficiency. *Am J Cardiol* 1992;70:616–621.

232. Wang PJ, Manolis A, Clyne C, et al. Accuracy of classification using a data log system in implantable cardioverter defibrillators. *PACE* 1991;14:1911–1916.

233. Luceri RM, Puchferran RL, Brownstein SL, et al. Improved

patient surveillance and data acquisitioning with a third-generation implantable cardioverter defibrillator. *PACE* 1991;14:1870–1874.

234. Stangl K, Sichart U, Wirtzfeld A, et al. Holter functions for the enhancement of the diagnosis and therapeutic capabilities of implanted pacemakers: Vitatext. The Netherlands: Vitatron Medical Inc., 1987; pp 1–6.

235. Hayes DL, Higano ST, Eisinger G. Utility of rate histograms in programming and follow-up of a DDDR pacemaker. *Mayo Clin Proc* 1989;64:495–502.

236. Lascault GR, Frank R, Himbert C, et al. Pacemaker Holter function and monitoring atrial arrhythmias. *Eur JCPE* 1992;2:285–293.

237. Ahern T, Nydegger C, McCormick DJ, et al. Incidence and timing of activity parameter changes in activity-responsive pacing systems. *PACE* 1992;15:762–770.

238. Levine PA, Young GH. Heart rate distribution assessed with the long-term monitoring capability of an implanted pacemaker: Implications for programming. *PACE* 1995;18:1739.

Antitachycardia Pacing and the Implantable Cardioverter-Defibrillator

Michael R. Gold

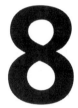

INTRODUCTION

The implantable cardioverter-defibrillator (ICD) has become standard therapy for the treatment of ventricular tachyarrhythmias. Clinical studies of these devices in humans began in 1980 and the Food and Drug Administration's (FDA) approval was granted in 1985. Since that time, annual implantation rates have increased more than 20-fold. The remarkable growth of the use of the ICD can be attributed both to the documented high efficacy in the prevention of sudden cardiac death[1,2] and to the disappointing outcomes and high arrhythmia recurrence rates with trials of antiarrhythmic drugs.[3,4]

The rapid increase and acceptance of the role of the ICD in the treatment of ventricular arrhythmias has been paralleled by an equally rapid evolution of technology. Initially, the pulse generators were large devices implanted in the abdomen and a thoracotomy was required for placement of defibrillation patches on the heart. The earliest versions of the ICD delivered only high-energy shocks to treat tachyarrhythmias and had simple counters to document activity. Now, thoracotomy is rarely needed as modern lead systems and improved shock waveforms allow for routine transvenous implantation. In addition, pulse generator size has been reduced sufficiently to permit pectoral placement, further simplifying the implantation process. All ICD systems at present have pacing capabilities and widely programmable shock therapy in addition to enhanced diagnostics and electrogram storage to facilitate therapy interpretation. In this chapter, the current use of the ICD will be summarized.

INDICATIONS

The indications for ICD implantation have not changed dramatically in the past decade. At present, implantation is approved for the treatment of cardiac arrest in the absence of reversible causes such as acute myocardial infarction, ischemia, or marked electrolyte imbalances. Other indications include sustained ventricular tachycardia and syncope that is thought to be secondary to a ventricular tachyarrhythmia.[5] The requirements for inducible sustained ventricular arrhythmias at electrophysiologic study or failure of multiple drug trials is no longer considered necessary for ICD placement. In fact, there has been a trend away from extensive electropharmacologic evaluation and toward earlier defibrillator placement. This appears to be a cost-effective approach for many high-risk patients.

Despite the documented efficacy of the ICD for the prevention of sudden cardiac death, only a minority of patients at risk for life-threatening arrhythmias meet present indications. This has led to the initiation of several studies evaluating prophylactic defibrillator use.[6] These include the evaluation of ICD use in patients with ischemic cardiomyopathy and nonsustained ventricular tachycardia (MUSTT and MADIT), in patients with left ventricular dysfunction and an abnormal signal-averaged electrocardiogram who are undergoing coronary artery bypass surgery (CABG Patch), and in patients with congestive heart failure (SCD-HEFT). These studies are evaluating ICD use in patients without a history of sustained arrhythmias and may increase the use of this technology if it is proven to be beneficial.

PULSE GENERATORS AND LEAD SYSTEMS

Early ICD pulse generators were relatively large and bulky. The size (115–145 cc) and weight (195–235 g) of these devices mandated abdominal implantation, typically in the left upper quadrant, either subcutaneously or under the rectus muscle. The surgical procedure for abdominal ICD implantation is more extensive than that for endocardial pacemakers in part because it requires tunneling leads from the chest. The abdominal location of the pulse generator and surgical procedure required is likely responsible for the higher complication rates observed with ICD implantation, particularly infection. Recently, however, pulse generator size has decreased significantly. With the downsizing of these devices (65–85 cc, 125–135 g) routine subcutaneous pectoral implantation is possible,[7] although the pulse generators are still significantly larger than pacemakers. This does not appear to be associated with any increased risk of complications, at least over the first year of follow-up.

Despite the large size of these early pulse generators, the battery life was only about two years. With improvement in battery design and reduction of monitoring circuit drain, the life span of many ICD pulse generators is now more than five years. This has obvious important implications for the cost-effectiveness of this therapy.[8]

There have been many changes in the programmability and internal circuitry of newer pulse generators. To assess ICD function, early defibrillators required placement of a temporary pacing catheter for arrhythmia induction. Now all pulse generators have noninvasive induction, most with the capabilities for programmed ventricular stimulation, greatly simplifying the testing process. The impedance and pacing thresholds of the ICD lead systems can be noninvasively measured as well, to aid in the monitoring of leads. The early pulse generators had only simple counters to document shocks. Now very detailed data logging is present, including precise measurements of arrhythmia rates, time of occurrence, and response to therapy. In addition, stored electrograms provide a recording of the arrhythmia at the time of device activity. This is most useful in assessing the appropriateness of therapy (i.e., shocks for atrial fibrillation vs. ventricular tachycardia) and any malfunctions of the system. Finally, the capacitors in the pulse generator need to be charged periodically to avoid very prolonged charging during spontaneous arrhythmias. Such capacitor reformation required office visits every 2 to 3 months for patients but is now performed automatically by the pulse generator.

The lead systems for sensing, pacing, and the delivery of shocks have also changed significantly over the past decade. Although transvenous defibrillation was developed by Mirowski in his pioneering studies of the ICD,[9] the initial commercial systems used epicardial sensing leads and patches placed on the heart. Subsequently, endocardial rate sensing leads and defibrillation coils were combined with epicardial patches as part of hybrid lead

431

systems. However, it was the development of integrated leads incorporating both rate-sensing electrodes and defibrillation coils that led to the routine use of nonthoracotomy lead systems. These have become the preferred lead system because a nonthoracotomy approach simplifies the surgical procedure, reducing perioperative complications compared with epicardial patch systems.[10–12] Initially, these leads were used with subcutaneous patches, but with the development of improved waveforms and with further experience with these leads, total transvenous lead systems have become the preferred approach to implantation. The pectoral placement of pulse generators allowed further improvement in lead technology because the pulse generator shell can serve as a subcutaneous electrode and actually become part of the lead system. The active pulse generator systems further simplify the implantation procedure while enhancing defibrillation efficacy.[13] A comparison of ICD lead systems is shown in Figure 8.1.

SENSING

A critical feature of proper ICD function is sensing. Appropriate sensing of ventricular fibrillation poses unique engineering challenges compared with sensing by pacemakers. Specifically, it is necessary to sense small amplitude signals to trigger therapy for tachyarrhythmias while not oversensing T waves or noise in sinus rhythm. For pacemakers, programmable fixed sensitivity can be used to sense ventricular electrograms (QRS complexes) reliably while not oversensing T waves. However, fixed sensitivity is inadequate for ICD systems because of the marked variability in electrogram amplitudes in different rhythms.[14] An example of the dangers of fixed sensitivity is shown in Figure 8.2. The patient is in ventricular fibrillation, but the ICD is treating the rhythm as asystole or bradycardia and responding with VVI pacing. This undersensing would obviously lead to cardiac arrest and likely death if not recognized and treated promptly.

To minimize undersensing, all present ICDs employ algorithms to change amplifier gain or sensitivity automatically. Following a sensed event, gain or sensitivity undergoes stepwise increases. The time course of the increase is designed to avoid oversensing of T waves while enabling sensitivity or gain to increase further to allow detection of small amplitude fibrillatory waves. Once a ventricular event is sensed, sensitivity or gain is decreased again. An example of automatic sensitivity is shown in

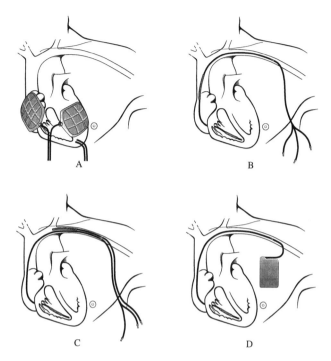

Figure 8.1 Schematic drawings of defibrillation lead system. (A) Epicardial system with two sensing leads on the left ventricle and patches on the left and right ventricles. (B) Integrated single-pass transvenous lead system (Endotak, Guidant Corp., St. Paul, MN) with a sensing electrode at the tip and two defibrillation coils, one in the right ventricle and the second at the right atrial-superior vena caval junction. (C) A two-lead transvenous lead system with bipolar sensing electrodes at the tip and coils in the right ventricle and superior vena cava. (D) Unipolar lead system (Medtronic Inc., Minneapolis, MN) with a right ventricular integrated lead (as in C) and an active pectoral pulse generator.

Figure 8.3. The automatic sensing algorithms have been shown to be extremely reliable.[12,15]

Despite automatic sensing algorithms, problems can still occur in several clinical situations. Redetection of ventricular fibrillation following a failed first shock can be prolonged particularly with integrated lead systems because the initial high-voltage shock results in diminished electrogram amplitudes, due to local "stunning" of myocardium from the large-voltage gradients near the defibrillation coils.

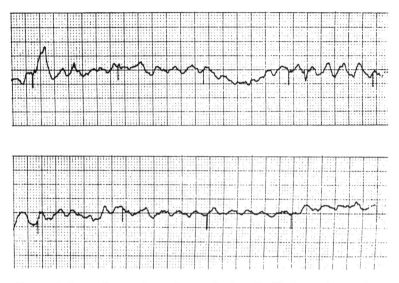

Figure 8.2 Undersensing of ventricular fibrillation. The patient had an ICD without automatic sensing and ventricular fibrillation developed while on telemetry monitor. Lower rate VVI pacing is noted, indicative of undersensing of ventricular fibrillation.

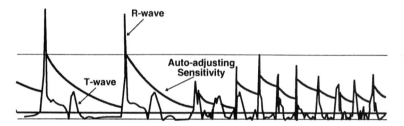

Figure 8.3 Automatic sensing algorithm. A schematic representation of automatic sensitivity during sinus rhythm and ventricular fibrillation. In sinus rhythm, sensitivity increases slowly to avoid oversensing T waves. However, with the onset of ventricular fibrillation, high sensitivity is maintained to minimize undersensing. (Reproduced with permission from Medtronic Inc., Minneapolis, MN.)

Another potential problem for ICD sensing occurs in patients with both pacemakers and defibrillators. Although less than 10 percent of patients require both devices, this poses a unique challenge for defibrillator sensing. Both undersensing and oversensing can occur due to device interactions. Frequently pacemakers will undersense ventricular fibrillation, resulting in lower rate asynchronous activity. Despite the inability to conduct impulses in ventricular fibrillation, the pacemaker spike can reset the sensitivity or gain of the ICD causing undersensing and delaying therapy. Oversensing can occur due to double or triple counting. This happens when both the pacemaker stimulus and the resulting conducted ventricular complex are sensed. For instance, with pacing at a rate of 90 beats/min, during moderate exercise and a rate-responsive pacemaker, the defibrillator may sense a rate of 180 beats/min and initiate a shock if both the stimulus artifact and ventricular electrogram are sensed. The short refractory periods of ICDs needed to sense rapid tachycardias make double counting possible. With dual-chamber pacemakers, the atrial stimulus, ventricular stimulus, and ventricular electrogram can all be sensed, which leads to triple counting.

To avoid pacemaker and defibrillator interactions, lead tips should be separated anatomically as much as possible, unipolar pacing avoided, and pacemaker outputs minimized. For early ICD systems, this often meant placing epicardial sensing leads on the left ventricle with standard endocardial pacemakers. However, with transvenous defibrillation leads such separation cannot be achieved as both pacing and defibrillation sensing leads are in the right ventricle. Nevertheless, these devices can be used safely if appropriate evaluation for interactions is performed.[16] This evaluation involves high output asynchronous pacemaker pacing during defibrillator testing. The defibrillator is monitored for double or triple counting during paced rhythms. In addition, it is mandatory to show appropriate detection of ventricular fibrillation despite pacing.[17]

PACING

As noted previously, all modern defibrillators have pacing capabilities. This always includes bradycardia pacing, and in many models antitachycardia pacing is also present. At this time, only ventricular pacing is available in ICD systems. For bradycardia pacing, VVI mode used as rate-responsive pacing is not available. Dual-chamber pacing capabilities are planned in future pulse generators. Frequent pacing is undesirable because it results in significant battery depletion and shortens the life span of these expensive devices. It may also be hemodynamically unfavorable, potentially leading to pacemaker syndrome or atrial arrhythmias, and can cause sensing problems. Pacing is most useful in patients with infrequent bradycardia or pauses after defibrillator shocks. If more frequent pacing is needed, then implantation of a separate pacemaker is usually preferred.

Antitachycardia pacing is used for the treatment of ventricular tachycardia. Pacing in this setting is useful only in the termination of reentrant arrhythmias. Evidence for reentry is the ability to initiate and terminate tachycardia with programmed stimulation and the demonstration of entrainment. The other mechanisms of tachycardia include enhanced automaticity and triggered activity. However, reentry is believed to be the predominant mechanism of monomorphic ventricular tachycardia, particularly in patients with ischemic heart disease.[18]

The pacing algorithms used to terminate ventricular tachycardia are adaptive; that is, the pacing rate is based on the tachycardia rate. For instance, the defibrillator can be programmed to deliver a train of stimuli at 85 percent of the cycle length of the tachycardia. This avoids the low efficacy rates of underpacing and reduces the incidence of pacing too rapidly and accelerating the tachycardia. Either burst or ramp pacing can be used. With burst pacing, the pacing rate or cycle length in the train is constant; with ramp pacing each successive paced beat has a shortened coupling interval. Examples of burst and ramp pacing to terminate ventricular tachycardia are shown in Figure 8.4. Randomized studies comparing these pacing modes have indicated that they have similar efficacies in terminating ventricular tachycardia and that both can cause acceleration and destabilization of rhythms.[19,20] Although testing of pacing algorithms with ventricular tachycardia induction is routinely performed, pace termination of spontaneous rhythms is more successful than that of induced rhythms. In fact, about 90 percent of spontaneous episodes of ventricular tachycardia can be pace terminated.[19-21]

There is considerable flexibility in the programming of ICD pulse generators for antitachycardia pacing. Typically, the number of trains of stimuli, the number of pulses in each train, the adaptive rates of pacing, the mode of stimulation (burst vs. ramp), and the stimulus output can be programmed in pacing algorithms. Moreover, different pacing schemes can be delivered in succession. An example of pacing schemes in a single patient is shown in Figure 8.5, in which burst followed by ramp pacing is delivered for slow tachycardias (150–190 beats/min) but only ramp pacing is used for rapid tachycardias. Care must be taken to avoid prolonged pacing

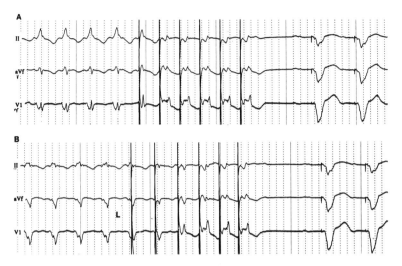

Figure 8.4 Antitachycardia pacing of ventricular tachycardia. Examples of burst (A) and ramp (B) pacing to terminate tachycardia in a patient. Note that the morphology and rate of ventricular tachycardia differ in two episodes in the same patient, illustrating the utility of adaptive rate pacing from the ICD. Bradycardia pacing is present at the termination of ventricular tachycardia.

during rapid or poorly tolerated arrhythmias. If pacing is unsuccessful, the efficacy of more definitive shock therapy may be compromised. For this reason, the duration of pacing can be limited in many ICDs (ATP Time-Out, Figure 8.5). Despite the theoretical concerns of the risks of failed antitachycardia pacing, there is no evidence of increased mortality with pulse generators with this capability.

DEFIBRILLATION

The primary and most important function of an ICD system is to terminate life-threatening rhythms with shocks. Shocks are achieved by capacitive discharges from the pulse generator. As such, they are exponentially declining waveforms that are terminated before full discharge or truncated in all ICD systems. The waveform for pulse generators used initially was a positive pulse that was truncated at 35 percent of the initial voltage. This is also known as a 65 percent tilt monophasic shock because only 65 percent of the initial voltage is delivered and the pulse had only one component

437

VT-1 Zone		

Initial detection:		
Rate Range	150 to 190 bpm	
Interval	400 to 316 ms	
Duration	7.0 sec	
Onset	19 %	
And/Or	AND	
Stability		
Inhibit if unstable	20 ms	
SRD	0:40 min:sec	

Redetection:	
Redetect Duration	1.0 sec
Post-Shock Duration	2.0 sec
Post-Shock Stability	22 ms
Post-Shock SRD	0:25 min:sec

ATP Therapy:	ATP1	ATP2
Scheme	Scan	Ramp/Scan
Number of Bursts	5	4
Pulses per Burst:		
Initial	5	6
Increment	1	1
Maximum	9	8
Coupling Interval	88 %	84 %
C.I. Decrement	0 ms	0 ms
Burst Cycle Length	81 %	84 %
Ramp Decrement	0 ms	10 ms
Scan Decrement	10 ms	10 ms
Minimum Interval	220 ms	220 ms
ATP Time-Out	1:00 min:sec	

Shock Therapy:	
Shock 1 Energy	1 J
Shock 2 Energy	10 J
Max Shock Energy	34 J

VT Zone		

Initial detection:		
Rate Range	190 to 240 bpm	
Interval	316 to 250 ms	
Duration	5.0 sec	
Stability		
Shock if unstable	18 ms	

Redetection:	
Redetect Duration	1.0 sec
Post-Shock Duration	1.0 sec

ATP Therapy:	ATP1	ATP2
Scheme	Ramp/Scan	Disabled
Number of Bursts	5	--
Pulses per Burst:		
Initial	6	--
Increment	0	--
Maximum	6	--
Coupling Interval	88 %	--
C.I. Decrement	8 ms	--
Burst Cycle Length	84 %	--
Ramp Decrement	6 ms	--
Scan Decrement	0 ms	--
Minimum Interval	220 ms	--
ATP Time-Out	0:30 min:sec	

Shock Therapy:	
Shock 1 Energy	10 J
Shock 2 Energy	25 J
Max Shock Energy	34 J

Figure 8.5 An example of programmed pacing parameters for ventricular tachycardia for an ICD (PRx III, Guidant Corp., St. Paul, MN). There are two zones for ventricular tachycardia. Burst and then ramp pacing is attempted; if tachycardia persists, low-energy cardioversion is performed in the lower rate zone (VT-1). Ramp pacing and then higher energy shocks are delivered in the upper rate zone (VT).

(Figure 8.6). The maximal shock that could be delivered was about 750 volts or 35 joules. For epicardial lead systems with two large patches, successful defibrillation could be achieved in nearly all patients with at least a 10-joule safety margin. Such a safety margin is considered necessary because implantation is performed under optimal conditions of a well-compensated patient under general anesthesia. At times of cardiac arrest, there are often electrolyte abnormalities, active ischemia, or decompensated congestive heart

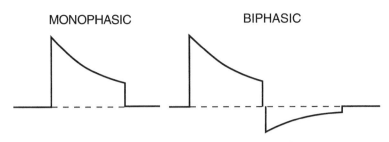

MONOPHASIC   BIPHASIC

Figure 8.6   Schematic representation of defibrillation waveforms. The time course of the delivered voltage for monophasic and biphasic shocks is shown. Note that shock waveforms are truncated, exponentially declining pulses.

failure, which would hinder defibrillation. In patients implanted with a safety margin less than 10 joules, sudden death remains high.[22] However, with an adequate defibrillation threshold, sudden death mortality is remarkably low, about 1 percent per year, in this high-risk patient population.[1,2,12,15] It is noteworthy that much less energy is required to cardiovert ventricular tachycardia compared with ventricular fibrillation (Figure 8.7). However, cardioversion is no more successful than antitachycardia pacing[23] and is often painful at the typical energies needed (≥ 0.5 joules). Consequently, cardioversion is rarely the primary therapy for monomorphic ventricular tachycardia that is hemodynamically tolerated.

Compared with epicardial patches, defibrillation thresholds are higher with nonthoracotomy lead systems.[12,24] The initial studies of these leads demonstrated an adequate defibrillation safety margin or satisfactory DFT with simple two-coil lead systems in only about one-half of patients.[25–27] With the addition of a subcutaneous patch, implantation success rates of 71 to 86 percent were reported.[26–30] The lowering of defibrillation thresholds with a subcutaneous patch is due to both a reduction of shock impedance resulting in higher peak currents and an improved current vector incorporating the left ventricle.

Despite the use of a subcutaneous patch and a three-lead configuration, thoracotomy was still required in about 20 percent of patients. The predictors of high defibrillation thresholds requiring thoracotomy were measures of cardiomegaly and increased cardiac mass by x-ray or echocardiography or the use of antiarrhythmic drugs at implantation, particularly amiodarone. Left ventricular ejection fraction does not correlate with defibrillation thresholds.[26,29,30]

439

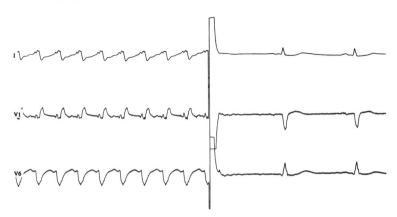

Figure 8.7 An example of low-energy cardioversion (0.5 joules) for the termination of ventricular tachycardia. The shock is shown by the high voltage artifact on the electrocardiographic recordings, which was followed by the restoration of sinus rhythm.

The need for thoracotomy has virtually been eliminated with further improvements in lead systems and waveforms. The testing of multiple lead configurations including defibrillation coils in the coronary sinus as well as placing the subcutaneous patch more posterior in an axillary position can enhance defibrillation efficacy.[25,31,32] Furthermore, the polarity of the defibrillation shock is an important determinant of defibrillation threshold. Traditionally, the right ventricular coil of a transvenous lead system was used as the cathode. However, by reversing polarity, or making the right ventricular coil the anode, defibrillation thresholds are decreased about 30 percent.[33] Our experience at the University of Maryland has been that an adequate defibrillation threshold for implantation can be achieved with a single, dual-coil lead in about 75 percent of patients with polarity reversal.

Although lead configuration, position, and shock polarity significantly affect defibrillation efficacy, it is the development of biphasic waveforms that has had the greatest impact on the success of transvenous defibrillation. With biphasic shocks, the polarity of the shock is reversed at the termination of the initial phase of the pulse and a second phase is delivered. In other words, the truncated positive phase is followed by a negative phase (see Figure 8.6). No additional battery voltage or stored energy is needed to deliver biphasic waveforms. The superiority of biphasic shocks has been consistently demonstrated with multiple waveforms and lead systems.[24,27,34-36] A paired comparison of monophasic and biphasic defibrillation thresholds in the same patients is shown in Figure 8.8. The benefit of biphasic shocks is not simply due to the delivery of the optimal polarity in each patient, as these waveforms are superior to the optimal monophasic waveform as shown in Figure 8.7. Despite the consistent observation across all lead systems that biphasic waveforms improve defibrillation efficacy, the mechanism for this effect is not well understood.

With biphasic shocks, transvenous defibrillation is adequate in >90 percent of patients, and with a subcutaneous patch or array, success rates >98 percent are achieved. As noted above, with the downsizing of pulse generators, pectoral implantation can be undertaken. In the left pectoral position the pulse generator shell can serve as an electrode for defibrillation. These active pulse generator lead systems are highly effective. With a single right ventricle coil, an adequate defibrillation threshold with this "unipolar" lead can be achieved in 98 percent of patients.[37] Again, left ventricular mass, not ejection fraction, is a predictor of defibrillation efficacy. With

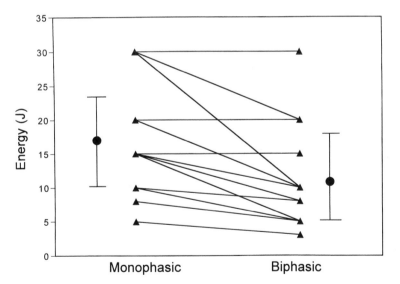

Figure 8.8 Paired comparisons of monophasic (65 percent tilt) and biphasic (60 percent first-phase tilt and 50 percent second-phase tilt) defibrillation thresholds in 20 patients. Reverse shock polarity was used with the right ventricular coil as the anode. Biphasic shocks significantly reduced defibrillation thresholds (18 ± 8 joules vs. 12 ± 7 joules, *p* < 0.01).

a dual-coil lead and an active shell, defibrillation thresholds are sufficiently low to consider pulse generators with lower maximal output and smaller capacitance, thus reducing device size because the two largest components in a pulse generator are the batteries and capacitors. Reducing capacitance does not affect the stored energy needed for defibrillation, although peak voltage at defibrillation threshold increases modestly.[38,39] Moreover, decreasing the pulse generator size has little effect on defibrillation thresholds with a unipolar lead system.[40] Thus, with the combination of efficient transvenous lead systems and an active pulse generator shell, implantable defibrillators may approach the size of pacemakers.

In all the measures of defibrillation efficacy mentioned above, assessment was performed at the time of lead implantation. With epicardial patch systems, defibrillation thresholds are stable over time and rise significantly only with the institution of anti-arrhythmic drug therapy.[41,42] However, with transvenous leads there is a significant rise of monophasic thresholds over the first six months. This can occasionally result in an inadequate safety margin requiring lead revision. Whether a similar rise occurs with biphasic shocks or active pulse generator lead systems is unknown.[43,44]

ICD IMPLANTATION

The implantation of an ICD system has changed dramatically with the development of nonthoracotomy lead systems. This has become the sole implantation approach in patients not undergoing concomitant cardiac surgery because, compared with epicardial patch systems, the placement of nonthoracotomy leads reduces surgical morbidity, mortality, duration of hospitalization, and costs.[10–12,45] The lead systems can be implanted safely by electrophysiologists, often without the use of an operating room or general anesthesia.[46–48] With the further simplification of lead systems and the downsizing of pulse generators to facilitate a subcutaneous pectoral approach, the implantation of an ICD system will approach that of a permanent pacemaker.

Whether implanted in an operating room or in an electrophysiology laboratory, and whether general anesthesia or conscious sedation is employed, the basic concepts of ICD surgery are the same. Meticulous sterile technique must be used and patients must receive perioperative intravenous antibiotics. The antibiotics chosen should provide adequate activity against *Staphylococcus* species, as these are the most common bacteria associated with device infections. Typically, vancomycin or a cephalosporin is used. A physiologic recorder is necessary for monitoring electrophysiologic signals, and heart rhythm, blood pressure, and respiration must be monitored. This can either be performed invasively with an arterial line and intubation or with electrocardiographic monitoring, a brachial cuff, and oximetry. Finally, the patient should be connected to a transthoracic defibrillator with skin pads for backup protection during defibrillation testing.

Unless contraindicated by a pacemaker, AV fistula, venous anomaly, severe dermatologic conditions, or scarring, a left-sided approach is preferred. Cutdown to the cephalic vein may be preferable to subclavian puncture to reduce the incidence of subclavian crush observed with these large leads. The transvenous defibrillator leads are implanted in the same fashion as pacemaker leads. Depending on the lead system employed (see Figure 8.1), this may entail one lead with the tip in the right ventricle or two leads. Adequate sensing (R waves >8mV) and pacing (threshold <1.0V) in sinus rhythm needs to be established.

Acute defibrillation testing is performed to ensure an adequate safety margin for the treatment of spontaneous arrhythmias. There are many testing algorithms to assess defibrillation efficacy, but typically the first shock is set to 10 joules less than the maximal output of the device. Ventricular fibrillation is induced by pacing through the right ventricular electrode, alternating current stimulation, or low-energy shock on the T wave. After an appropriate time in the ventricular arrhythmia to mimic sensing and charging of a pulse generator (about 10 sec), a shock is delivered. If this shock fails, a high-output internal or transthoracic shock should be given immediately for arrhythmia termination. If the first shock is successful, it can be repeated at the same energy for minimal testing to establish adequate acute defibrillation efficacy. Alternatively, shock energy can be decreased progressively on each trial until a missed first shock to establish a defibrillation threshold.[49] At least two minutes should be allowed between defibrillation episodes to allow full hemodynamic recovery and minimize any cumulative effects of multiple shocks. Acute defibrillation testing is performed with an external defibrillator that delivers identical shocks as the pulse generator. Other testing algorithms involving assessing shock energies to induce ventricular fibrillation (upper limit of vulnerability),[50] lower initial shock energies (binary search), and device-based testing are being evaluated to simplify acute testing.

If an adequate safety margin cannot be demonstrated, further testing is necessary. The simplest change is to reverse the polarity of the shocks. Other changes that can be made include repositioning leads, particularly if a second coil is part of the system, or placement of a subcutaneous patch or array. Once defibrillation testing is completed, the pulse generator is connected to the leads and normal ICD function is demonstrated. This includes sensing, pacing, and defibrillation, so one additional defibrillation trial is performed. It is noteworthy that pacing and sensing thresholds often rise modestly following defibrillation testing. If the lead system is otherwise functioning normally and no gross macroscopic movement is noted fluoroscopically, lead repositioning is not necessary for 10 to 40 percent changes of threshold measurements.

ICD PROGRAMMING

Appropriate programming of the pulse generator is critical for proper function. There are many programmable parameters in modern ICD systems, and this presents a challenge to optimize therapy. Bradycardia pacing is programmed to provide rate support either at rest or following shocks. As noted previously, only the VVI mode is available with current pulse generators. The rate is programmed as low as possible to minimize pacing, which depletes the ICD battery, and to avoid sensing problems during pacing. Typically, rates of 35 to 50 beats/min are used.

For patients with ventricular fibrillation as their clinical arrhythmia, only a single tachycardia zone is necessary. The rate cutoff is usually programmed above 170 beats/min to avoid shocks for sinus tachycardia and atrial fibrillation, but below 210 beats/min to avoid delays in therapy with undersensing of ventricular fibrillation. The first shock delivered should be at least 10 joules above the defibrillation threshold. Subsequent shocks are usually at maximal output. Of note, all pulse generators deliver only a finite number of consecutive shocks, typically four to seven, to avoid battery depletion due to inappropriate therapy secondary to atrial arrhythmias or lead malfunction. If therapy is for ventricular fibrillation, additional shocks are unlikely to be of benefit. Some pulse generators can also be programmed for committed or noncommitted shocks. Committed shocks indicate that therapy will be delivered when detection criteria are met, even if the arrhythmia terminates spontaneously. This is useful for patients with ventricular fibrillation when undersensing may result in a delay of therapy. With noncommitted shocks, arrhythmia monitoring continues during charging, and the shock is not delivered if the arrhythmia terminates spontaneously. Noncommitted shocks are preferable in patients with nonsustained ventricular tachycardia and atrial fibrillation. In general, unless sensing of ventricular fibrillation is problematic, then noncommitted shocks should be used.

For patients with spontaneous or inducible ventricular tachycardia, multiple tachycardia zones can be programmed. All new pulse generators have tiered therapy; that is, different therapies are initiated for different arrhythmia rates. The rate cutoff should be at least 15 beats/min less than the rate of inducible arrhythmias because spontaneous arrhythmias tend to be slower than those initiated with programmed stimulation. To improve diagnostic accuracy, enhanced detection algorithms are available in tachycardia zones such as sudden onset or stability. Programming of sudden onset will prevent therapy for a gradual increase in heart rate consistent with sinus tachycardia during exercise. With the stability feature, programmed therapy is withheld for irregular cycle lengths consistent with atrial fibrillation. If enhanced detection algorithms are activated, then testing of their response during ventricular tachycardia should be tested whenever possible.

COMPLICATIONS

Complications associated with ICD implantation remain a significant problem. With the advent of nonthoracotomy lead systems, serious perioperative complications have been reduced, although lead-related problems may be increased (Table 8.1). Mortality associated with ICD implantation is about 1 percent when a nonthoracotomy approach is employed.[12,15] This may be reduced further with improvements in shock waveforms and lead systems to simplify the implantation, reduce the number of defibrillation trials needed, and shorten surgical times. Other serious perioperative complications such as myocardial infarction and stroke occur in less than 1 percent of procedures.

Infection remains an important problem associated with ICD placement. Reported infection rates are 0 to 4.0 percent with nonthoracotomy ICD systems.[12,15,26,28,29,51] These overall rates are significantly higher than rates for patients with pacemakers. The reasons for this difference are unclear but may be related to longer procedure times and abdominal pulse generator placement associated with ICD implantation. It is noteworthy that infection rates

Table 8.1 ICD Complications

Inappropriate or asymptomatic shocks
Presentation
  Asymptomatic but appropriate due to sustained VT
  Asymptomatic but appropriate due to committed device and nonsustained VT
  SVT; atrial fibrillation; atrial flutter; PAT
  T-wave oversensing; P-wave oversensing
  Sensing of single- or dual-chamber pacing spikes during DDD or VVI pacing
  Sinus tachycardia
  Lead or adaptor failure due to fracture of insulation breakdown; loose set screws; lead dislodgment near the tricuspid valve
Response
  Inactivate device while the patient is being continuously monitored; make a diagnosis

Failure to deliver therapy
Presentation
  Inability to sense VT/VF due to lead or adaptor problems; inappropriate programming of sensitivity or detection algorithm; undersensing due to pacemaker spikes
  Slowing of tachycardia by antiarrhythmic drugs below rate cutoff
Response
  Reprogram device or deliver appropriate therapy immediately (e.g., cardioversion or more antiarrhythmic drugs)

Ineffective therapy
Presentation
  Outside interference and inhibition of ICD
  Inadvertent device deactivation or device shutdown
  Fracture of patch or defibrillation coil
  Device end of life
  Rise in defibrillation threshold due to drugs or change in substrate
Response
  Deliver appropriate therapy as if device were not present

are similar with abdominal pulse generator replacements or new implants. Infection rates will likely decline with routine pectoral pulse generator use and simplification of lead systems. Superficial cellulitis associated with ICD placement can often be treated with intravenous antibiotics and local wound care. However, deep infections involving the pulse generator pocket or leads require removal of the whole ICD system.

ICD pulse generators are extremely reliable and component

malfunctions are rare. Other problems associated with pulse generator placement include seroma and hematoma formation. A seroma is diagnosed clinically by the formation of a fluid collection in the pulse generator pocket in the absence of signs of infection or ecchymosis. Typically this develops within the first month postoperatively and can be managed conservatively with restricted mobility and pressure dressings. Prophylactic antibiotics are given only if there is discharge and thus a risk of superficial contamination. Hematoma is diagnosed by a fluid collection with ecchymosis. A small hematoma can also be managed conservatively, but a large hematoma, particularly if rapidly expanding, indicates active bleeding. These fluid collections should be explored. Needle aspiration of any ICD pocket fluid collection should be avoided because it increases the infection risk and only rarely is therapeutic. Hematoma formation is often associated with anticoagulation so full anticoagulation should be avoided for 48 hours postoperatively, if possible.

Mechanical complications associated with ICD leads remain a common problem. Early lead dislodgment has been reported in up to 10 percent of transvenous implantations[29,31,51–53] but very infrequently with epicardial leads. This was most frequent with coils in the coronary sinus, which fortunately are rarely needed with present pulse generators using biphasic shocks. With integrated leads placed in the right ventricle, dislodgment rates less than 2 percent have been noted. Many of these problems are due to poor anchoring at the subclavian or cephalic vein insertion site. With more secure anchoring, primarily with two lead sleeves and interposed loose lead for tension relief, dislodgment rates are very low. With these relatively large integrated leads subclavian thrombosis can occur. Subclavian thrombosis associated with ipsilateral arm swelling is treated with anticoagulation.

Mechanical lead problems resulting in oversensing have been observed in 1.5 to 3.5 percent of ICD systems.[52,54–57] Oversensing presents clinically as multiple asymptomatic shocks (Figure 8.9). This complication rate may be even higher when connectors are used between the lead and pulse generator and are observed with comparable frequency for epicardial and transvenous leads.[56] The most common problem is sensing lead insulation breaks, which typically occur distally near the pulse generator. The incidence of these problems is much greater when these leads are used as part of ICD systems than in pacemaker systems, despite similar design and construction. The mechanisms for this high complication rate are

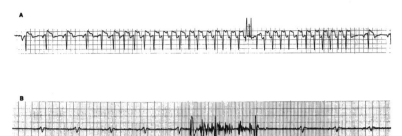

Figure 8.9 Stored electrograms during ICD activity. (A) Electrogram during a short episode of atrial flutter. The arrhythmia was detected but no shock was delivered because the pulse generator was programmed to the noncommitted mode. The patient had received multiple other shocks for longer episodes of atrial fibrillation and flutter. Note the unchanged electrogram morphology (QRS complex) indicative of a supraventricular arrhythmia and the atrial activity in both sinus rhythm and atrial flutter that can be observed with far-field electrograms that are recording signals between the atrial and ventricular coils. **(B)** Noise due to an insulation break from an electrogram from the rate sensing bipolar lead (near field). The patient experienced multiple shocks without preceding symptoms and a shock in sinus rhythm was documented.

probably related to the mechanical stresses placed on the lead by the abdominal cavity, tunneling, and the heavy pulse generator.[57] Mechanical problems will likely decrease by avoiding connectors, by not coiling excess lead under the pulse generator, and with pectoral placement of downsized pulse generators. With large integrated leads, insulation breaks can also occur at the subclavian insertion site. This subclavian crush syndrome may be reduced with cephalic vein access.[58]

Defibrillation patches are also subjected to mechanical stresses that can cause dislodgment, albeit at a lower rate than with transvenous leads. Crinkling can occur, which decreases the effective lead surface area and may compromise defibrillation function. Finally, with subcutaneous patches, hematoma formation has been reported, often associated with early postoperative anticoagulation.[28]

FOLLOW-UP

The follow-up of patients after ICD implantation includes both perioperative and chronic care. The initial postoperative care involves cardiac monitoring with frequent assessment of vital signs similar to that done with other procedures in sedated or anesthetized patients. Traditionally a predischarge ICD test is performed with the induction of ventricular tachyarrhythmias. However, with patients often being discharged within 24 hours following transvenous pectoral implants, the utility and feasibility of this test are less clear. At a minimum, sensing and pacing should be documented to rule out a macroscopic lead dislodgment, and the wound should be inspected. Patients are instructed on wound care and to restrict activity during the initial postoperative period. Normal activity can be resumed after the initial follow-up visit. However, motor vehicle driving is often restricted for six months following episodes of syncope or cardiac arrest. The initial follow-up visit is two to four weeks postimplantation and is primarily for wound assessment. Thereafter, patients are seen routinely every three to six months for ICD evaluation. This usually entails interrogation of the pulse generator and assessment of battery status, lead impedance, pacing thresholds, and sensing. In addition to the medical assessment of the patient, many electrophysiology services have organized ICD support groups to provide education and emotional support.

For patients with a lot of device activity, more frequent evaluations are needed. Patients should be instructed to report multiple device discharges immediately. The history preceding device firings can be useful in determining the arrhythmia involved. Asymptomatic discharges during extreme exertion are suggestive of sinus tachycardia, while syncope and near syncope are most likely associated with ventricular tachyarrhythmias. Often no clear prodrome or change of activity occurred before shocks. In these instances, the advanced data logging capabilities, and particularly stored electrograms, are very useful.[59,60] Examples of stored electrograms during tachycardia detection during atrial flutter and with oversensing due to an insulation break in the ICD sensing lead are shown in Figure 8.9. Obviously, a correct arrhythmia determination is necessary to treat frequent device activity appropriately.

SUMMARY

There have been remarkable changes in ICD therapy during the past 10 years. Integrated lead systems, which include pacing, rate sensing, and defibrillation elements, are reliable and efficacious. With improvement in shock waveforms, primarily with the use of biphasic shocks and an active pectoral pulse generator, total transvenous systems can be implanted in virtually all patients. The downsizing of pulse generators and improvement of lead design allow the simplicity of defibrillator implantation to approach that of pacemakers. Routine outpatient ICD implantation is now possible and will increase in frequency only if prophylactic trials of defibrillators prove beneficial. With advanced data logging and stored electrograms, the art of shock interpretation has been replaced by a detailed characterization of arrhythmias. With further advances in lead technology and arrhythmia-discrimination algorithms, the efficacy and reliability of therapy should improve further.

REFERENCES

1. Lehmann MH, Steinman RT, Schuger CD, Jackson K. The automatic implantable cardioverter defibrillator as antiarrhythmic treatment modality of choice for survivors of cardiac arrest unrelated to acute myocardial infarction. *Am J Cardiol* 1988;62:803–805.
2. Winkle RA, Mead RH, Ruder MA, et al. Long-term outcome with the automatic implantable cardioverter-defibrillator. *J Am Coll Cardiol* 1989;13:1353–1361.
3. Steinbeck G, Andersen D, Bach P, et al. A comparison of electrophysiologically guided antiarrhythmic drug therapy with beta-blocker therapy in patients with symptomatic, sustained ventricular tachyarrhythmias. *N Engl J Med* 1992;327:987–992.
4. Mason JW. A comparison of electrophysiologic testing with holter monitoring to predict antiarrhythmic-drug efficacy for ventricular tachyarrhythmias. *N Engl J Med* 1993;329:445–451.
5. Dreifus LS, Fisch C, Griffin JC, et al. Guidelines for implantation of cardiac pacemakers and antiarrhythmia devices. *J Am Coll Cardiol* 1991;18:1–13.
6. Buxton AE, Fisher JD, Josephson ME, et al. Prevention of sudden death in patients with coronary artery disease: The multicenter unsustained tachycardia trial (MUSTT). *Prog Cardiovasc Dis* 1993;36:215–226.
7. Stanton MS, Hayes DL, Munger TM, et al. Consistent subcutaneous prepectoral implantation of a new implantable cardioverter defibrillator. *Mayo Clin Proc* 1994;69:309–314.
8. Larsen GC, Manolis AS, Sonnenberg FA, et al. Cost-effectiveness of the implantable cardioverter-defibrillator: Ef-

fect of improved battery life and comparison with amiodarone therapy. *J Am Coll Cardiol* 1992;19:1323–1334.

9. Mirowski M, Mower MM, Gott VL, Brawley RK. Feasibility and effectiveness of low-energy catheter defibrillation in man. *Circulation* 1973:47:79–85.

10. Saksena S. The PCD Investigators. Defibrillation thresholds and perioperative mortality associated with endocardial and epicardial defibrillation lead systems. *PACE* 1993;16:202–207.

11. Kleman JM, Castle LW, Kidwell GA, et al. Nonthoracotomy-versus thoracotomy-implantable defibrillators. Intention-to-treat comparison of clinical outcomes. *Circulation* 1994;90: 2833–2842.

12. Zipes DP, Roberts D. Results of the international study of the implantable pacemaker cardioverter-defibrillator. A comparison of epicardial and endocardial lead systems. *Circulation* 1995;92:59–65.

13. Bardy GH, Johnson G, Poole JE, et al. A simplified, single-lead unipolar transvenous cardioversion-defibrillation system. *Circulation* 1993;88:543–547.

14. Singer I, Adams L, Austin E. Potential hazards of fixed gain sensing and arrhythmia reconfirmation for implantable cardioverter defibrillators. *PACE* 1993;16:1070–1079.

15. Hauser RG, Kurschinski DT, McVeigh K, et al. Clinical results with nonthoracotomy ICD systems. *PACE* 1993;16: 141–148.

16. Blanck Z, Niazi I, Axtell K, et al. Feasibility of concomitant implantation of permanent transvenous pacemaker and defibrillator systems. *Am J Cardiol* 1994;74:1249–1253.

17. Clemo HF, Ellenbogen DA, Belz MK, et al. Safety of pacemaker implantation in patients with transvenous (nonthoracotomy) implantable cardioverter defibrillators. *PACE* 1994;17:2285–2291.

18. Josephson ME, Almendral JM, Buxton AE, et al. Mechanisms of ventricular tachycardia. *Circulation* 1987;75:III-41–III-47.

19. Gillis AM, Leitch JW, Sheldon RS, et al. A prospective randomized comparison of autodecremental pacing to burst pacing in device therapy for chronic ventricular tachycardia secondary to coronary artery disease. *Am J Cardiol* 1993; 72:1146–1151.

20. Newman D, Dorian P, Hardy J. Randomized controlled comparison of antitachycardia pacing algorithms for termination of ventricular tachycardia. *J Am Coll Cardiol* 1993;21:1413–1418.

21. Trappe H-J, Fieguth H-G, Pftizner P, et al. Epicardial and nonthoracotomy defibrillation lead systems combined with a cardioverter defibrillator. *PACE* 1995;18:127–132.

22. Epstein AE, Ellenbogen KA, Kirk KA, et al. Clinical characteristics and outcomes of patients with high defibrillation thresholds: A multicenter study. *Circulation* 1992;86:1206–1216.

23. Bardy GH, Poole JE, Kudenchuk PJ, et al. A prospective randomized repeat-crossover comparison of antitachycardia pacing with low-energy cardioversion. *Circulation* 1993; 98:1889–1896.

24. Bardy GH, Troutman C, Johnson G, et al. Electrode system influence on biphasic waveform defibrillation efficacy in humans. *Circulation* 1991;84:665–671.

25. Jordaens L, Trouerbach J-W, Vertongen P, et al. Experience of cardioverter-defibrillators inserted without thoracotomy: evaluation of transvenously inserted intracardiac leads alone or with a subcutaneous axillary patch. *Br Heart J* 1993;69:14–19.

26. Brooks R, Garan H, Torchiana D, et al. Determinants of successful nonthoracotomy cardioverter-defibrillator implantation: Experience in 101 patients using two different lead systems. *J Am Coll Cardiol* 1993;22:1835–1842.

27. Block M, Hammel D, Bocker D, et al. A prospective randomized cross-over comparison of mono- and biphasic defibrillation using nonthoracotomy lead configurations in humans. *J Cardiovasc Electrophysiol* 1994;5:581–590.

28. Block M, Hammel D, Isbruch F, et al. Results and realistic expectations with transvenous lead systems. *PACE* 1992;15: 665–670.

29. Sra JS, Natale A, Axtell K, et al. Experience with two different nonthoracotomy systems for implantable defibrillator in 170 patients. *PACE* 1994;17:1741–1750.

30. Kopp DE, Blakeman BP, Kall JG, et al. Predictors of defibrillation energy requirements with nonepicardial lead systems. *PACE* 1995;18:253–260.

31. Bardy GH, Hofer B, Johnson G, et al. Implantable transvenous cardioverter-defibrillators. *Circulation* 1993;87:1152–1168.

32. Saksena S, DeGroot P, Krol RB, et al. Low-energy endocardial defibrillation using an axillary or a pectoral thoracic electrode location. *Circulation* 1993;88:2655–2660.

33. Strickberger SA, Hummel JD, Horwood LE, et al. Effect of shock polarity on ventricular defibrillation threshold using a transvenous lead system. *J Am Coll Cardiol* 1994;24:1069–1072.

34. Saksena S, An H, Mehra R, et al. Prospective comparison of biphasic and monophasic shocks for implantable cardioverter-defibrillators using endocardial leads. *Am J Cardiol* 1992;70:304–310.

35. Wyse DG, Kavanagh KM, Gillis AM, et al. Comparison of biphasic and monophasic shocks for defibrillation using a nonthoracotomy system. *Am J Cardiol* 1993;71:197–202.

36. Swartz JF, Fletcher RD, Karasik PE. Optimization of biphasic waveforms for human nonthoracotomy defibrillation. *Circulation* 1993;88:2646–2654.

37. Raitt MH, Johnson G, Dolack GL, et al. Clinical predictors of the defibrillation threshold with the unipolar implantable defibrillation system. *J Am Coll Cardiol* 1995;25:1576–1583.

38. Bardy GH, Poole JE, Kudenchuk PJ, et al. A prospective randomized comparison in humans of biphasic waveform 60-μF and 120-μF capacitance pulses using a unipolar defibrillation system. *Circulation* 1995;91:91–95.

39. Block M, Hammel D, Bocker D, et al. Internal defibrillation with smaller capacitors: A prospective randomized crossover comparison of defibrillation efficacy obtained with 90-μF and 125-μF capacitors in humans. *J Cardiovasc Electrophysiol* 1995;6:333–342.

40. Jones GK, Poole JE, Kudenchuk PJ, et al. A prospective randomized evaluation of implantable cardioverter-defibrillator size on unipolar defibrillation system efficacy. *Circulation* 1995;92:2940–2943.

41. Wetherbee JN, Chapman PD, Troup PJ, et al. Long term internal cardiac defibrillation threshold stability. *PACE* 1989;12:443–450.

42. Guarnieri T, Levine J, Veltri EP, et al. Success of chronic defibrillation and the role of antiarrhythmic drugs with the automatic implantable cardioverter/defibrillator. *Am J Cardiol* 1987;60:1061–1064.

43. Venditti FJ, Martin DT, Vassolas G, Bowen S. Rise in chronic defibrillation thresholds in nonthoracotomy implantable defibrillator. *Circulation* 1994;89:216–223.

44. Poole JE, Bardy GH, Dolack GL, et al. Serial defibrillation

threshold measures in man: A prospective controlled study. *J Cardiovasc Electrophysiol* 1995;6:19–25.
45. Venditti FJ, O'Connell M, Martin DT, Shahian DM. Transvenous cardioverter defibrillators: Cost implications of a less invasive approach. *PACE* 1995;18:711–715.
46. Strickberger SA, Hummel JD, Daoud E, et al. Implantation by electrophysiologists of 100 consecutive cardioverter defibrillators with nonthoracotomy lead systems. *Circulation* 1994; 90:868–872.
47. Fitzpatrick AP, Lesh MD, Epstein LM, et al. Electrophysiological laboratory, electrophysiologist-implanted, nonthoracotomy-implantable cardioverter/defibrillators. *Circulation* 1994;89:2503–2508.
48. Tung RT, Bajaj AK. Safety of implantation of a cardioverter-defibrillator without general anesthesia in an electrophysiology laboratory. *Am J Cardiol* 1995;75:908–912.
49. Singer I, Lang D. Defibrillation threshold: Clinical utility and therapeutic implications. *PACE* 1992;15:932–949.
50. Hwang C, Swerdlow CD, Kass RM, et al. Upper limit of vulnerability reliably predicts the defibrillation threshold in humans. *Circulation* 1994;90:2308–2314.
51. Schwartzman D, Nallamothu N, Callans DF, et al. Postoperative lead-related complications in patients with nonthoracotomy defibrillation lead systems. *J Am Coll Cardiol* 1995;26:776–786.
52. Raviele A, Gasparini G. Italian Endotak Investigator Group. Italian Multicenter clinical experience with endocardial defibrillation: Acute and long-term results in 307 patients. *PACE* 1995;18:599–608.
53. Yee R, Klein GJ, Leitch JW, et al. A permanent transvenous lead system for an implantable pacemaker cardioverter-defibrillator. *Circulation* 1992;85:196–204.
54. Almassi GH, Olinger GN, Wetherbee JN, Fehl G. Long-term complications of implantable cardioverter defibrillator lead systems. *Ann Thorac Surg* 1993;55:888–892.
55. Saksena S, Poczobutt-Johanos M, Castle LW, et al. Long-term multicenter experience with a second-generation implantable pacemaker-defibrillator in patients with malignant ventricular tachyarrhythmias. *J Am Coll Cardiol* 1992;19:490–499.
56. Stambler BS, Wood MA, Damiano RJ, et al. Sensing/pacing lead complications with a newer generation implantable cardioverter-defibrillator: Worldwide experience from the

guardian ATP 4210 clinical trial. *J Am Coll Cardiol* 1994;23: 123–132.

57. Peters RW, Foster AH, Shorofsky SR, et al. Spurious discharges due to late insulation break in endocardial sensing leads for cardioverter defibrillators. *PACE* 1995;18:478–481.

58. Roelke M, O'Nunain SS, Osswald S, et al. Subclavian crush syndrome complicating transvenous cardioverter defibrillator systems. *PACE* 1995;18:973–979.

59. Hook BG, Callans DJ, Kleinman RB, et al. Implantable cardioverter-defibrillator therapy in the absence of significant symptoms: Rhythm diagnosis and management aided by stored electrogram analysis. *Circulation* 1993;87:1897–1906.

60. Marchlinski FE, Callans DJ, Gottlieb CD, et al. Benefits and lessons learned from stored electrogram information in implantable defibrillators. *J Cardiovasc Electrophysiol* 1995;6:832–851.

Follow-up of the
Pacemaker Patient

Mark H. Schoenfeld

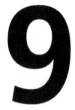

THE GOALS OF PACEMAKER FOLLOW-UP

The follow-up of a pacemaker patient begins with the immediate postimplantation period and extends throughout the life of the patient, rather than throughout the life of the pacemaker system per se. This is the case even in those unusual circumstances in which it is elected not to replace a depleting generator. The original indications for pacemaker insertion require periodic review, and new indications for ongoing pacemaker therapy or for modifications of the existing system also warrant continuing evaluation. The pacemaker physician needs to assess those symptoms not satisfactorily treated by the pacemaker as well as those symptoms potentially *caused by* the pacemaker. Pacer follow-up is important in documenting actual pacer-system malfunction. It is also essential in identifying *potential* sources of pacer system malfunction *before* they result in patient compromise, so that appropriate preemptive corrective measures may be undertaken. Systematic record keeping is an important part of this process, particularly in following end-of-life parameters and in tracking patients whose systems may be subject to product recall or failure. It remains a challenge to optimize the functioning and longevity of a pacemaker system in the face of constantly changing patient needs, whether due to changes in lifestyle, medical circumstances, cardiac function, or electrophysiologic milieu. The issue of who should perform such pacer follow-up remains an ongoing debate—what is clear is that these skills must be continuously and finely maintained.[1,2] It is the purpose of this chapter to explore these issues and examine the methodology of pacemaker follow-up.[3–7]

THE IMMEDIATE POSTIMPLANTATION PERIOD

Following the implantation of a new pacemaker system, the patient is generally observed on a cardiac monitor for one to two days to confirm adequate pacemaker functioning. The roles of ambulatory pacemaker implantation and shorter hospital stays remain controversial. Most patients receive prophylactic antibiotic coverage for 24 hours following pacer insertion, although this has not been established as a clinical necessity. Follow-up posteroanterior (PA) and lateral chest x-rays are obtained to confirm satisfactory positioning of the pacer lead(s) and to serve as a baseline for subsequent comparisons. Twelve-lead electrocardiograms both with and without a magnet are obtained immediately before discharge; the magnet tracings are particularly important to confirm capture in patients whose pacemaker activity is predominantly suppressed by their overriding intrinsic rhythm. Most essential in the immediate postimplantation period is education of the patient. The importance of always carrying a temporary pacemaker identification card (later replaced with a permanent registration card provided by the manufacturer) is stressed. Identification bracelets are often recommended as well. The patient is asked to refrain from vigorous activity for a period of four to six weeks to minimize the possibility of lead dislodgment. One of the questions most commonly asked by patients prior to discharge is whether microwave ovens need to be avoided—with modern-day generators the answer is "no." Plans are then made for outpatient wound evaluation and/or suture removal, generally within two weeks. Patients are asked to be attentive to any signs of potential fever or infection such as pain, redness, swelling, or drainage at the incision site.

SETTING UP FOR PACEMAKER FOLLOW-UP: EQUIPMENT, RECORD KEEPING, AND PRODUCT ADVISORIES

To accomplish the various goals of pacemaker follow-up delineated in the introduction to this chapter, the site of pacemaker follow-up should allow history taking and patient examination and should be fully equipped to allow demonstration of appropriate pacemaker function (Table 9.1). This includes capabilities for 12-lead electrocardiography (with and without a magnet), x-rays (and fluoroscopy, if possible), transtelephonic and ambulatory electrocardiographic monitoring, and availability of a programmer and physicians manual

Table 9.1 Pacemaker Clinic
Pacemaker Clinic Organization
Routine schedule for pacemaker follow-up
Separate location for pacemaker records
Pacemaker Data
Patient's name, age, identification, address, phone number
Pacemaker generator data: model, serial number
Pacemaker lead(s): model, serial number
Operative note from implant with implant data
Examination of incision
Chest radiograms (baseline and repeated as necessary)
Serial 12-lead ECGs of paced/nonpaced rhythm
Serial rhythm strips (± magnet)
Interrogation of pulse generator
Measurement of sensing/pacing thesholds
Recording of real-time telemetry data
Measurement of sensor-related data (histograms, etc.)
Printout of final values

for every model of pacemaker encountered. Depending on the number of different pacer models employed, the last requirement may necessitate extensive familiarity with a wide variety of programming devices because of the present lack of universal programming.[8]

Record keeping is an indispensable component of a pacemaker clinic. Its purpose is to accurately reflect such patient demographics as name and address, to identify specifics of the pacer system employed (model and serial numbers, implant values), to track patient symptoms and various parameters of pacemaker function (e.g., sensing and pacing thresholds, identified changes in magnet rate), and to update any changes in programmed parameters. Such records may, in some facilities, be computer-stored and retrievable, and allow for the generation of comprehensive updated reports (Figure 9.1).[9] Record keeping also allows for organization and maintenance of strict schedules for patient follow-up. This promotes identification of potential problems with pacer function well before they are actualized, rather than having patients drop in only after the problem is manifest.

The establishment of a federal pacemaker registry is now mandated by Medicare guidelines, wherein specifics of such pacer data as patient demographics and model and serial numbers are reported at the time of implantation. This, coupled with

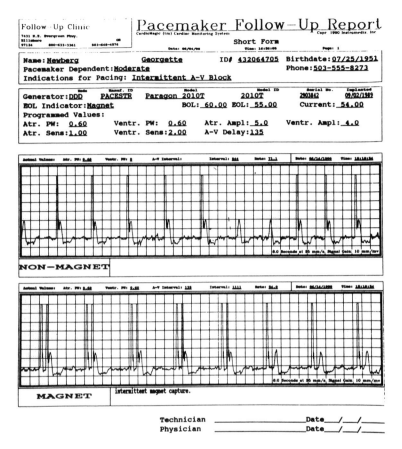

Figure 9.1 Computerized report of pacemaker-related data. (Courtesy of Instromedix, Inc.)

manufacturer-generated patient lists and accurate record keeping by the pacer physician, should facilitate contacting patients if a systematic problem with a particular type of pacer system is identified or if a product advisory/recall is issued. If the physician has observed such a problem, such as premature battery depletion, the manufacturer can then be consulted to determine whether others may have similar observations. However, independent of a formally issued recall, it is the responsibility of the pacer physician to decide whether corrective measures are warranted in a particular case. If such a recall or advisory on a particular pacer product *has* been issued, the nature of the potential malfunction should determine the timing of the pacer-system revision, if required at all. If reported component failure is random and unpredictable, then replacement should be undertaken more rapidly, especially in those patients deemed to be significantly "pacer dependent." Unfortunately, as of this writing, there is no manufacturer-independent large-scale national device/lead database that allows for the timely notification of pacemaker system malfunction to physicians and their patients.[10] As such, the pacer physician must be ever-vigilant as to trends of potential pacer malfunction in his or her own practice as well as to reports from others, whether via other physicians or manufacturers' notifications.

THE OUTPATIENT VISIT
The first outpatient visit

The first visit, approximately two weeks subsequent to implantation, is primarily directed toward evaluation of the healing wound. This is particularly important in diabetic patients prone to slower healing and patients requiring anticoagulation, in whom pocket hematomas can prove catastrophic.[11] Symptoms are reviewed as with any visit. Chest x-ray (PA and lateral) and electrocardiograms with and without a magnet should be performed. Most acute problems arising within two weeks of implantation relate to either lead malposition or healing of the incision and/or pocket, and the pacemaker physician directs attention to these issues in particular, as will be discussed later. Arrangements for transtelephonic monitoring according to preset guidelines are made, as well as for a three-month checkup. At that point, the inflammation associated with the tissue–electrode interface has generally resolved, allowing for assessment of chronic pacing and sensing thresholds. After the three-month checkup, patients are generally seen twice yearly, or as otherwise dictated by their clinical needs.

Subsequent outpatient visits: history

The elicitation and evaluation of symptomatology requires careful sleuthing on the part of the pacemaker physician. Perceptions of pain, well-being, or vigor may vary widely from patient to patient depending on an individual's "threshold" for discomfort or malaise. These may also be a function of a patient's fears and expectations. If the patient does not feel "100 percent better" after pacer insertion, does this reflect malfunction, or were the patient's original symptoms multifactorial in etiology and not preventable by antibradycardia pacing alone? As such, it is sometimes difficult to distinguish symptoms that warrant only reassurance from those symptoms that may be subtle clues to underlying pacemaker malfunction, malprogramming, or "patient–pacer mismatch." In the last two cases (pacemaker malprogramming and "patient–pacer mismatch"), the pacer system may be functioning perfectly appropriately but fails to result in optimal *patient* functioning and indeed may even *produce* symptoms. For example, a previously vigorous patient who receives a dual-chamber system for complete heart block may be exertionally limited with an upper tracking rate of only 120 ppm, especially if electrical Wenckebach or 2 : 1 heart block develops at the pacemaker's upper rate limit (Figure 9.2). Such pacemaker "malprogramming" is easily corrected by adjusting the upper rate limit upward. On the other hand, a patient with marked sinus bradycardia who develops hypotension and consequent malaise from well-intended single-chamber ventricular pacing may require actual revision to a dual-chamber system because of nonprogrammable "patient–pacer mismatch" due to pacemaker syndrome.

Cardiac symptoms of angina or congestive heart failure may arise unrelated to the pacer or to the arrhythmia prompting its original implantation. Pacer adjustments may, however, result in alleviation of these symptoms in some cases. The lower rate limit may be increased in patients with so-called "rate-limited cardiac output" to minimize congestive heart failure. There may also be an "optimal" AV interval to maximize cardiac output in certain patients with dual-chamber systems; this interval may be determined by Swan-Ganz catheter measurements or Doppler measurements of cardiac output. Recently, the potential benefit of dual-chamber

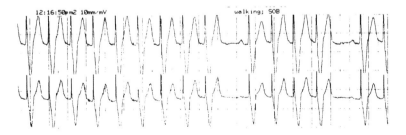

Figure 9.2 Holter transmission in a dual-chamber system with ventricular tracking at the upper rate of 120 ppm associated with electrical Wenckebach phenomenon. This vigorous patient reported exercise limitation and dyspnea in association with this upper rate limitation.

461

pacing in patients with hypertrophic cardiomyopathy has been demonstrated, and in such patients optimization of the AV interval may be critical in alleviating symptoms of outflow obstruction. Patients with angina requiring increased time for diastolic coronary perfusion may benefit from a reduction in their lower rate limit. Symptoms reminiscent of the bradyarrhythmia for which a pacer was inserted may reappear, either because of pacemaker malfunction or, paradoxically, because of appropriate cardiac pacing that is poorly tolerated by the patient.[12] Reported symptoms may include dizziness, presyncope, or syncope but may extend to more subtle concerns such as weakness, fatigability, and dyspnea. The appearance of these symptoms in the apparent presence of a well-functioning pacer system is referred to as the "pacemaker syndrome."[13-15] This typically reflects the loss of atrioventricular synchrony resulting from single-chamber ventricular pacing and may produce systemic hypotension, atrioventricular valvular regurgitation, reduction in cardiac output, pulmonary congestion, and unpleasant neck pulsations (cannon A waves due to atrial contraction against a closed atrioventricular valve). In the worst-case scenario of atrioventricular dyssynchrony, actual retrograde 1:1 ventriculoatrial conduction may occur. Retrograde VA conduction is observed in approximately 80 percent of patients with sick sinus syndrome and even in a small minority of patients (15 percent) with antegrade heart block. Knowledge of this phenomenon may prompt the physician, when possible, to reduce pacer dependence by lowering the lower rate limit or to consider upgrading to a dual-chamber system. On rare occasions, single-chamber atrial pacing in patients with abnormal AV nodal conduction and "early" Wenckebach points may result in prolongation of the PR interval and thus depart from a more ideal atrioventricular timing sequence (with the "ideal" AV delay thought to be 150–175 msec). Echo studies have shown that the optimal AV interval during DDD pacing with P-wave tracking is about 25 msec less than during right atrial pacing. In such cases, reduction of the atrial paced rate will reduce the resulting PR interval; in other cases revision to a dual-chamber system may be considered so that the AV delay can actually be programmed.

Symptoms that are noncardiac but pacer-related may include myopectoral stimulation (most common in unipolar systems in which the generator case serves as the anode), diaphragmatic stimulation (reflecting pacing either through a thin right ventricular wall or via a lead displaced toward the vicinity of the right phrenic nerve), or concerns related to the pacemaker wound itself (pain, overt erosion). These will be addressed in a later section.

Physical examination

Most attention will be directed toward the healing incision and pacer pocket, looking for erythema, tenderness, incipient or overt erosion, or pocket hematoma. Patients may note caudal migration of the generator or superficiality of the pacemaker leads, but these phenomena are frequent and of concern only rarely. Erosion of a generator or a lead is potentially quite serious and may result in systemic infection (see Figure 9.3). A variety of approaches to "salvaging" an eroded system have been advocated, although ideally the entire system should be explanted and replaced with a new system after an appropriate period of intravenous antibiotics.

Myopectoral stimulation may be appreciated at the pocket site most commonly in unipolar systems. Rarely, this may be attributed to incorrect placement of the generator can with the uncoated side down, leading to anodal stimulation of the pectoral muscles; it may thus be corrected by inversion of the generator. It may also indicate lead fracture close to the muscle layer. Frequently no problem is identifiable, but the situation may be corrected by reprogramming to a lower output in order to avoid invasive revision to a bipolar system. Reduction of current or voltage is often effective in eliminating muscle stimulation—far more so than reduction of pulse width duration.

Diaphragmatic stimulation may be apparent on physical examination and rarely requires fluoroscopy for confirmation. As mentioned previously, it may indicate direct stimulation of the diaphragm (left-sided) through a thin ventricular wall or, less commonly, through a perforated ventricle. In the former case, reduction of output may alleviate the problem. Another etiology for diaphragmatic stimulation (right-sided) is phrenic nerve stimulation with a displaced atrial or ventricular lead. Depending on which lead is responsible, the corrective approach may entail inactivation of the atrial channel, reduction of atrial output, or repositioning of the displaced lead.

Other important aspects of the physical examination include vital signs, with particular emphasis on pulse and blood pressure. The latter may vary significantly as a function of pacing mode (e.g., VVI versus DDD) or pacing rate. Neck veins should be evaluated for the presence of cannon A waves; cardiac examination should confirm paradoxical splitting of the second heart sound in most

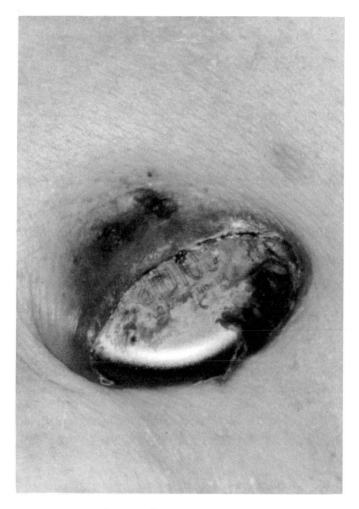

Figure 9.3   Pacemaker erosion.

cases of right ventricular pacing, and should exclude the presence of a pericardial friction rub suggestive of cardiac perforation. The arm ipsilateral to the lead insertion site should be examined for edema, perhaps reflecting venous thrombosis, usually a spontaneously resolving phenomenon and rarely responsible for thromboembolism. Edema coupled with inflammation may, less commonly, represent a gouty attack precipitated by the recent surgical implantation of a pacer system.

Physical manipulation of the pacer system should be undertaken to evaluate the integrity of the leads and their connections to the generator can. Rarely, inversion of the generator can lead to myopectoral stimulation and/or loss of capture in unipolar systems. This may result because the generator was inadvertently implanted with the uncoated side down or because the patient has reversed the can by "twiddling." In rate-adaptive systems dependent on sensing muscular activity, the can may be tapped to demonstrate appropriate increases in the pacing rate. Traction applied to the generator may expose a previously unsuspected malconnection or lead fracture and result in loss of capture or myopectoral stimulation (Figure 9.4). In some cases these maneuvers should be undertaken with fluoroscopic visualization. Confirmation of continued capture should be made with the patient in erect as well as supine position in cases where inadequate or insufficient lead "slack" may be present. Myopotential inhibition in single-chamber systems or myopotential triggering of ventricular pacing in dual-chamber systems may be elicited by various movements such as abduction of the arm ipsilateral to the generator. If myopotential inhibition is elicited and clinically significant, reprogramming to reduce sensitivity, asynchronous pacing, or triggered modes may be undertaken to ensure continuous pacing in the pacer-dependent patient. Alternatively, consideration of changing the unipolar system to a bipolar system is another option. Carotid sinus massage is another physical maneuver that may be employed to induce slowing to the lower rate limit, thereby confirming the ability of the pacemaker to capture. Rarely, carotid massage-induced slowing of the sinus node may be useful in dual-chamber systems to differentiate supraventricular tachycardia from physiological sinus tachycardia with ventricular tracking near the upper rate limit.

Radiography

The chest x-ray (PA/lateral using the dorsal spine technique) remains an important feature of pacemaker follow-up, conveying a wealth of information.[16] Early following implant it serves to delineate lead positioning and screw-tip advancement (in active fixation leads); lead dislocation is rare beyond the first month postimplantation. Subsequent films should be performed generally on a yearly basis or if specific questions are to be addressed. In particular, lead conductor fractures may be identified in cases of failure to sense or capture in the setting of elevated lead impedance. These typically occur at sites of more acute angulation or at sites of

BROKEN EPICARDIAL ELECTRODE

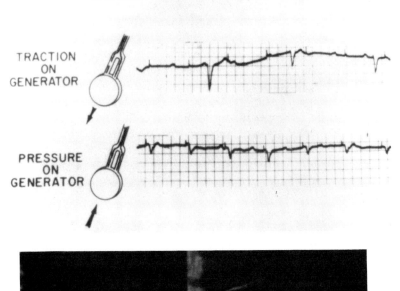

TRACTION
ON
GENERATOR

PRESSURE
ON
GENERATOR

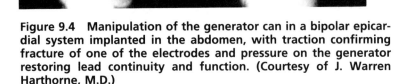

Figure 9.4   Manipulation of the generator can in a bipolar epicardial system implanted in the abdomen, with traction confirming fracture of one of the electrodes and pressure on the generator restoring lead continuity and function. (Courtesy of J. Warren Harthorne, M.D.)

anchoring if a protective sleeve was not applied at the time of implant. Fluoroscopy, in conjunction with traction on the lead and generator, may be required to delineate the fracture. (More recently, a manufacturer's advisory on potential fracture of an inner J-shaped retention wire has recommended periodic fluoroscopy to evaluate for fracture in certain active fixation J-shaped atrial leads.) The venous insertion site may be apparent on the film; jugular venous cutdown, for example, entails lead entry superior to the clavicle. Anatomic variants (such as persistent left superior vena cava) may also be appreciated and, in previously unknown patients, raise unnecessary concern over the unorthodox placement of the ventricular lead. Polarity of the lead(s) may also be appreciated, though whether the generator is actually *programmed* to bipolar or unipolar remains to be determined. Examination of the connector block may disclose an insecure or incomplete lead connection or inadequate tightening of a set screw. The generator may also be examined for position and, very importantly, to identify the specific model in patients with an unknown system. Various radiographic identification codes exist that are manufacturer-specific and facilitate recognition of the specific device in question (Figure 9.5). Older systems not employing such radiographically apparent codes may be identified on the basis of generator shape or battery configuration on the x-ray.

Electrocardiography and magnet application

It is beyond the scope of this chapter to provide a detailed discussion of pacemaker electrocardiography. Rather, a general approach to the use of electrocardiography in following pacemakers will be addressed. The 12-lead electrocardiogram, both with and without magnet application, is an essential component of each visit. Aside from confirming the pacer's ability to sense and capture, the elec-

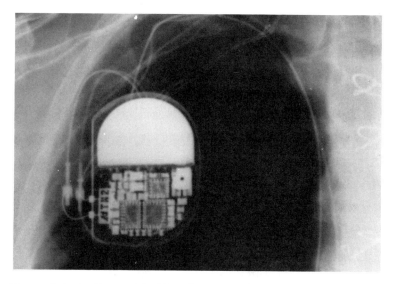

Figure 9.5 Radiographic identification of a pacer generator has been facilitated by the use of device-specific identification codes.

trocardiogram can provide important information on lead integrity and position.[17] Thus, for example, the typical morphology of a right ventricular paced complex is that of left bundle branch block, whereas right bundle branch block morphology may suggest left ventricular pacing, whether intentional (e.g., epicardial wires) or otherwise (e.g., perforation). If appropriate equipment is used, analysis of pacemaker spike axis and amplitude may on occasion be helpful in disclosing such problems as insulation defects (usually increased spike amplitude in bipolar systems) or partial electrode fractures (spike attenuation with prolongation of spike-to-spike interval exactly by a multiple of the automatic interval).

With regard to interpretation of pacemaker electrocardiograms, whether simple or complex, the best rules of thumb are:

Rule 1. The pacemaker system is (almost) always right—we just haven't figured out why it's doing what it's doing!

Rule 2. The exception to Rule 1 is when the pacemaker system is malfunctioning.

Magnet application with electrocardiographic monitoring confirms the ability to capture a cardiac chamber during asynchronous pacing at the programmed output settings. This may be otherwise inapparent if the patient's endogenous rhythm inhibits pacer firing. Magnet responses vary widely among manufacturers and even among various models of a single manufacturer (Table 9.2). Thus, for example, magnet application in single-chamber systems may result in asynchronous pacing at the standard rate or programmed rate, ventricular demand pacing at a fast rate, or ventricular triggered pacing. Magnet application in dual-chamber systems may result in dual-chamber asynchronous pacing at a programmed rate or at a standard rate, at a programmed rate plus 14 percent, or even in asynchronous single-chamber ventricular pacing at a standard rate.

"End-of-life" (or more correctly, elective replacement) indicators (ERTs) may in some models be available only in the magnet mode. In such instances, routine magnet application may be especially important to determine the need for replacement of a depleting pacer generator.

The application of a magnet over the generator is a procedure rarely associated with adverse effects. On occasion ventricular ectopy may result from asynchronous ventricular pacing, but this is seldom sustained. Caution is warranted if the patient has both a

Table 9.2 End-of-Life Characteristics for Selected Pacemakers

Cardiac Pacemakers, Inc.

Model Name and Number	ICHD Code	Rate		Magnet Rate		ERT Indication and Behavior
		BOL	EOL	BOL	EOL	
445 VistaT	VVI	70[a]	70	100	85	A
925 Delta	DDD	65[a]	65	96		
1124 Triumph VR	VVIR	70[a]	20% dec.	85 (VOO)	65 (VOO)	
1224 Triumph DR	DDDR	70[a]	65 (VVI)	85 (DOO)	75 (DOO)	C
					65 (VOO)	
1226 Prelude DR	DDDR	70[a]	65 (VVI)	85 (DOO)	65 (VOO)	
1230 Vigor DR	DDDR	70[a]	65 (VVI)	85 (DOO)	65 (VOO)	

Intermedics

Model Name and Number	ICHD Code	Rate		Magnet Rate		ERT Indication and Behavior
		BOL	EOL	BOL	EOL	
282-02 Nova	SSI	a	65 (SSI)	d	90/65	B: 65 ppm
282-04 Nova II	SSI	a	c	d	90/80	C: 90–80 ppm
284-02 Cosmos	DDD	a	65 (VVI)	d	90/65	B: 65 ppm
284-05 Cosmos II	DDD	a	c	d	90/80	C: 90–80 ppm
292-03 Dash	SSIR	a		d	90/80	C
292-05 Dart	SSIR	a		d	90/80	C
294-03 Relay	DDDR	a		d	90/80 (VOO)	C

Table 9.2 Continued.

Medtronic

Model Name and Number	ICHD Code	Rate BOL	Rate EOL	Magnet Rate BOL	Magnet Rate EOL	ERT Indication and Behavior
8420 Spectrax SXT	VVI	70ᵃ	63	70ᵃ	63	D: 10%, E
8438 Classix	VVI	70ᵃ	63	70ᶜ	63	D: 10%, E
8416 Legend	VVIR	70ᵃ	65			
Synergist II	DDDR	70ᵃ	70	85	75 (DOO)	C: 85–75–65, E
			65 (VVI)		65 (VOO)	
	VVIR	70ᵃ	70	70ᵃ	75 (VOO)	C:
7076 Elite	DDDR	70ᵃ	65 (VVI)	85 (DOO)	65 (VOO)	
	SSIR	70ᵃ	65 (SSI)	85 (SOO)	65 (SOO)	
7940 Thera DR	DDDR	70ᵃ	65 (VVI)	85 (DOO)	65 (VOO)	

Pacesetter

Model Name and Number	ICHD Code	Rate BOL	Rate EOL	Magnet Rate BOL	Magnet Rate EOL	ERT Indication and Behavior
250-6 Phoenix	VVI	70ᵃ	63	70ᶜ	63	F
262 AFP	VVI	70ᵃ	70	80	62	
2028L Synchrony	DDDR	72ᵃ	63	70ᵇ	63	F
2250L Trilogy SR	SSIR			70ᵇ	62.7	F
2350L Trilogy DR	DDDR			70ᵇ	62.7	F

Telectronics Model Name and Number	ICHD Code	Rate		Magnet Rate		ERT Indication and Behavior
		BOL	EOL	BOL	EOL	
528C Optima MPT II	VVI	70[a]	56	99	85	H
528D Optima MPT III	VVI	70[a]	70	99	95	I
1202 Meta MV	VVIR	70[a]	70	99	93	
1250 Meta	DDDR	70[a]	63.3 VVI	>85	<78	
1254 Meta	DDDR	70[a]	63.3 VVI	>85	<78	

[a] Programmable parameter.
[b] Same as programmed rate.
[c] Reverts to VVI STAT 1 mode, which is VVI at 65 and disables magnet mode.
[d] Four cycles of asynchronous pacing at 90 ppm, then asynchronous at the programmed rate.
A = gradual decline in magnet rate *only*.
B = a sudden decrease in paced and/or magnet rate.
C = a two-step change in magnet rate.
D = a sudden 10 percent decrease in pacing and/or magnet rate.
E = Pulse-width stretching of 40 to 85 percent at EOL.
F = a 100 msec interval increase in paced and magnet rate.
G = at BOL, magnet rate is 14 percent above programmed rate. At EOL, magnet rate is 11 percent below programmed rate.
H = a gradual decline in paced and/or magnet rate: 20 percent decrease in paced rate, 14 bpm decrease in magnet rate.
I = a gradual decrease in magnet rate only (by 4 bpm); and 20 percent rate decrease is a secondary elective replacement indicator.
J = a gradual decline in magnet rate only.

pacer and an implantable cardioverter-defibrillator; implanted defibrillators may be inactivated by prolonged magnet exposure.

Because most devices respond to magnet application by asynchronous pacing, magnets may also be employed, both diagnostically and therapeutically, in cases where potential pacer malfunction is attributed to sensing problems (Table 9.3). Thus, for example, pacemaker-mediated tachycardia may occur in dual-chamber systems because of sensing of retrogradely conducted atrial activity that in turn triggers ventricular paced beats; application of a magnet will prevent atrial sensing and thereby interrupt the tachycardia. In addition, if pacer spike-to-spike intervals are prolonged or pacer pauses are present because of oversensing (of P waves, T waves, myopotentials, polarization voltage, or false signals), magnet application will prevent undue inhibition of pacer output. In cases of pacemaker dependence, magnet conversion to asynchronous pacing may be critical in preventing asystole due to such oversensing or, in dual-chamber systems, due to crosstalk inhibition (particularly if the appropriate pacemaker programmer is unavailable).

DETERMINATION OF THE UNDERLYING RHYTHM AND PACER DEPENDENCE

Pacemaker dependency connotes a condition in which cessation of pacemaker function may result in significant symptomatic bradycardia or ventricular asystole, thereby endangering the patient. The term is problematic for a variety of reasons. First, it is often misused in cases where 100 percent pacing is observed. In this sense any pacer patient may be rendered "pacer dependent" by having the device programmed to a rate greater than her or his intrinsic heart rate. Second, in patients with conduction abnormalities such as atrioventricular block, the degree of impairment may vary from one point in time to another. That is, the ability to conduct 1:1 from atrium to ventricle may be somewhat "whimsical" and, further, may also vary with the application of various medications that facilitate or depress conduction (Figure 9.6). Last, with reprogramming of pacers to slower rates, *gradual* slowing of the pacer rate is more likely to allow the emergence of an escape rhythm than is a sudden cessation of pacing. In this case, abrupt termination of pacing may result in ventricular asystole and thereby define a state of pacemaker dependence (Figure 9.7).

Table 9.3 Uses of Magnets

1. Device identification—each model has characteristic response.
2. Determination of single-chamber or dual-chamber pacing modes in patient with spontaneous normal sinus rhythm that inhibits pacer output.
3. Elective replacement indicators—characteristic of each device.
4. Necessary for programming in some devices—reed switch actuation by magnet in programming head.
5. Threshold margin test in some devices.
6. Assesses pacing capture capabilities at programmed output.
7. Diagnosis of some problems related to sensing, e.g., far-field signals, T-wave sensing, crosstalk inhibition.
8. Termination of pacemaker-mediated tachycardias.
9. Underdrive pacing to terminate some arrhythmias, e.g., ventricular tachycardia.
10. Ensures pacing in certain situations where electromagnetic interference may inhibit output, e.g., electrocautery.
11. Inactivates/activates certain ICDs, allows assessment of R-wave synchronization in certain ICDs ("beepogram").

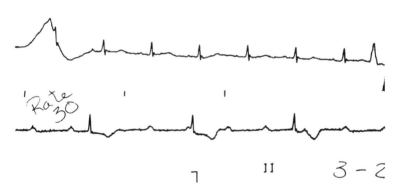

Figure 9.6 (top) Intact AV conduction in a pacer patient with resulting inhibition of pacer output. Pacemaker was originally inserted for complete heart block. (bottom) Underlying rhythm in the same patient several months later demonstrating recurrent complete heart block.

In patients in whom gradual reprogramming of the generator to slower rates still results in 100 percent pacing at the slowest programmable rate, it is still possible to determine the presence (or absence) of an underlying rhythm if output is programmable to subthreshold values. Alternatively, chest wall stimulation may be

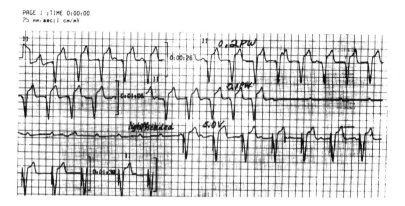

Figure 9.7 Abrupt cessation of ventricular pacing achieved by decrements in pulse-width output without first attempting to reduce ventricular paced rate gradually. A gradual reduction in rate may have allowed the demonstration of an escape rhythm but symptomatic ventricular asystole resulted instead.

applied with alligator clip cables from a temporary pacing device via skin electrodes (one situated directly over the generator can) in an effort to produce electromagnetic interference and thereby inhibit pacer output. This technique is particularly well suited to unipolar systems with limited programming capabilities for rate or output. Some devices have programmable inhibition of pacemaker output as a temporary mode.

It is unclear whether the choice of a lower programmed pacer rate will "discourage" the emergence of chronic pacer dependency in patients with varying degrees of atrioventricular block.

PROGRAMMABILITY AND THE DETERMINATION OF SENSING AND PACING THRESHOLDS

The application of multiprogrammability to a variety of clinical situations, such as for troubleshooting, has been discussed in Chapter 7 and will not be reviewed in great detail here. Pacemaker programmers are poorly understood devices with which the pacemaker physician must become increasingly familiar.[8] Pacemaker programmers enable both programmability and telemetry of a host of data including programming commands, administrative data, programmed data, measured data, and diagnostic data. Programmability of output, whether of pulse width or amplitude (current or voltage) or both, is available in most currently available pacemaker systems and allows for the determination of chronic pacing thresholds. Very importantly, in the setting of higher chronic thresholds it allows for programming to higher effective outputs so as to ensure safe pacing often without the need of secondary (invasive) intervention such as lead repositioning. Some devices have programmable features allowing for automatic threshold determination by sequential decrements in voltage output; in some cases this is a "vario" feature requiring application in order to be performed. In other systems, pulse width or amplitude must be individually programmed to lower values to determine at what point loss of capture occurs. Programming to *subthreshold* values will allow for assessment of underlying rhythm but, as indicated earlier, should be undertaken cautiously, because it may result in abrupt cessation of pacing with ventricular asystole in certain patients.

The threshold determination is an important feature of pacer follow-up because generator longevity may be significantly enhanced if the output can be programmed to the lowest value that will provide an adequate safety margin for effective pacing. Calculation of strength–duration curves for stimulation requirements enables the pacer physician to determine what this lowest value might be. In general, at short pulse durations, small changes in pulse width will effect large differences in voltage/current thresholds. Shorter pulse widths will result in lower impedances and increased stimulation efficiency. For devices with fixed output voltage and programmable pulse durations, satisfactory margins can be achieved by tripling the pulse-width threshold if this value is less than 0.4 msec; four times threshold should be considered for higher pulse-width thresholds. For devices with programmable voltage, pulse-duration thresholds can be determined at 2.5 V and programmed to that pulse duration at 5 V to provide an adequate safety margin, as suggested by Furman. Others advocate that if pulse duration is very low (less than 0.1 msec) at a given output voltage, voltage may be reduced while extending the pulse width somewhat. In general, output voltage less than 2.5 V will not significantly reduce battery drain and is applied only in cases where unwanted myopectoral or diaphragmatic stimulation is of concern. On the other hand, if pulse-duration threshold is high, increasing the output voltage will be required to ensure safe pacing because higher pulse widths approaching rheobase will be neither effective nor energy efficient.

Determination of pacing thresholds should be made for both chambers where applicable.[18] In many dual-chamber devices the atrial and ventricular channels have outputs that are separately programmable.[3] The programmed rate is set to a value greater than the intrinsic rate. Determination of *atrial* capture at progressively lower atrial outputs is usually easily made in patients with intact conduction to the ventricle, by determining whether the responding QRS complexes occur at the programmed rate. In patients with AV block, programmed rates required to confirm atrial capture may be fast enough to produce even higher degree block to the ventricle with prolonged periods of ventricular asystole; as such, atrial pacing thresholds may be more difficult to determine in patients without intact AV conduction.

Ventricular *sensing* thresholds may be determined by programming the ventricular inhibited mode to a rate slower than the intrinsic rate and, by decreasing sensitivity (i.e., increasing the millivolt values), to determine at what value pacer output is no longer appropriately inhibited. The same approach may be applied for establishing atrial sensing thresholds. The triggered modes may also be used in their respective chambers to determine sensing thresholds. The inappropriate triggering of a pacemaker spike at a given programmed value either may diagnose a problem with undersensing (Figure 9.8) or, alternatively, may coincide with other signals that are being *oversensed*, such as T waves or myopotentials. In dual-chamber systems, atrial sensing can be confirmed by programming to a P-wave synchronous ventricular triggered mode, shortening the AV interval so as to trigger ventricular pacing, and reducing atrial sensitivity progressively until paced ventricular events no longer result. The need for programming chronically to

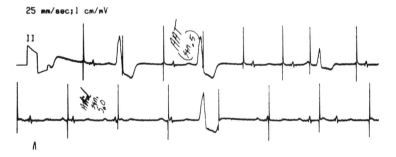

Figure 9.8 Atrial triggered pacing mode. (top) Maximal sensitivity of 0.5 mV atrial sensing is appropriate. (bottom) With reduction of atrial sensitivity to 5.0 mV there is a failure of atrial sensing with atrial spikes that do not coincide with native P waves.

higher sensitivity is quite common in atrial pacing in view of the small atrial electrograms often observed. Decreasing sensitivity, or reprogramming to a purely triggered mode, is sometimes required in single-chamber systems—either atrial or ventricular—where unwanted *oversensing* (of far-field signals, electromagnetic interference, myopotentials, etc.) results in undue inhibition of pacemaker output. The possibility of myopotential inhibition of ventricular output should be examined by increasing the programmed VVI rate so as to require 100 percent pacing and progressively increasing ventricular sensitivity; this will rule out this problem. In some dual-chamber systems, the problem of myopotential inhibition may be treated by reprogramming to the DAD mode. Likewise, the possibility of myopotential *triggering* of ventricular pacing in dual-chamber systems should be evaluated by having the patient perform deltopectoral isometric exercises at increasing atrial sensitivities.

Programmability of polarity has become increasingly available in current pacemakers and, unfortunately, increasingly required. Problems with insulation defects in certain polyurethane leads subject to the "subclavian crush" syndrome, resulting in low impedance values, may be temporarily addressed by reprogramming from bipolar to unipolar mode. This maneuver generally will increase the lead impedance in these situations and prevent loss of capture and possible undersensing, but will not prevent oversensing from make/break electrical transients arising from contact between the two conductors. Ultimately, lead replacement is required in the pacer-dependent patient.

PROGRAMMABILITY: SPECIAL CONSIDERATIONS IN DUAL-CHAMBER SYSTEMS

In dual-chamber systems, the potential for crosstalk inhibition and pacemaker-mediated tachycardia should be explored. The possibility of crosstalk can be assessed by programming the ventricular channel to highest sensitivity and the atrial output to its highest value. The programmed rate should exceed the native rate so as to require continuous atrial pacing, and the programmed AV interval should be shorter than the native PR interval. The absence of crosstalk inhibition at maximal atrial output and ventricular sensitivity suggests that this problem is not likely to be encountered at usual settings. Assessment of this phenomenon should be undertaken cautiously in patients with heart block, because ventricular asystole may occur. Identification of crosstalk warrants reprogramming, where possible, to lower atrial output or ventricular sensitivity, or consideration of another mode such as VDD.

The propensity for pacemaker-mediated tachycardia (PMT) in the DDD mode may be explored by shortening the atrial refractory period to its minimum. If retrograde ventriculoatrial conduction is present, PMT may be observed if it is triggered by a spontaneous PVC or if atrial output is programmed to subthreshold values. In the latter case, AV sequential paced rhythm fails to capture the atrium but captures the ventricle, with the possibility of retrograde conduction leading to activation of a nonrefractory atrium and setting up PMT. Identification of PMT may then be approached by limiting the upper ventricular tracking rate, extending the postventricular atrial refractory period, or changing to a different mode such as DDI.

Not infrequently, a patient with a dual-chamber device will present with new-onset atrial fibrillation or flutter. The atrial fibrillation or flutter waves may be sensed and trigger rapid ventricular responses, often irregularly (Figure 9.9). Although the upper rate limit may be reduced to minimize rapid ventricular tracking, it is usually advisable to reprogram to the VVI mode and plan to reprogram back to DDD once cardioversion to sinus rhythm, if feasible, has been accomplished. In some devices, atrial flutter may be converted to sinus rhythm by temporary burst pacing from the atrial channel (Figure 9.10).

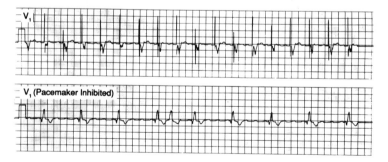

Figure 9.9 Simultaneous rhythm strips V₁ and V₅ showing ventricular tracking of atrial flutter/atrial fibrillation resulting in irregular ventricular pacing near the upper rate limit (rate 100 ppm) in the DDD mode. When the pacemaker was temporarily inhibited, the ventricular rate was 40 ppm, with high-grade atrioventricular block.

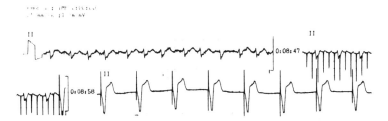

Figure 9.10 Interruption of atrial flutter by burst atrial pacing at a rate greater than 300 ppm with resultant junctional bradycardia and the need for ventricular pacing at the lower rate limit.

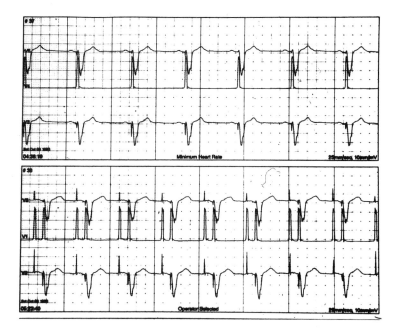

Figure 9.11 Pacemaker programmed with circadian function, allowing for slower pacemaker rates at night to simulate physiologic nocturnal bradycardia and conserve on device longevity (upper tracing) 4:23 A.M., slower rate allowed; (lower tracing) one hour later with AV pacing at a faster baseline rate.

With advances in both pacemaker generators and their associated programmers, growth in programmability features has been exponential. Thus, for example, the ability to physiologically adapt the atrioventricular delay interval to a patient's rate (shortening

479

with faster rates), the capability of changing the AV interval as a function of whether the atrial activity is sensed or paced, and the option of slowing the pacer rate at night to minimize pacing (circadian function) are all recently appreciated advances (Figure 9.11). Search hysteresis in certain dual–chamber models allows the patient's rate to dip down to a low value before kicking in at a fast-paced rate, with automatic scanning of when the endogenous rhythm returns to normal. This feature has been of use in many patients with "malignant" vasovagal syncope (Figure 9.12).

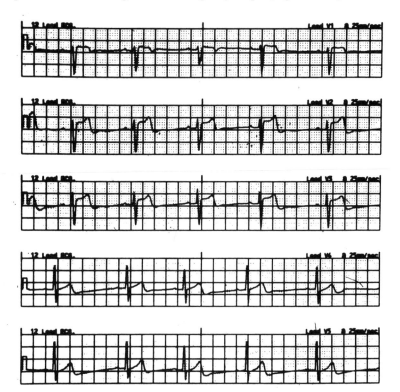

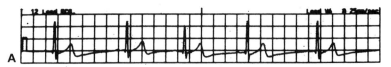

Figure 9.12 A 15-year-old patient with vasovagal syncope refractory to medications, with pacemaker "search hysteresis" feature activated. (A) baseline; (B) AV pacing activated.

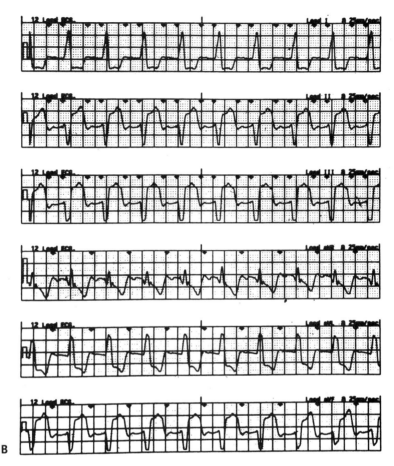

B

Fig. 9.12 (*Continued*)

Automatic mode switching is a very important programmable feature newly incorporated into certain dual-chamber models (Figure 9.13). It allows reversion from dual-chamber pacing to single-chamber ventricular pacing when atrial fibrillation is recognized, and a return to dual-chamber mode when sinus rhythm has been restored. Recognizing the growing versatility of these pacemakers is a challenge to the pacer physician, both in selecting the appropriate device at the time of implant and in prescribing the appropriate program in follow-up.

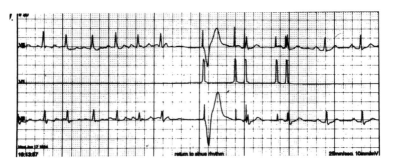

Figure 9.13 Reversion from VVI pacing during paroxysmal atrial fibrillation to dual-chamber pacing once the sinus mechanism has returned, in a pacer programmed to allow automatic mode switching.

TELEMETRY: SETTINGS, MEASURED DATA, HISTOGRAMS, ELECTROGRAMS, MARKER CHANNELS

Even before any reprogramming is undertaken or thresholds are determined, the device should be interrogated to document the present programmed settings. Most current devices have such telemetry available. It should be emphasized that independent confirmation of such parameters as mode and rate should be made electrocardiographically after all interventions because telemetry will not always reflect true programmed settings, although this is rare. This is particularly true in the case of pacer systems that have come into contact with extreme environmental noise (such as electrocautery or defibrillation) causing subsequent resetting of the device or pacer malfunction—in these cases, "what you see" (via telemetry) is not always "what you get." The ability to undertake telemetry, as in the case of programming, is device-specific and requires manufacturer-specific programmers and/or modules. Inability to perform telemetry suggests either that the wrong programmer or module has been used or that the device is an older model incapable of providing telemetry. The importance of knowing the correct device model is clear when attempting telemetry; if the patient is previously unknown, the pacemaker identification card and radiographic identification become indispensable. Recent technologic advances in some programmers have, however, allowed identification of the model of a generator when at least the manufacturer is known.

Real-time telemetry of *measured data* such as battery voltage or lead impedance, where obtainable, may prove quite useful in diagnosing problems with impending battery depletion or lead integrity, respectively.[19–21] A very low telemetered impedance may suggest problems with lead insulation, for example, whereas a very high telemetered impedance may indicate conductor fracture or a loose set screw, which may be inapparent radiographically (Figures 9.14 and 9.15). With time, battery voltage declines and battery impedance rises, allowing projections of device longevity.

Historical information, such as initial implant values, may also be recorded in some systems and be available for recall at a later date

```
294-03 SN 001777            JAN 26 '93  5:12 PM
            RELAY       TELEMETRY DATA
    PACING RATE                      70 PPM
    PACING INTERVAL                 857 MSEC
    CELL VOLTAGE                    2.72 VOLTS
    CELL IMPEDANCE                  2.67 KOHMS
    CELL CURRENT                    17.3 UA
                    ATRIAL(Uni)   VENTRICULAR( Bi )
    SENSITIVITY         1.0          5.0 MV
    LEAD IMPEDANCE      635         1815 OHMS
    PULSE AMPLITUDE    3.99         4.03 VOLTS
    PULSE WIDTH        0.35         0.35 MSEC
    OUTPUT CURRENT      6.1          2.2 MA
    ENERGY DELIVERED    8.1          3.0 UJ
    CHARGE DELIVERED   2.15         0.77 UC

                                     [ RETURN ]
```

Figure 9.14 Telemetry indicated an elevated ventricular impedance of 1815 ohms in this patient with a lead conductor fracture.

```
            (      MEASURED DATA      )

    Pacer Rate _____ 70.5 ppm

    Ventricular:
      Pulse Amplitude _____ 2.7 Volts
      Pulse Current _____ 12.2 mAmperes
      Pulse Energy _____ 10 µJoules
      Pulse Charge _____ 4 µCoulombs
      Lead Impedance _____ <250 Ohms

    Atrial:
      Pulse Amplitude _____ 5.3 Volts
      Pulse Current _____ 9.2 mAmperes
      Pulse Energy _____ 25 µJoules
      Pulse Charge _____ 5 µCoulombs
      Lead Impedance _____ 582 Ohms

    Battery Data: (W.G. 8077 - NOM. 1.8 AHR)
      Voltage _____ 2.73 Volts
      Current _____ 41 µAmperes
      Impedance _____ <1 KOhms
```

Figure 9.15 A ventricular impedance of less than 250 ohms was demonstrated by telemetry in this patient with a polyurethane insulation failure.

via telemetry. Some models allow both programmers and generators to have actual times displayed, important in programming certain circadian features indicated previously, as well as identifying when certain events, such as automatic mode switching, have occurred since the last interrogation. Other features that may be telemetered include nominal programmed values for certain models and a screen indicating the full array of programmability inherent in a particular device (Figure 9.16).

Aside from identifying programmed settings and measured data (Figure 9.17), telemetry of event counters is usually possible with current systems. These may be further subdivided into event histograms/event counts, sensor-indicated rate histograms and event records. In some cases, the frequency of pacing since the last visit may be determined to address the question of pacer-dependence at the present programmed settings (event histogram/event count). Histograms may be obtainable to demonstrate how often different rates occur during rate-adaptive pacing at a particular activity-sensing threshold.[13–15] The determination of such events (or predicted events) may enable the physician to reprogram the device settings so as to achieve rates thought to be more appropriate or "physiologic" for the patient (sensor-indicated rate histogram) (Figure 9.18). Histograms of "event records" are now available in some models, allowing for precise determination of when some event occurred, symptomatic or otherwise, and at what rate (Figure 9.19). In this fashion, episodes of rapid heart action/tachycardia and other events, such as automatic mode switching or search hysteresis episodes, may be assessed in some models. Pacer generators may thus serve as their own mini-Holter monitors.

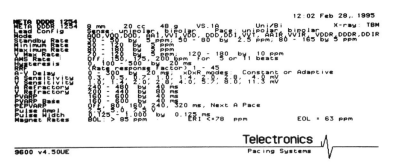

Figure 9.16 Telemetry of the full range of programmable features for one pacemaker model (Telectronics Pacing Systems).

(PROGRAMMED PARAMETERS)

Mode	AAI	
Sensor	ON	
Rate	70	ppm
Atr. Pulse Config.	BIPOLAR	
A. Pulse Width	.4	msec
A. Pulse Amplitude	3.5	Volts
A. Sense Config.	BIPOLAR	
A. Sensitivity	.75	mVolts
A. Refractory	400	msec
Magnet	TEMPORARY OFF	
Threshold	4.0	
Slope	7	
Maximum Sensor Rate	110	ppm
Reaction Time	Medium	
Recovery Time	Slow	

(MEASURED DATA)

Pacer Rate	70.6	ppm

Atrial:

Pulse Amplitude	3.4	Volts
Pulse Current	4.1	mAmperes
Pulse Energy	5	μJoules
Pulse Charge	2	μCoulombs
Lead Impedance	843	Ohms

Battery Data: (W.G. 8074 - NOM. 2.3 AHR)

Voltage	2.80	Volts
Current	28	μAmperes
Impedance	< 1	KOhms

(TEST RESULTS)

Atrial Capture Threshold	2.0	Volts
Test Pulse Width	.4	msec
Safety Margin	1.8 : 1	

Figure 9.17 Telemetered programmed settings, measured data, and threshold measurement test in a patient programmed to the AAI mode.

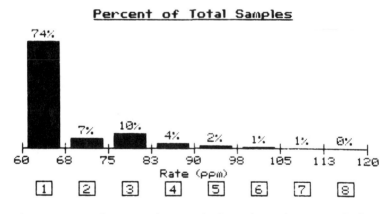

SENSOR INDICATED RATE HISTOGRAM

Total Time Sampled: 36d 22h 8m 29s
Sampling Rate: 1.6 seconds
Slope: 8 (Normal) **Threshold:** 2.0

Bin Number	Range (ppm)	Sample Counts
1	60 — 68	1,452,812
2	68 — 75	136,130
3	75 — 83	203,072
4	83 — 90	78,315
5	90 — 98	47,937
6	98 — 105	24,809
7	105 — 113	16,055
8	113 — 120	4,014
	Total:	1,963,144

Percent of Total Samples

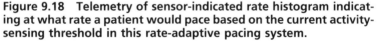

Figure 9.18 Telemetry of sensor-indicated rate histogram indicating at what rate a patient would pace based on the current activity-sensing threshold in this rate-adaptive pacing system.

Real-time intracardiac electrograms and marker channels may be available, depending on the system used; they facilitate the physician's ability to diagnose appropriate, or inappropriate, pacer function.[22] The size of the intracardiac electrograms may give the pacer physician a rough idea of the sensing capabilities of the system and may also delineate the strength of far-field signals.

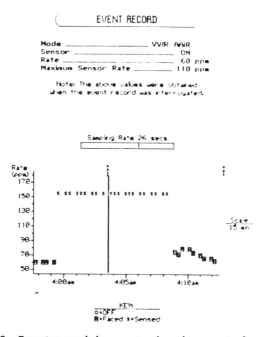

Figure 9.19 Event record demonstrating the onset of palpitations in a patient with a pacer, consistent with spontaneous paroxysmal supraventricular tachycardia (Courtesy of Dr. Paul A. Levine; Pacesetter Systems, Sylmar, CA).

The clinical utility of intracardiac electrograms includes the identifying retrograde conduction, measuring ventriculoatrial conduction time, assisting rhythm identification, evaluating unusual sensing phenonema, evaluating lead connector integrity, assisting threshold determinations, and evaluating myopotential sensing. Potentially more useful are marker channels, which denote when a particular channel (atrial or ventricular) is sensing activity or emitting a paced output (Figure 9.20). By telling the physician what the pacer is "seeing and doing," certain phenomena, such as crosstalk inhibition, may be more easily defined. Event markers do, however, have their limitations. They describe pacer behavior but not its (in)appropriateness; a stimulus output report does not necessarily imply capture; and the markers apply only to real-time (as opposed to stored) events.

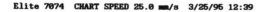

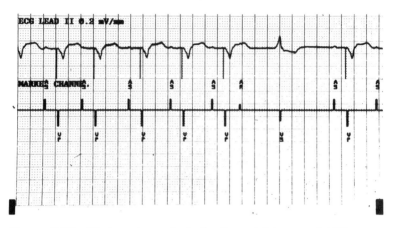

Figure 9.20 Marker channels indicating atrial sensed (AS), ventricular sensed (VS), and ventricular paced (VP) events as well as events that are refractory on the atrial channel (AR) (Medtronics, Inc., Minneapolis, MN).

AMBULATORY ELECTROCARDIOGRAPHIC RECORDING: TRANSTELEPHONIC MONITORING, HOLTER MONITORING, TREADMILL TESTING

A variety of electrocardiographic techniques enable ambulatory determinations of pacemaker function. The most important of these is transtelephonic monitoring of the patient's free-running and magnet rates.[23,24]

This technique does *not* totally supplant the direct outpatient visit with the pacer physician, during which time physical examination and programming manipulations already described are essential. It does, however, reduce the frequency of outpatient visits; these visits may be particularly burdensome for patients who are frail, are in nursing homes, or are unable to travel. Specific Medicare guidelines designated for follow-up schedules are as follows:

> *Guideline I*: Applies to most pacers, with either inability to demonstrate or insufficient exposure to demonstrate:
> 1. A five-year longevity of greater than 90 percent, and
> 2. Nonabrupt decline of output over three or more months, of less than a 50 percent drop in output voltage/less

than 20 percent magnet deviation or a drop by 5 ppm or less.

Single-chamber pacers—First month: Every two weeks. Second to thirty-sixth month: Every eight weeks. Thereafter: Every four weeks.

Dual-chamber pacers—First month: Every two weeks. Second to sixth month: Every four weeks. Seventh to thirty-sixth month: Every eight weeks. Thereafter: Every four weeks.

Guideline II: The minority of pacers that *do* meet the criteria for longevity indicated above.

Single-chamber pacers—First month: Every two weeks. Second to forty-eighth month: Every twelve weeks. Forty-ninth to seventy-second month: Every eight weeks. Thereafter: Every four weeks.

Dual-chamber pacers—First month: Every two weeks. Second to thirtieth month: Every twelve weeks. Thirty-first to forty-eighth month: Every eight weeks. Thereafter: Every four weeks.

Despite its limitation (insufficient voltage depending on the lead used, 60-Hz interference, telephone noise, motion artifact), transtelephonic monitoring enables the pacer physician to determine changes in free-running or magnet pacing rates indicative of battery depletion and may indicate problems with pacemaker sensing or capture. Patients experiencing symptoms potentially related to pacer function or malfunction are encouraged to transmit their rhythm when they are symptomatic, independent of the above scheduling guidelines. Occasionally other arrhythmias, not related to the pacemaker or bradyarrhythmia necessitating its insertion, may be revealed.

Twenty-four-hour Holter monitoring may be useful as an extension of this approach to disclose problems with pacer malfunction potentially responsible for a patient's symptoms (Figures 9.21 and 9.22).[25] The approach is limited by sampling error in the patient with infrequent symptoms in that no abnormalities may be identified if the patient is "having a good day." Rather, the technique is more often useful in demonstrating previously *unsuspected* and *asymptomatic* malfunctions, such as intermittent undersensing or myopotential triggering. Activity-related rate trends warranting reprogramming, particularly with dual-chamber or rate-adaptive pac-

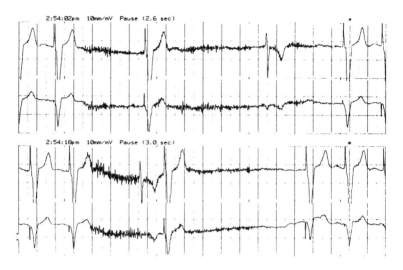

Figure 9.21 Two-channel Holter (simultaneous V$_1$ and modified V$_5$) showing symptomatic inhibition of pacing by myopotentials.

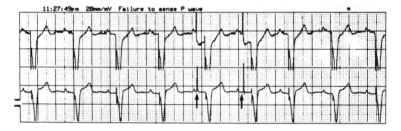

Figure 9.22 Routine Holter (simultaneous V$_1$ and modified V$_5$) recorded in a patient with a DDD pacemaker and no symptoms. The arrow highlights two P waves that were not sensed.

ing, may be observed with Holter monitoring. The degree of pacer dependence at a given set of programmed parameters on a "sample day" may also be evaluated.

Treadmill testing may, on occasion, be useful in assessing exercise tolerance, chronotropic competence, and maximal heart rates achievable, either independent of pacing or in the setting of specifically programmed parameters. In rate-adaptive systems it is particularly useful to assess activity-sensing thresholds as well as the rapidity of pacing rate increases and declines with activity. For example, in an older patient who develops angina it may be important to make the system less sensitive to activity, lower the upper rate limit, and have a relatively quicker decline of pacing rate once activity ceases. Upper rate behavior in dual-chamber systems may also be appreciated with exercise testing (e.g., Wenckebach versus 2 : 1 block periodicity); exercise-induced arrhythmias potentially contributing to pacer-mediated tachycardias may rarely be observed.

ELECTIVE REPLACEMENT INDICATORS

It is important to distinguish end-of-life from recommended replacement times. The former connotes gross pacemaker malfunction or lack of function; the latter strives to indicate a time when generator replacement should be considered well in advance of end of life.[26,27] Elective replacement indicators (ERI or ERT) may be reached (and are preferably reached) in the absence of patient symptoms or electrocardiographically demonstrated abnormalities in free-running pacer function. Indeed, changes in the generator, such as in magnet rates, may occur years in advance of true end of life. Elective replacement indicators are used to recommend generator change within a period of a few weeks to months. They are device specific and may be found by consulting with the manufacturer or the physicians manual (see Table 9.2). Various indicators have been used, including gradual or stepwise declines in free-running or magnet pacing rates, and rate drops to a preset value. Other indicators have included pulse-width stretching and automatic changes in pacing modes, such as from DDD to VVI or from VVIR to VVI (designed to reset for energy conservation). The diversity of strategies among (and even within) pacemaker companies for ERT indicators is striking, as Table 9.2 shows. When it is available, real-time telemetry of available battery voltage and impedance may be particularly useful in confirming battery depletion, particularly as progressive increases in battery impedance are observed. In most systems, however, changes in pacing rate are the predominant indicators of the need for elective replacement.

To complicate interpretation of this phenomenon, the mechanism governing it may be latched or unlatched.[15] If the battery voltage falls below a minimum trip point voltage responsible for triggering the ERI, a decline in pacing rate will be observed (either free-running or magnet). If the mechanism is latched, the newer slower rate is permanent even if the fall in available battery voltage is transient or momentary. In contrast, in unlatched systems, the generator may return to the original higher rate if the current drain on the battery diminishes and available battery voltage increases. In the latter case, therefore, sudden changes in pacing rate may be observed as a function of changes in available voltage and may thus be misconstrued as pacer malfunction. Clearly, an understanding of this behavior, of resetting phenomena, and of specific elective replacement indicators is imperative for the pacer physician so he or she can determine impending pacer battery depletion before gross end of life occurs.

SPECIAL SITUATIONS ENCOUNTERED BY THE PACEMAKER PHYSICIAN: THE HOSPITALIZED PREOPERATIVE PATIENT, INTERRUPTION OF TACHYARRHYTHMIAS, SPECIALIZED MEDICAL PROCEDURES, RADIOLOGIC TESTS, AND THE PACER PATIENT WITH RECURRENT SYNCOPE

The pacer physician is often asked to evaluate a patient with a pacemaker prior to general or cardiac surgery. In addition to obtaining details from the history and physical examination outlined previously, it is most essential to establish the degree of pacer dependence and, via telemetry, the current programmed settings. Electrocautery and defibrillation, often required intraoperatively, may result in a variety of pacemaker phenomena. Electrocautery may cause transient inhibition of pacer output because of oversensing of electromagnetic interference. This is particularly of concern in the patient whose underlying rhythm is ventricular asystole. If 100 percent pacer dependence has been demonstrated preoperatively, the device may be programmed to either an asynchronous mode or a triggered mode to preempt undue inhibition of pacer output. If such programming is not possible, then a magnet may be taped over the generator during the period of cautery. It is ideal to avoid electrocautery entirely if at all possible, especially near the pacer generator. The cautery electrode should be placed as far as possible from the generator. In addition, short bursts of cautery are recommended.

Both electrocautery and defibrillation may produce irreversible damage to the generator. They may also result in resetting of the generator to a backup or noise-reversion mode that is device specific. It is essential to be aware of the reset mode for the pacer under consideration. Postoperative electrocardiograms with and without a magnet are required to rule out this phenomenon, lest the physicians caring for the patient presume, wrongly, that the device is operating under its preoperatively programmed specifications (Figure 9.23).

Transient undersensing and both acute and chronic rises in pacing threshold have also been observed with defibrillation and cardioversion.[28] Some of this may relate to transmission of current down the lead(s) causing a burn at the tissue–electrode interface resulting in the potential for exit block. The majority of problems are encountered with unipolar pacemakers implanted in the right pectoral fossa (Figure 9.24). To minimize the above phenomena, it is recommended that cautery and defibrillation be used sparingly,

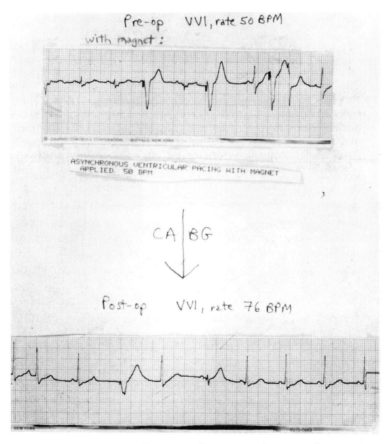

Figure 9.23 Example of Intermedics pacemaker reset by CABG to VVI pacing, 76 bpm.

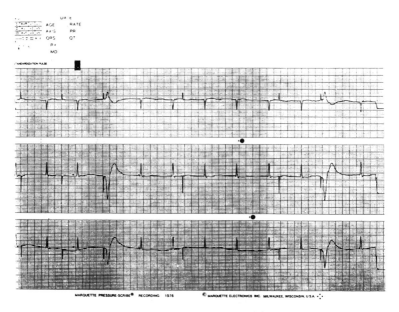

Figure 9.24 Transient and episodic undersensing by the ventricular channel in a patient after cardioversion from atrial fibrillation to normal sinus rhythm. This occurred in conjunction with transient elevation of pacing thresholds, despite the use of anteroposterior paddles. The return to baseline pacing and sensing thresholds occurred 30 minutes after cardioversion.

remote from the pacer system, with the least amount of energy feasible, and, in the case of cardioversion–defibrillation, via anteroposterior rather than anteroapical paddles. In addition, pacing and sensing thresholds should be checked following external defibrillation. Finally, equipment for temporary pacing should be nearby, especially in a pacemaker-dependent patient.

Other sources of electromagnetic interference encountered in the hospital setting are magnetic resonance imaging (MRI), extracorporeal shock-wave lithotripsy, and radiation therapy. Exposure to MRI should be avoided until more details become available about the risks of this technique to the pacer.[29] One study has shown that reversion to asynchronous pacing (VOO or DOO) may occur, but other potential hazards, such as rapid pacing or resetting to back-up mode, remain to be explored. However, in this study none of the pulse generators exhibited any changes in their programmed parameters or any changes in their ability to be reprogrammed following MRI.

In the case of lithotripsy, distancing of the pacer from the focal point of the lithotripsy is recommended to avoid potential problems with undue inhibition of pacer output or irregular sensing.[30] This is particularly true in activity-sensing devices dependent on piezoelectric crystals. These crystals may be capable of over-sensing shock waves and result in increased pacing rates; alternatively, they may be susceptible to damage (e.g., crystal is shattered) from the shock waves. Current recommendations in this procedure are:

1. Patients with piezoelectric activity-sensing rate-responsive pacemakers should not undergo lithotripsy if the device is implanted in the abdomen;
2. Patients with activity-sensing rate-adaptive pacemakers implanted in the thorax should have their rate-responsive features turned off;
3. Patients with single-chamber ventricular devices can safely undergo lithotripsy; and
4. Patients with implanted dual-chamber devices in the thorax should be programmed to the VVI mode before lithotripsy.

Radiation therapy (e.g., for breast or lung cancer) to the chest may be unavoidable in certain patients with pacemakers. To minimize the risk of pacer system failure or random component damage from the ionizing radiation, appropriate methods of shielding the generator and limiting the field of radiation should be discussed with the radiation therapist. Damage to the pacemaker generator is both random and cumulative. Damage may result in sudden loss of output, alterations in programmed parameters, and rate runaway. If adequate shielding is not possible, repositioning the generator should be considered.

Patients with pacers used to treat bradycardias may also be susceptible to tachyarrhythmias. In some patients, if tachyarrhythmias exist or are anticipated at the time of implantation, a device capable of subsequent noninvasive programmed cardiac stimulation may be selected.[31] Thus, for example, a patient with sick sinus syndrome and a strongly positive signal–averaged electrocardiogram may warrant a device allowing for noninvasive electrophysiologic studies. In many systems, the generator may be reprogrammed to the ventricular triggered mode, and programmed stimulation may be performed with chest wall stimulation (see Chapter 8). If the triggered mode is used, extrastimuli may be introduced, allowing for the induction and/or termination of ventricular arrhythmias. Noninvasive electrophysiologic studies in patients with permanent pacemakers facilitate both diagnosis and pharmacologic testing for tachyarrhythmias and preempt many of the concerns related to catheter placement for invasive studies—namely, procedural complications and patient tolerance.[30] They require, nonetheless, monitoring in a electrophysiology laboratory with the capability of defibrillator backup.

The pacer physician may be called upon to terminate tachyarrhythmias acutely, preferably without the need for cardioversion or defibrillation. Some devices allow for temporary increases in the upper rate of atrial pacing to greater than 300 ppm, allowing for the possibility of burst pacing to terminate atrial flutter. Rarely, application of a magnet with resultant synchronous pacing may be successful in terminating a tachyarrhythmia. Reprogramming the device to faster rates for overdrive pacing, or using the triggered mode with chest wall stimulation to "program in" extrastimuli, may also prove useful. In all cases, the intervention should be undertaken cautiously with defibrillator backup. The physician should also be aware of potential pacer interactions with antiarrhythmic drugs, notably flecainide, which may result in increased pacing thresholds.

The patient with a pacer may occasionally return with new or current episodes of presyncope and syncope. This may reflect pacer-system malfunction and requires the careful evaluation already discussed—namely, determination of sensing and pacing thresholds and the possibility of pacer inhibition by myopotentials or other electromagnetic interference. Other potentially symptomatic arrhythmias such as ventricular tachycardia, revealed on ambulatory Holter monitoring or provoked via programmed stimulation, may co-exist. Pacemaker-mediated tachycardias may also arise and generate symptoms, and the potential for this should be evaluated as addressed earlier. Tilt testing may prove useful in revealing the presence of vasodepressor syncope; it will not preempt symptoms if significant hypotension occurs. Under such circumstances, medical therapy with fludrocortisone and/or beta blockers may prove useful.

A surprising number of patients may experience severe symptoms of presyncope, syncope, malaise, palpitations, or dyspnea from pacemaker syndrome discussed previously; one such pacer patient evaluated by the author actually had an automobile crash on the Connecticut Turnpike as a result of this syndrome. This phenomenon, observed during single-chamber ventricular pacing, results in hemodynamic compromise from retrograde activation of the atria in some cases and from cyclic losses of synchrony between the atria and ventricles in other cases (see Chapter 3 for a detailed discussion). The presence of retrograde ventriculoatrial conduction should be ascertained with electrocardiography, particularly in the inferior leads (e.g., II, III, and aVf) and/or telemetered intracardiac electrograms (Figure 9.25). Blood pressure determinations should be made in the supine and erect positions with both ventricular pacing and nonpaced rhythm if possible. Rarely, cardiac output determinations may also be required to demonstrate hemodynamic compromise associated with ventricular pacing. If pacemaker syndrome is identified, consideration should be given to reprogramming the pacer to reduce pacer dependence (e.g., decrease the lower rate), but ultimately revision to a dual-chamber system may be required.

SUMMARY

The physician caring for the pacemaker patient is confronted with both challenging and exciting responsibilities. In part these consist of identifying problems, where they exist, that are not satisfactorily treated by the pacer system or that actually are caused by it. Pacer evaluation also entails anticipation of problems *before* they occur. Most difficult is the optimization of pacer performance so as to achieve both maximal pacer longevity and feelings of well being in the patient. To accomplish the above goals, a detailed appreciation of the pacer system under consideration is required as

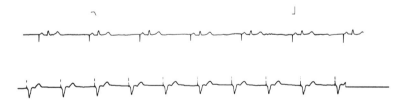

Figure 9.25 (top) The pacemaker is programmed to the DDD mode and there is 100 percent atrial pacing and no cardiac symptoms. When the pacemaker was reprogrammed to the VVIR mode (bottom), the patient was dyspneic and became presyncopal despite rate-responsive pacing. Retrograde VA conduction is apparent with ventricular pacing. In some pacemakers with intracardiac electrograms, or marker channels, the VA conduction time can be measured at different heart rates.

well as "sleuthing" to unravel the mysteries of the patient–pacer relationship.

REFERENCES

1. Schoenfeld MH. Quality assurance in cardiac electrophysiology and pacing: A brief synopsis. *PACE* 1994;17:267–269.
2. Schoenfeld MH. Manpower concerns in cardiac electrophysiology and pacing. *PACE* 1995;18:1977–1979.
3. Furman S. Cardiac pacing and pacemakers: VIII. *Am Heart J* 1977;94:795–804.
4. Griffin JC, Schuenenemyer TD. Pacemaker follow up: An introduction and overview. *Clin Prog Pacing Electrophysiol* 1983;1:30.
5. Griffin JC, Schuenenemyer TD, Hess KR, et al. Pacemaker follow up: Its role in the detection and correction of pacemaker system malfunction. *PACE* 1986;9:387–391.
6. Furman S. Pacemaker follow-up. In S Furman, DL Hayes, DR Holmes (eds.), *A Practice of Cardiac Pacing* (2nd ed.). Mount Kisco, NY: Futura, 1989.
7. Levine PA. Proceedings of the policy conference of the North American Society of Pacing and Electrophysiology on programmability and pacemaker follow-up programs. *Clin Prog Pacing Electrophysiol* 1984;2:145–191.
8. Schoenfeld MH. A primer on pacemaker programmers. *PACE* 1993;16:2044–2052.
9. MacGregor DC, Covvey HD, Noble EJ, et al. Computer-assisted reporting system for the follow-up of patients with cardiac pacemakers. *PACE* 1980;3:568–588.
10. Schoenfeld MH. Recommendations for implementation of a North American multicenter arrhythmia device/lead database. *PACE* 1992;15:1632–1636.
11. Byrd CL, Schwartz SJ, Gonzalez M, et al. Pacemaker clinic evaluations: Key to early identification of surgical problems. *PACE* 1986;9:1259–1264.
12. Hoffman A, Jost M, Pfisterer M, et al. Persisting symptoms despite permanent pacing. Incidence, causes, and follow-up. *Chest* 1984;85:207–210.
13. Ausubel K, Furman S. The pacemaker syndrome. *Ann Intern Med* 1985;103:420–429.

14. Ellenbogen KA, Thames MD, Mohanty PK. New insights into pacemaker syndrome gained from hemodynamic, humoral and vascular responses during ventriculoatrial pacing. *Am J Cardiol* 1990;65:53–59.
15. Kenny RS, Sutton R. Pacemaker syndrome. *BMJ* 1986;293:902–903.
16. Steiner RM, Morse D. The radiology of cardiac pacemakers. *JAMA* 1978;240:2574–2576.
17. Mugica J, Henry L, Rollet M, et al. The clinical utility of pacemaker follow-up visits. *PACE* 1986;9:1249–1251.
18. Luceri RM, Hayes DL. Follow-up of DDD pacemakers. *PACE* 1984;7:1187–1194.
19. Levine PA, Sholder J, Duncan JL. Clinical benefits of telemetered electrograms in assessment of DDD function. *PACE* 1984;7:1170–1177.
20. Sanders R, Martin R, Fruman H, Goldberg MK. Data storage and retrieval by implantable pacemakers for diagnostic purposes. *PACE* 1984;7:1228–1233.
21. Sholder J, Levine PA, Mann BM, et al. Bidirectional telemetry and interrogation. In SS Barold, J Mugica (eds.), *Cardiac Pacing. The Third Decade of Cardiac Pacing.* Mount Kisco, NY: Futura, 1982; pp 145–166.
22. Duffin EG Jr. The marker channel: A telemetric diagnostic aid. *PACE* 1984;7:1165–1169.
23. Strathmore NF, Mond HG. Noninvasive monitoring and testing of pacemaker function. *PACE* 1987;10:1359–1370.
24. Zinberg A. Transtelephonic follow-up. *Clin Prog Pacing Electrophysiol* 1984;2:177.
25. Famularo MA, Kennedy HL. Ambulatory electrocardiography in the assessment of pacemaker function. *Am Heart J* 1982;104:1086–1094.
26. Barold SS, Schoenfeld MH. Pacemaker elective replacement indicators: Latched or unlatched? *PACE* 1989;12:990–995.
27. Barold SS, Schoenfeld MH, Falkoff MD, et al. Elective replacement indicators of simple and complex pacemakers. In SS Barold, J Mugica (eds.), *New Perspectives in Cardiac Pacing* (2nd ed.). Mount Kisco, NY: Futura, 1991; pp 493–526.
28. Levine PA, Barold SS, Fletcher RD, Talbot P. Adverse acute and chronic effects of electrical defibrillation and cardioversion of implanted unipolar cardiac pacing systems. *J Am Coll Cardiol* 1983;1:1413–1422.

29. Holmes DR, Hayes DL, Gray JE, Merideth J. The effects of magnetic resonance imaging on implantable pulse generators. *PACE* 1986;9:360–370.

30. Cooper D, Wilkoff B, Masterson M, et al. Effects of extracorporeal shock wave lithotripsy on cardiac pacemakers and its safety in patients with implanted cardiac pacemakers. *PACE* 1988;11:1607–1616.

31. Friehling TD, Marinchak RA, Kowey PR. Role of permanent pacemakers in the pharmacologic therapy of patients with reentrant tachyarrhythmias. *PACE* 1988;11:83–92.

Index

A
AAI pacing, 283–285
AAIR pacing, 286
AAI-T, 62
Abbreviations, in timing cycle, 279–281
Ablation, of AV node-His bundle, 20
ACC/AHA guidelines for pacemaker implantation, 5, 21
Accelerometers, 99–100
Action potential, 38, 39
Activation, of electrodes, 69, 70
Active fixation leads, 73–74, 75, 235
Activity sensors, 96, 97, 98–99
Afterpotentials, 63, 91
Air embolism, from pacemaker implantation, 249–250
Ambulatory electrocardiographic recording, 488–491
American College of Cardiology/ American Heart Association (ACC/AHA) guidelines for pacemaker implantation, 5, 21
AMS (automatic mode switching), 313–315, 481–482
Anatomy, of cardiac conduction system, 1–3

Angina, postimplantation, 461–462
Anodal stimulation, stimulation threshold with, 49, 50
ANP (atrial natriuretic peptide), 143
Antibiotic prophylaxis, for pacemaker implantation, 224
Anticoagulants, and pacemaker implantation, 224
Antitachycardia pacing, 435–437
AOO pacing, 281
AOOR pacing, 287–288
ARP (atrial refractory period), 294–295, 296
Arrhythmia, from pacemaker implantation, 250–251
Artifacts, 357–358, 359, 360
failure to capture due to
with pacing stimuli absent, 377
with pacing stimuli present, 357–358, 359, 360
ASW (atrial sensing window), 323–325
Asynchronous pacing
atrial, 281
AV sequential, 281, 282
dual-chamber rate-modulated, 287–288
single-chamber rate-modulated, 287–288

501

Myocardial stimulation threshold.
    See Stimulation threshold
Myopectoral stimulation, 462, 463
Myopotential(s), 60–61
Myopotential inhibition, 477

N
Naloxone, to reverse sedation, 225
Native signal, change in, 364–365
NBG code, 280
Neurocardiogenic syncope, 16–18
Noise mode operation, 367
Noise reversion circuits, 92–93
Noise-sampling period, 94
Noncapture
    atrial, 380–384
    functional, 358, 359, 361
    pacing stimuli absent with, 368–377
    pacing stimuli present with
        in dual-chamber system, 379–384
        in single-chamber system, 337–358
    ventricular, 379–381
Noncommitted shocks, 445
Nonphysiologic AV delay, 298–299, 300, 389

O
Obstructive hypertrophic
    cardiomyopathy, 18–19
    AV synchrony with, 134–135
Open circuit
    failure to capture due to, 351–357
    sensing failure due to, 374–376
OPG-Gee, 378
Orders, preimplantation, 224–225
Orthogonal electrode array, 63
Orthostatic hypotension, idiopathic, 20
Outpatient visit(s), 460–472
    electrocardiography and magnet
        application in, 467–472
    first, 460
    history in, 460–463

physical examination in, 463–465
radiography in, 465–467
Output circuits, of pulse generator, 89–92
Oversensing
    in dual-chamber pacing system, 386, 387
    with implantable cardioverter-defibrillator, 435, 447–448
    in single-chamber pacing system, 371–374
Oversensing drive, 386, 387
Overshoot potential, 38
Oxygen consumption, work and, 152, 153
Oxygen saturation, mixed venous, 104–106

P
Paced ventricular atrial refractory
    period (PVARP), 296, 297
    DDDR pacing during, 318, 319
    and endless-loop tachycardia, 394–395
Pacemaker, 333–334
    and implantable cardioverter-defibrillator, 434–435
    migration of, 260–261
Pacemaker circus movement
    tachycardia, 327–328
Pacemaker clinic, 457–458
Pacemaker dependence,
    determination of, 472–474
Pacemaker diagnostics, 399–410
    electrograms in, 401–404
    event counters in, 404–410
    event markers in, 400–401
    measured data in, 399–400
Pacemaker eccentricities, 397–399
Pacemaker follow-up, 456–498
    ambulatory electrocardiographic
        recording in, 488–491
    determination of underlying
        rhythm and pacer
        dependence in, 472–474